2014

The Year Book of VASCULAR SURGERY®

Editor-in-Chief

David L. Gillespie, MD, RVT, FACS

Chief, Department of Vascular and Endovascular Surgery, Cardiovascular Care Center, Southcoast Health Systems, Charlton Hospital, Fall River, Massachusetts

ELSEVIER
MOSBY

ELSEVIER
MOSBY

Vice President, Global Medical Reference: Mary E. Gatsch
Associate Publisher: John Vassallo
Developmental Editor: Stephanie Carter
Production Supervisor, Electronic Year Books: Donna M. Skelton
Electronic Article Manager: Mike Sheets
Illustrations and Permissions Coordinator: Dawn Vohsen

2014 EDITION

Composition by TNQ Books and Journals Pvt Ltd, India

Editorial Office:
Elsevier
Suite 1800
1600 John F. Kennedy Blvd.
Philadelphia, PA 19103-2899

International Standard Serial Number: 0749-4041
International Standard Book Number: 978-0-323-26493-8

Associate Editors

Ruth L. Bush, MD, JD, MPH
Interim Vice Dean, Bryan/College Station Campus, Professor of Surgery, Texas A&M Health Science Center College of Medicine, Bryan, Texas

Marc A. Passman, MD
Professor of Surgery, Section of Vascular Surgery and Endovascular Therapy, University of Alabama at Birmingham, Birmingham, Alabama

Benjamin W. Starnes, MD
Professor of Surgery and Chief, Division of Vascular Surgery; University of Washington, Seattle, Washington

Michael T. Watkins, MD
Director, Vascular Surgery Research Lab, Massachusetts General Hospital, Boston, Massachusetts

Contributors

James H. Black, III, MD, FACS
The Bertram M. Bernheim, MD Associate Professor of Surgery, Chief, Division of Vascular Surgery and Endovascular Therapy, Johns Hopkins Hospital, Baltimore, Maryland

Matthew A. Corriere, MD, MS
Assistant Professor, Department of Vascular and Endovascular Surgery, Wake Forest University School of Medicine, Winston-Salem, North Carolina

John P. Cullen, PhD
Research Associate Professor, Division of Vascular Surgery, University of Rochester School of Medicine and Dentistry, Rochester, New York

Brian G. Peterson, MD, FACS
Associate Professor of Surgery, St. Louis University School of Medicine, St Louis, Missouri

Joseph D. Raffetto, MD, FACS, FSVM
Associate Professor of Surgery, Harvard Medical School, Brigham and Women's Hospital; Chief, Vascular Surgery Division, VA Boston Healthcare System, West Roxbury, Massachusetts

Table of Contents

Journals Represented

Journals represented in this Year Book are listed below.

American Journal of Cardiology
American Journal of Kidney Diseases
Annals of Surgery
Annals of Vascular Surgery
Canadian Journal of Anaesthesia
Cardiovascular and Interventional Radiological
Circulation
European Journal of Radiology
European Journal of Vascular and Endovascular Surgery
International Journal of Cardiology
International Journal of Oral and Maxillofacial Surgery
Journal of Surgical Research
Journal of the American College of Cardiology
Journal of the American College of Surgeons
Journal of the American Medical Association Surgery
Journal of the American Society of Nephrology
Journal of Thoracic and Cardiovascular Surgery
Journal of Vascular Surgery
Journal of Vascular Surgery Venous and Lymphatic Disorders
Medicine and Science in Sports and Exercise
Stroke

Standard Abbreviations

The following terms are abbreviated in this edition: acquired immunodeficiency syndrome (AIDS), cardiopulmonary resuscitation (CPR), central nervous system (CNS), cerebrospinal fluid (CSF), computed tomography (CT), deoxyribonucleic acid (DNA), electrocardiography (ECG), health maintenance organization (HMO), human immunodeficiency virus (HIV), intensive care unit (ICU), intramuscular (IM), intravenous (IV), magnetic resonance (MR) imaging (MRI), ribonucleic acid (RNA), and ultrasound (US).

Note

The Year Book of Vascular Surgery® is a literature survey service providing abstracts of articles published in the professional literature. Every effort is made to assure the accuracy of the information presented in these pages. Neither the editors nor the publisher of the Year Book of Vascular Surgery® can be responsible for errors in the original materials. The editors' comments are their own opinions. Mention of specific products within this publication does not constitute endorsement.

To facilitate the use of the Year Book of Vascular Surgery® as a reference tool, all illustrations and tables included in this publication are now identified as they appear in the original article. This change is meant to help the reader recognize that any illustration or table appearing in the YEAR BOOK OF VASCULAR SURGERY® may be only one of many in the original article. For this reason, figure and table numbers will often appear to be out of sequence within the YEAR BOOK OF VASCULAR SURGERY®.

1 Basic Considerations

Shock wave treatment induces angiogenesis and mobilizes endogenous CD31/CD34-positive endothelial cells in a hindlimb ischemia model: Implications for angiogenesis and vasculogenesis

Tepeköylü C, Wang F-S, Kozaryn R, et al (Innsbruck Med Univ, Austria; Chang Gung Memorial Hosp, Kaohsiung, Taiwan; et al)

J Thorac Cardiovasc Surg 146:971-978, 2013

Objectives.—Shock waves have been shown to induce recruitment of intravenously injected endothelial progenitor cells to ischemic hind limbs in rats. We hypothesized that shock wave treatment as sole therapy would induce angiogenesis in this ischemia model and would lead to mobilization of endogenous endothelial (progenitor) cells.

Methods.—A total of 18 rats, aged 5 weeks old, were subdivided into 3 groups: sham (n = 6), ischemic muscle with shock wave treatment (shock wave treatment group, n = 6), and without shock wave treatment (control, n = 6). Hind limb ischemia was induced by ligation of the femoral artery. Three weeks later, shock wave treatment (300 impulses at 0.1 mJ/mm^2) was applied to the adductor muscle; the controls were left untreated. Muscle samples were analyzed using real-time polymerase chain reaction for angiogenic factors and chemoattractants for endothelial progenitor cell mobilization. Fluorescence activated cell sorting analysis of the peripheral blood was performed for CD31/CD34-positive cells. Perfusion was measured using laser Doppler imaging. Functional improvement was evaluated by walking analysis.

Results.—Angiogenic factors/endothelial progenitor cell chemoattractants, stromal cell-derived factor-1 and vascular endothelial growth factor, were increased in the treatment group, as shown by real-time polymerase chain reaction, indicating the mobilization of endothelial progenitor cells. Fluorescence activated cell sorting analysis of the peripheral blood revealed high numbers of CD31/CD34-positive cells in the treatment group. Greater numbers of capillaries were found in the treated muscles. Blood perfusion increased markedly in the treatment group and led to functional restoration, as shown by the results from the walking analysis.

Conclusions.—Shock wave therapy therefore could develop into a feasible alternative to stem cell therapy in regenerative medicine, in particular for ischemic heart and limb disease (Figs 1-5).

▶ Cell-based therapies have potential to expand treatment options for peripheral arterial disease (PAD), particularly among "no-option" patients who are poor

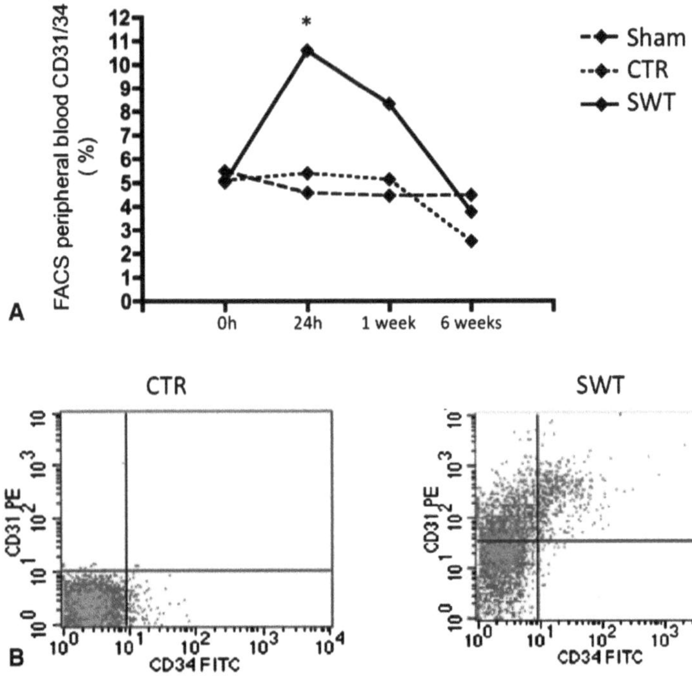

FIGURE 1.—Circulating CD31/CD34-positive endothelial cells. A, Fluorescence activated cell sorting *(FACS)* analysis of peripheral blood revealed significantly greater numbers of circulating CD31/CD34-positive endothelial cells 24 hours after shock wave treatment *(SWT)*, indicating early mobilization of endothelial progenitor cell, most probably from bone marrow. Number of endothelial progenitor cells still elevated after 1 week; however, 6 weeks after SWT, no difference found between treatment and control *(CTR)* group. *$P < .05$. B, Representative views from fluorescence activated cell sorting 24 hours after SWT showing greater numbers of endothelial progenitor cells in treatment group. *FITC*, Fluorescein isothiocyanate. (Reprinted from Tepeköylü C, Wang F-S, Kozaryn R, et al. Shock wave treatment induces angiogenesis and mobilizes endogenous CD31/CD34-positive endothelial cells in a hindlimb ischemia model: Implications for angiogenesis and vasculogenesis. *J Thorac Cardiovasc Surg*. 2013;146:971-978, Copyright 2013, with permission from The American Association for Thoracic Surgery.)

candidates for conventional treatment interventions. This study explored effects of shock-wave treatment (SWT) on neovascularization and functional gait outcomes in a rat hindlimb ischemia model. After SWT, the authors observed significant but transient increases in circulating CD31- or CD34-positive endothelial progenitor cells (EPC) (Fig 1). Within treated muscle, SWT was also associated with increases in messenger RNA levels of angiogenic factors that recruit EPC (HIF-1α, SDF-1) and their receptor (C-X-C chemokine receptor type 4) as well as upregulation of vascular endothelial growth factor (VEGF)-A at 24 hours and at 6 weeks (Fig 2). VEGF protein was also increased following SWT versus controls, although no specific time point for this comparison was provided. These changes in angiogenic factors were accompanied by increases in capillary density and cell proliferation (Fig 3), as well as improvements in laser Doppler perfusion (Fig 4). Importantly, these molecular, cellular, and

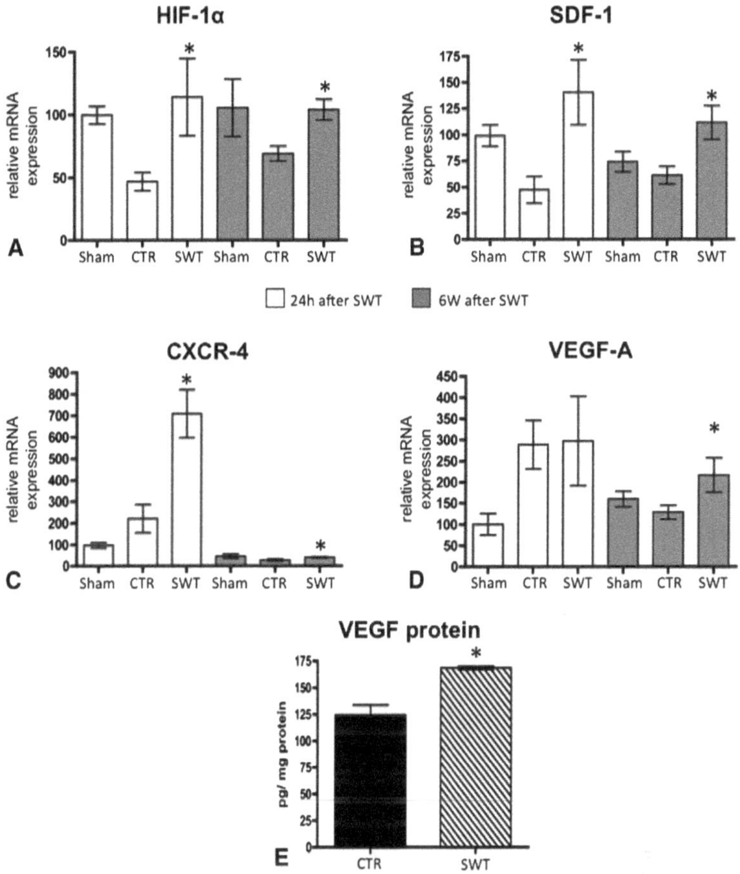

FIGURE 2.—Increase of angiogenic and chemoattractive factors in treated muscle. A, Expression of hypoxia-inducible factor 1*α* (*HIF-1α*) regulating stromal cell-derived factor-1 (*SDF-1*) significantly elevated in treatment group 24 hours and 6 weeks after shock wave therapy (*SWT*). In line with these findings, B, SDF-1 and C, its receptor C-X-C chemokine receptor type 4 (*CXCR-4*) also significantly upregulated. Vascular endothelial growth factor (*VEGF*)-A mRNA showed increased levels at 24 hours after treatment in treatment and control (*CTR*) groups. D, However, levels remain elevated in treatment group even at 6 weeks after SWT. E, VEGF protein concentration (given as pg/mg protein) showed significant increase in treatment group compared with untreated controls. $^{*}P < .05$. (Reprinted from Tepeköylü C, Wang F-S, Kozaryn R, et al. Shock wave treatment induces angiogenesis and mobilizes endogenous CD31/CD34-positive endothelial cells in a hindlimb ischemia model: Implications for angiogenesis and vasculogenesis. *J Thorac Cardiovasc Surg*. 2013;146:971-978, Copyright 2013, with permission from The American Association for Thoracic Surgery.)

tissue-level changes were accompanied by recovery of gait assessment measures at 6 weeks (Fig 5). Together, these findings suggest that SWT may have promise as a treatment for PAD, although it should be noted that the hindlimb ischemia model used does not also model the systemic effects of atherosclerosis. Given

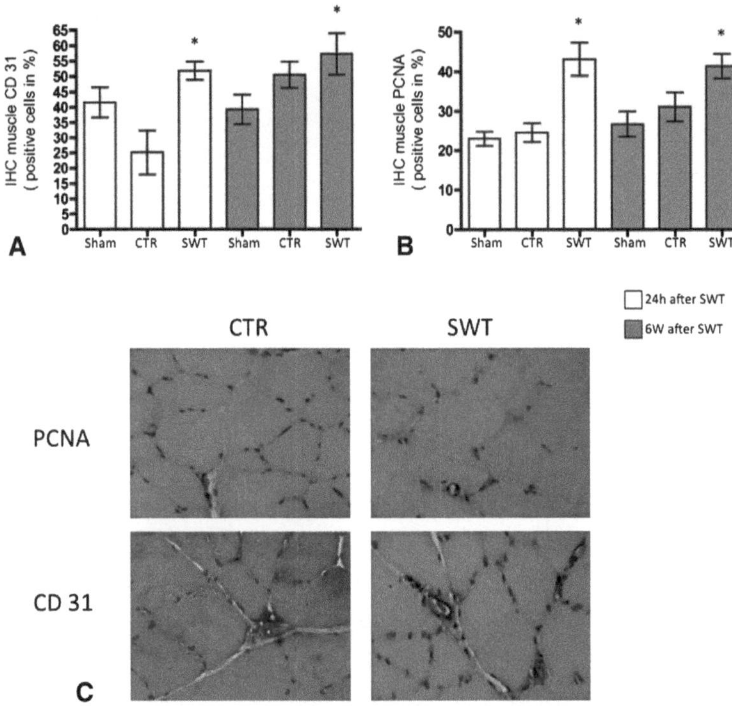

FIGURE 3.—Increase of capillary density in treated ischemic muscle. A, Immunohistochemical staining for CD31-positive cells revealed significantly greater numbers of capillaries 24 hours and 6 weeks after shock wave therapy *(SWT)*. Data presented as percentage of total cells per high power field. B, Significantly more proliferating cells found in treatment group, as shown by proliferating cell nuclear antigen *(PCNA)*. In addition to hypothesis of endothelial progenitor recruitment for vasculogenesis, this indicates additional vessel sprouting in parallel. C, Representative views of immunohistochemical *(IHC)* staining for CD31 (endothelial cells) and PCNA (proliferating cells). Magnification ×400. $^*P < .05$. *CTR*, Control. (Reprinted from Tepeköylü C, Wang F-S, Kozaryn R, et al. Shock wave treatment induces angiogenesis and mobilizes endogenous CD31/CD34-positive endothelial cells in a hindlimb ischemia model: Implications for angiogenesis and vasculogenesis. *J Thorac Cardiovasc Surg*. 2013;146:971-978, Copyright 2013, with permission from The American Association for Thoracic Surgery.)

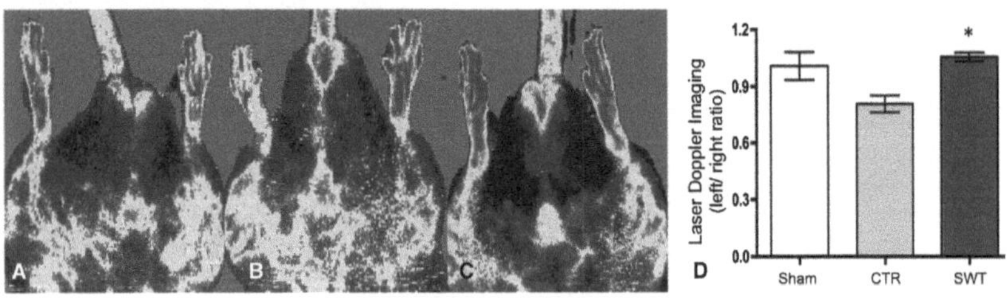

FIGURE 4.—Restoration of blood perfusion. Blood perfusion of hind limbs measured by laser Doppler perfusion imaging 6 weeks after treatment. A, Blood perfusion of sham-operated rat; B, Representative view of perfusion in untreated control *(CTR)*; and C, representative view of perfusion of shock wave therapy *(SWT)* rat. Blood perfusion clearly restored in treatment group. D, Quantification of measurements expressed as ratio of right (operated, ischemic) leg to left (nonoperated, nonischemic) leg revealing significant improvement in treatment group compared with untreated controls. $^*P < .05$. (Reprinted from Tepeköylü C, Wang F-S, Kozaryn R, et al. Shock wave treatment induces angiogenesis and mobilizes endogenous CD31/CD34-positive endothelial cells in a hindlimb ischemia model: Implications for angiogenesis and vasculogenesis. *J Thorac Cardiovasc Surg*. 2013;146:971-978, Copyright 2013, with permission from The American Association for Thoracic Surgery.)

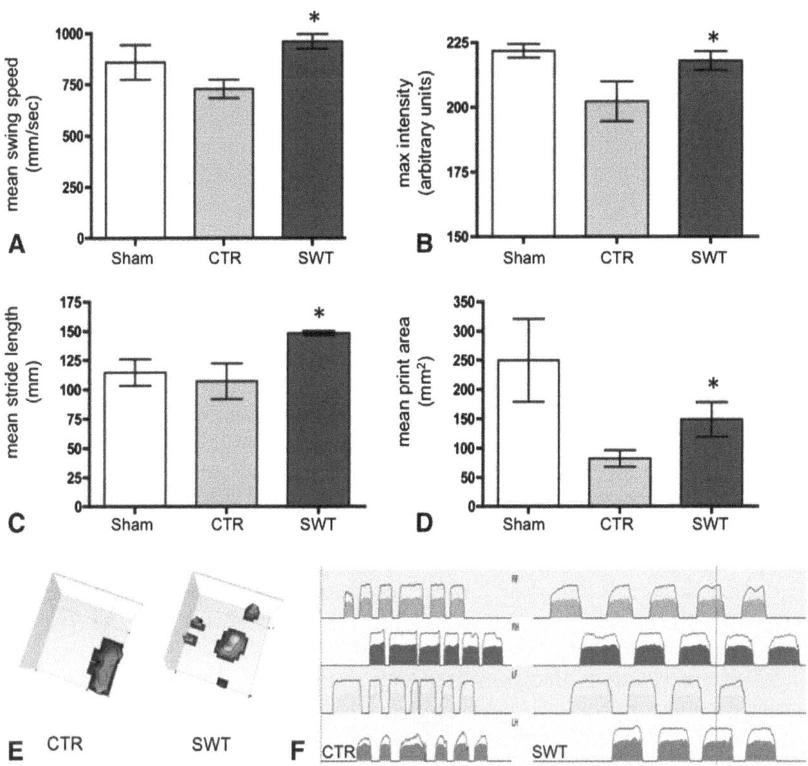

FIGURE 5.—Functional recovery of ischemic limbs. Functional assessment performed by catwalk gait analysis 6 weeks after treatment showing restored blood perfusion resulted in recovery of walking pattern in shock wave therapy *(SWT)* group. Significant improvement found in A, swing speed of hind limbs and B, their maximum print intensity. Recovery also seen in C, mean stride length and D, mean print area. E, More physiologic footprint of treatment animal *(Right)* compared with typically malfunctioning step of control *(CTR)* animal *(Left)*. F, Walking regularity clearly restored 6 weeks after SWT. $^*P < .05$. (Reprinted from Tepeköylü C, Wang F-S, Kozaryn R, et al. Shock wave treatment induces angiogenesis and mobilizes endogenous CD31/CD34-positive endothelial cells in a hindlimb ischemia model: Implications for angiogenesis and vasculogenesis. *J Thorac Cardiovasc Surg*. 2013;146:971-978, Copyright 2013, with permission from The American Association for Thoracic Surgery.)

that SWT was only applied to the adductor muscle in these experiments, it also remains to be seen whether this treatment in humans may have practical limitations related to technical factors.

M. Corriere, MD, MS

Design considerations for studies of the biomechanical environment of the femoropopliteal arteries

Ansari F, Pack LK, Brooks SS, et al (Univ of California, Berkeley; Ctr for Devices and Radiological Health, Silver Spring, MD)

J Vasc Surg 58:804-813, 2013

Objective.—The purpose of this study was to review the available literature regarding the biomechanics of the superficial femoral artery (SFA) and popliteal artery (PA) in patients with peripheral arterial disease (PAD). Stents are one of many available therapies used to treat patients with PAD. Because stents are permanent implants, they undergo a variety of deformations as patients go about their daily activities such as walking, sitting in a chair, or climbing stairs. As a part of the marketing application for United States Food and Drug Administration approval, stents need to be evaluated for long-term durability under a variety of loading modes. The information available in the literature provides direction for such evaluation.

Methods.—We performed a literature search of the PubMed database looking for "key vessel" and "mechanics" (all fields) or "deformation" (all fields) or "flexion" (all fields) or "mechanical environment" (all fields) or "tortuosity" (all fields) or "dynamics" (all fields) or "forces" (all fields), where the "key vessel" was "Femoral Artery," "Superficial Femoral Artery," "Popliteal Artery," and "Femoropopliteal."

Results.—Using a decision tree, we found 12 relevant articles that focused solely on the nonradial cyclic deformations associated with musculoskeletal motion. Despite the many limitations associated with combining these studies, we learned that under walking conditions, the proximal and mid-SFA deforms, on average, by shortening in the axial direction 4.0%, by twisting 2.1°/cm, and by bending 72.1 mm; the distal SFA and proximal PA deform by shortening in the axial direction 13.9%, by twisting 3.5°/cm, and by being pinched such that the aspect ratio of the lumen changes 4.6%. The distal PA deforms by shortening in the axial direction 12.3%, by twisting 3.5°/cm, by bending 22.1 mm, and by being pinched such that the aspect ratio of the lumen changes 12.5%.

Conclusions.—A review of the current literature reveals heterogeneous study designs that confound interpretation. Studies included different physiologic settings from young to mature participants, participants with and without disease, and cadavers. Investigators used a range of imaging modalities and definitions of arterial segments, which affected our ability to compile the data as we learned that deformations vary according to the specific anatomic location within the SFA/PA. As a result of this analysis, we identified design considerations for future studies, because although this work has been valuable and significant, there are many limitations with the currently available data such that all we know about the SFA/PA environment is that we don't know (Figs 1 and 4-6, Tables 2 and 3).

▶ This review summarizes biomechanical characteristics of the superficial femoral artery (SFA) and popliteal artery (PA) among patients with peripheral

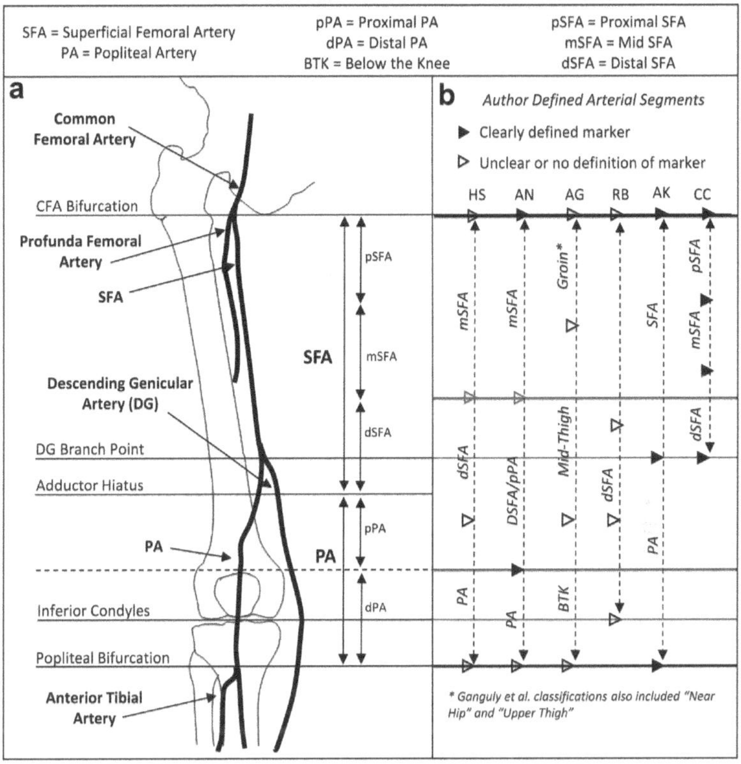

FIGURE 1.—Illustration summarizing (a) anatomic markers used to clinically define superficial femoral artery (*SFA*) and popliteal artery (*PA*) and subsets and (b) author-defined arterial segments from the authors cited in this review. See Table I for the author acronym key. See reference 28 for additional breakdown of the popliteal artery. *CFA*, Common femoral artery. (Reprinted from Ansari F, Pack LK, Brooks SS, et al. Design considerations for studies of the biomechanical environment of the femoropopliteal arteries. *J Vasc Surg*. 2013;58:804-813, Copyright 2013, with permission from The Society for Vascular Surgery.)

arterial disease (PAD) from a stent-design perspective. With the overall goal of understanding how daily activities of patients with PAD impose deformations on SFA/PA stents, the authors focused on nonradial cyclic deformations (ie, deformations other than those resulting from cyclic distension due to blood flow) by excluding the following types of studies: those performed in vitro, focused on arteries other than the SFA and/or PA, primarily assessed hemodynamics, or not including quantitative outcomes related to nonradial deformation. Twelve articles and 3 related conference presentations meeting these criteria were identified through a PubMed search and then analyzed.

The authors summarized a diverse set of anatomic definitions into a set of markers applied to all studies (Fig 1) and categorized nonradial deformation modes into 4 categories with specific definitions: (1) axial shortening and elongation (defined as normalized change in length during flexion; Fig 4) and (2) bending (defined relative to the tortuosity of the vessel and fulcrum about which it bends; Fig 5), (3) twisting (defined as the change in angular distance

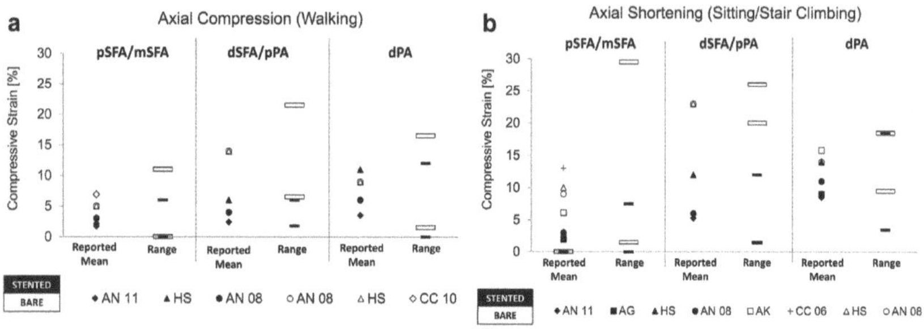

FIGURE 4.—Summary of axial shortening data for (**a**) walking and (**b**) sitting/stair climbing positions from the literature database reports values from each article, as well as the maximum value for stented and bare artery data from the entire literature database. See Table I for the author acronym key. *dPA*, Distal popliteal artery; *dSFA*, distal superficial femoral artery; *mSFA*, midsuperficial femoral artery; *pPA*, proximal popliteal artery; *pSFA*, proximal superficial femoral artery. (Reprinted from Ansari F, Pack LK, Brooks SS, et al. Design considerations for studies of the biomechanical environment of the femoropopliteal arteries. *J Vasc Surg*. 2013;58:804-813, Copyright 2013, with permission from The Society for Vascular Surgery.)

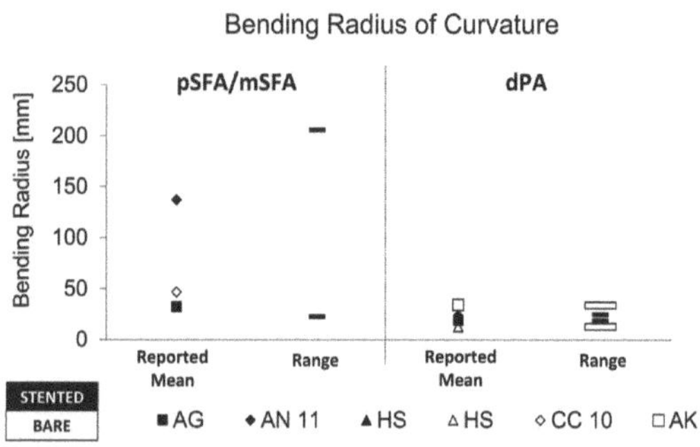

FIGURE 5.—Bending data are summarized for stented and bare vessels. Adjustments were made to the data to produce centerline bending radius magnitude, as discussed in the text. Only AG provided maximum and minimum measurements, with a minimum measured radius of curvature of 17 mm in the "mid-thigh" region. Also note that the ranges of the magnitudes for the stented and bare overlap were the same. See Table I for the author abbreviation key. *dPA*, Distal popliteal artery; *mSFA*, midsuperficial femoral artery; *pSFA*, proximal superficial femoral artery. (Reprinted from Ansari F, Pack LK, Brooks SS, et al. Design considerations for studies of the biomechanical environment of the femoropopliteal arteries. *J Vasc Surg*. 2013;58:804-813, Copyright 2013, with permission from The Society for Vascular Surgery.)

between the profunda femoris and descending genicular artery branches; Fig 6), and (4) pinching (radial compression during muscle contraction that deforms the cross-section from a circular to elliptical shape). These forces, which act in combination during walking, sitting, and climbing stairs, vary considerably between anatomic locations (Table 2) and underscore the unique biomechanical environment of the SFA/PA. Considering all of these factors, it is a wonder that SFA/PA stents perform as well as they do. Although these deformation data are considered primarily from the perspective of stent fracture and/or durability, they may also be of value for comparing stenting with other endovascular treatments such as balloon angioplasty or atherectomy at specific locations.

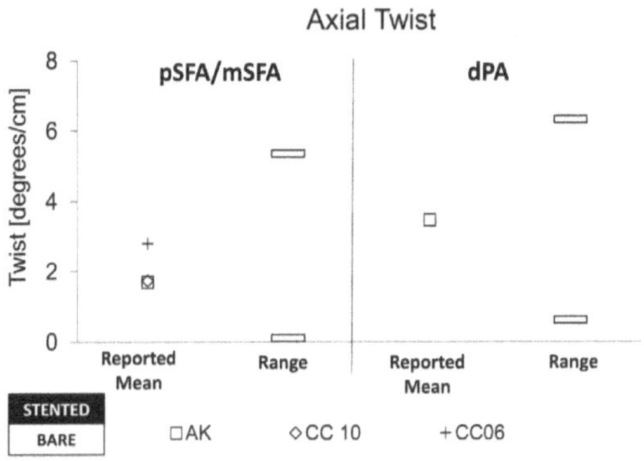

FIGURE 6.—Summary of axial twist data for the femoropopliteal artery includes mean values for each source and maximum measured values from all sources. Only bare artery data are available at this time. See Table I for the author abbreviation key. *dPA*, Distal popliteal artery; *mSFA*, midsuperficial femoral artery; *pSFA*, proximal superficial femoral artery. (Reprinted from Ansari F, Pack LK, Brooks SS, et al. Design considerations for studies of the biomechanical environment of the femoropopliteal arteries. *J Vasc Surg*. 2013;58:804-813, Copyright 2013, with permission from The Society for Vascular Surgery.)

TABLE 2.—Summary of all Nonradial Deformation Data[a]

Variable	pSFA/mSFA	dSFA/pPA	dPA	References[b]
Axial shortening, %				
Sitting/stair climbing	6.14 (0.4-29.5)	13.9 (1.5-26.0)	12.3 (3.5-18.5)	AN 11, AG, HS, AN 08, AK, HS, CC 06
Walking	4.0 (0-11.0)	8.1 (1.8-21.5)	7.7 (0-16.5)	HS, AN 08, CC 06, AK, HS, AN 08, AN 11, AG 11
Axial twist, °/cm	2.1 (0.1-5.4)	-	3.5 (0.6-6.3)	AK, CC 10, CC 06
Bending radius of curvature, mm	72.1 (19-206)	-	22.1 (13.0-33.8)	AG, AN 11, HS, CC 10, AK
Local compression (percent change in aspect ratio), %	-	4.6 (4.5-4.7)	12.5 (12.4-12.6)	RB

dPA, Distal popliteal artery; *dSFA*, distal superficial femoral artery; *mSFA*, midsuperficial femoral artery; *pSFA*, proximal superficial femoral artery.

[a]The mean and range are reported, with maximum and minimum values inclusive of all reported values and mean values ± 1.5 standard deviations.

[b]See Table I for author key.

TABLE 3.—Suggested Elements for Future Imaging Studies Involving Arterial Deformations

- Use of a single stent design with known mechanical properties
- Evaluation of the effect of overlapping stents
- Inclusion of data from patients requiring stents
- Use of three-dimensional imaging modalities
- Standardized approach to applying limb motion
- Segmenting the data by specific anatomic location

Although the results themselves are fascinating, the amount of work that was required to categorize the heterogenous study results for comparative purposes is perhaps even more impressive, underscoring the challenges imparted by inconsistent imaging techniques, physiologic models, limb positioning, and anatomic definitions between studies despite use of detailed inclusion and exclusion criteria. The authors have synthesized these study design issues into a list of suggested elements for future imaging studies of arterial deformation (Table 3) that will provide valuable guidance for investigators seeking to maximize the reproducibility and generalizability of future studies.

M. Corriere, MD, MS

Epigallocatechin-3-gallate is a potent phytochemical inhibitor of intimal hyperplasia in the wire-injured carotid artery

Orozco-Sevilla V, Naftalovich R, Hoffmann T, et al (Englewood Hosp and Med Ctr, NJ; et al)

J Vasc Surg 58:1360-1365, 2013

Objective.—Epigallocatechin-3-gallate (EGCG), a catechin gallate ester, is the major component of green tea and has been demonstrated to inhibit tumor growth as well as inhibit smooth muscle cell migration. We evaluated the effect of the phytochemicals resveratrol, allicin, sulforaphane (SFN), and EGCG on intimal hyperplasia in the carotid artery injury model.

Methods.—Intimal hyperplasia was induced in carotid arteries of adult Sprague-Dawley rats with a wire injury. Experimental animals received intraperitoneal injections of one of the four phytochemicals daily beginning 1 day prior to surgery and continued for up to 4 weeks. Control animals were administered saline. Carotid specimens were harvested at 2 weeks and subjected to quantitative image analysis. In addition, EGCG specimens were analyzed for cell proliferation, immunohistochemistry, and Western blot analysis.

Results.—Quantitative image analysis showed significant phytochemical suppression of intimal hyperplasia at 2 and 4 weeks postoperatively with EGCG (62% decrease in intimal area). Significant decreases were also noted at 2 weeks for SFN (56%) and resveratrol (44%), whereas the decrease with allicin (24%) was not significant. Quantification of intimal hyperplasia by intima:media ratio showed similar results. Cell proliferation assay of specimens demonstrated suppression by EGCG. Immunohistochemical staining of EGCG-treated specimens showed extracellular signal-regulated kinase (ERK) suppression but not of the c-jun *N*-terminal kinase or p38 pathways. Western blot analysis confirmed reduced ERK activation in arteries treated with EGCG.

Conclusions.—Intraperitoneal injection of the phytochemicals EGCG, SFN, resveratrol, and allicin have suppressive effects on the development of intimal hyperplasia in the carotid artery injury model, with maximal effect due to EGCG. The mechanism of EGCG action may be due to inhibition of ERK activation. EGCG may affect a common pathway underlying either neoplastic cellular growth or vascular smooth muscle cellular proliferation.

▶ Percutaneous coronary intervention with stenting is the most common procedure for the treatment of symptomatic coronary and peripheral artery disease; however, 30% to 50% of stent-based coronary and peripheral interventions will fail during the first year because of the development of neointimal hyperplasia and restenosis. Studies have demonstrated that many phytochemicals, chemical compounds that occur naturally in plants, are effective natural remedies for the treatment of various disease processes.

Epigallocatechin-3-gallate (EGCG), the major catechin in green tea, has been shown to be anticarcinogenic as well as an antioxidant with antithrombotic and anti-inflammatory effects. The present study examined the effect of the phytochemicals resveratrol, allicin, sulforaphane (SFN), and EGCG on intimal hyperplasia in a rat carotid artery injury model. Although all of these phytochemicals inhibited intimal hyperplasia after 2 and 4 weeks, EGCG had the most profound effect with a 62% reduction observed compared with control animals. In addition, EGCG treatment demonstrated an inhibitory effect on cell proliferation, and it was also shown to inhibit extracellular signal-regulated kinase activation. Although there are some limitations to this study, including the fact that the compounds were delivered by intraperitoneal injection and therefore it is not an exact mimic of the oral consumption route, including postabsorption metabolism, of human consumers of green tea, these are promising results given the extent of inhibition caused by EGCG and definitely warrant further investigation.

J. Cullen, PhD

Diversity in vascular surgery

Woo K, for the Society of Vascular Surgery Diversity and Inclusion Committee (Univ of Southern California and Keck School of Medicine, Los Angeles, CA; et al)

J Vasc Surg 56:1710-1716, 2012

A growing body of literature in vascular surgery demonstrates disparities in the type of health care that racial/ethnic minorities receive in the United States. Numerous recommendations, including those of the Institute of Medicine, have been set forth, which identify increasing the number of minority health professionals as a key strategy to eliminating health disparities. The purpose of this study is to compare the racial/ethnic distribution of the Society for Vascular Surgery (SVS) membership, the SVS leadership, vascular surgery trainees, and medical students. The results demonstrate that the racial/ethnic distribution of the SVS membership reflects a considerable lack of diversity with a paucity of diversity among the SVS leadership. An increasing rate of racial/ethnic diversity among vascular surgery trainees may indicate that the SVS will see an improvement in diversity in the future.

▶ Even though many of us assume we live in a society that is diverse and culturally sensitive, many health care disparities still exist for racial and ethnic minorities. The Institute of Medicine has been a staunch advocate of bringing health care equality to all and has released multiple reports over the past few years that highlight the health disparities still faced today by many minorities, as defined by race, ethnicity, sexual orientation, and gender identity. As the population of the United States becomes more diverse and less "white," so do the demographics of vascular patients. Also, the implementation of the Affordable Care Act (ACA) will allow more individuals, including those from racial and ethnic minorities, to avail themselves of the health care system. In addition, the Health Care and Education Reconciliation component of the ACA provides important incentives and requirements to create a more equitable health care system that include increasing diversity among health professionals. This study compared the racial/ethnic distribution of the Society for Vascular Surgery (SVS) membership, the SVS leadership, vascular surgery trainees, and medical students and evaluated the status of the SVS's effort to increase the number of minority vascular surgeons. Overall, of a total of 3129 SVS members who responded, 93% identified as men and 81% as Caucasian. This does not in any way reflect the diversity of the patient population SVS serves, and it is imperative that these discrepancies are eliminated. It is well known that minority physicians are more likely to serve a minority population, and furthermore patients with a racially/ethnically concordant physician also report greater satisfaction in their participation in the health care decision-making process. Diversity in health care is imperative, and if we consider vascular surgery to be a caring and compassionate profession, then we are obligated to change to address the disparities faced by racial and ethnic minorities. This not only calls for the racial and ethnic identities of the providers to become more diverse but also for existing providers to become more aware of the disparities that minority groups face on a daily basis. Training providers to be culturally competent may be considered the next step; however this type of training focuses only on the patient. We need to move to a training model of cultural humility that focuses on both the patient and the provider, with the goal of training the health care provider to practice self-awareness and reflection.

J. Cullen, PhD

Zinc finger protein 191 deficiency attenuates vascular smooth muscle cell proliferation, migration, and intimal hyperplasia after endovascular arterial injury

Lv L, Zhang J, Wang P, et al (Shanghai Jiaotong Univ, China)
J Vasc Surg 59:500-509, 2014

Objective.—Restenosis engenders surgical vascular intervention failure. Zinc finger protein 191 (ZFP191) is a novel member of the SCAN domain family of Krüppel-like zinc finger transcription factors. Previous work reveals that ZFP191 is a pleiotropic factor that plays important roles in hematopoiesis, brain development, and tumor growth. Here, we sought to determine whether intimal hyperplasia was affected by the activity of ZFP191 and to investigate the molecular mechanisms that may underpin the process.

Methods.—Intimal hyperplasia was induced by guidewire injury in mouse femoral arteries. The arteries were harvested for morphometric assessment and determination of ZFP191 expression. Next, ZFP191 knockdown in cultured mouse aortic vascular smooth muscle cells (VSMCs) was achieved by lentiviral transduction of short-hairpin RNA. MTT (3-[4,5-dimethylthiazol-2-yl]-2,5-diphenyltetrazolium bromide) assay, [^{3}H]thymidine incorporation assay, scratch assay, and transwell migration assay were used to evaluate the effects of ZFP191 knockdown on VSMC growth and migration. In addition, β-catenin, c-myc, cyclin D1, matrix metalloproteinase (MMP) 9, MMP2, and MMP7 were measured by Western blotting in the absence of ZFP191 in vitro and in vivo. Zymography was used to evaluate MMP activity in cell culture-conditioned media. Lastly, artery injury was performed in wild-type (WT) and heterozygous ZFP191 knockout (KO) mice, and morphometric analysis of the arteries was determined.

Results.—Guidewire injury was associated with development of intimal hyperplasia, and ZFP191 expression was enhanced by 51% in the injured arteries. Cultured primary VSMCs transfected with lentiviral shZFP191 displayed reduced proliferation and migration compared with controls. Mechanically, ZFP191 knockdown potently decreased the level of β-catenin and its downstream targets c-myc and cyclin D1. ZFP191 knockdown downregulated the expression of MMP9, MMP2, and MMP7, and zymography confirmed that ZFP191 knockdown reduced the activity of MMPs. Consistent with the in vitro data, elevated expression of β-catenin, c-myc, cyclin D1, MMP9, MMP2, and MMP7 accompanied upregulation of ZFP191 after injury in the femoral arteries of mice, and these levels were downregulated in ZFP191 KO vessels. Finally, intimal hyperplasia was greatly blocked in heterozygous ZFP191 KO mice compared with WT mice (intima/media ratio, 0.124 vs 0.412; $P < .05$).

Conclusions.—ZFP191 played an essential role in aggressive proliferation and migration of VSMCs, which in turn facilitated intimal hyperplasia. Our findings offer the first genetic evidence of ZFP191 as a potential therapeutic target to prevent restenosis.

► The most common treatment of symptomatic coronary and peripheral artery disease is percutaneous coronary intervention with stenting. However, 30% to 50% of stent-based coronary and peripheral interventions will fail during the first year because of the development of neointimal hyperplasia and restenosis. The main cause of this is the migration and proliferation of vascular smooth muscle cells (VSMC) in the intima of the vessel wall. The exact mechanisms through which this migration and proliferation occurs has not been completely elucidated; however, inhibition of these processes is considered a general therapeutic strategy for restenosis. Zinc finger factors participate in a variety of cellular activities, including development and differentiation, and play a role in human disease. The presence of zinc finger protein 191 (ZFP191) expression in multiple tissues and at multiple stages of development implies that the gene may have important biologic functions. The present study tested the hypothesis that ZFP191 participates in VSMC proliferation and migration and is involved in neointima formation. The 2 major findings were that genetic deficiency of ZFP191 in mice results in almost complete inhibition of restenosis after endothelial denudation and that ZFP191 exerts important effects on the proliferation and migration of VSMCs, which may be due to regulation of the Wnt/β-catenin pathway and effects on their downstream matrix metalloproteinase targets. This animal study has yielded exciting results; however, investigation into the pathobiology of restenosis and a better understanding of pathophysiological mechanisms underlying vascular smooth muscle cell migration and proliferation, especially the role of ZFP191, is required before therapeutic applications of ZFP191 inhibition can be investigated.

J. Cullen, PhD

2 Epidemiology

A Review of Current Reporting of Abdominal Aortic Aneurysm Mortality and Prevalence in the Literature

Stather PW, Sidloff DA, Rhema IA, et al (Univ of Leicester, UK)

Eur J Vasc Endovasc Surg 47:240-242, 2014

Background.—It is common for authors to introduce a paper by demonstrating the importance of the clinical condition being addressed, usually by quoting data such as mortality and prevalence rates. Abdominal aortic aneurysm (AAA) epidemiology is changing, and therefore such figures for AAA are subject to error. The aim of this study was to analyse the accuracy of AAA prevalence and mortality citations in the contemporaneous literature.

Methods.—Two separate literature searches were performed using PubMed to identify studies reporting either aneurysm prevalence or mortality. The first 40 articles or those published over the last 2 years were included in each search to provide a snapshot of current trends. For a prevalence citation to be appropriate, a paper had to cite an original article publishing its own prevalence of AAA or a national report. In addition, the cited prevalence should match that published within the referenced article. These reported statistics were compared with the most recent data on aneurysm-related mortality.

Results.—The prevalence of AAA was reported to be as low as 1% and as high as 12.7% (mean 5.7%, median 5%). Only 47.5% of studies had referenced original articles, national reports or NICE, and only 32.4% of cited prevalences matched those from the referenced article. In total 5/40 studies were completely accurate. 80% of studies cited aneurysm mortality in the USA, with the majority stating 15,000 deaths per year (range 9,000 to 30,000). Current USA crude AAA mortality is 6,289 (2010).

Conclusion.—References for AAA mortality and prevalence reported in the current literature are often inaccurate. This study highlights the importance of accurately reporting mortality and prevalence data and using up-to-date citations.

▶ This study importantly identified inaccuracies in secondary reporting for abdominal aortic aneurysm (AAA) prevalence and aneurysm mortality with the majority of recent articles reviewed overreporting the burden of disease.

The most commonly quoted mortality statistic from the United States was 15 000 deaths per year, with this statistic cited from 11 sources between 1995 and 2011. The most up-to-date mortality statistic in the United States, however, is 6289 in 2010, less than half of previously quoted numbers. Current crude AAA mortality from 4 developed countries is as follows:

United States: 6289;

United Kingdom: 5251;

Germany: 1251; and

Italy: 2073.

The range of reported prevalence was from 1.7% to 12.7%. Actual and accurate prevalence are as follows:

Svensjö: 2.2%[1];

Nordon: 4.0%–8.0%[2]; and

Lederle: 4.2%.[3]

This study provides an important benchmark and snapshot of current reported AAA prevalence and mortality data and draws attention to the inaccuracies therein. The good news is, the prevalence and mortality are declining!

B. W. Starnes, MD

References

1. Svensjö S, Björck M, Gürtelschmid M, Djavani Gidlund K, Hellberg A, Wanhainen A. Low prevalence of abdominal aortic aneurysm among 65-year-old Swedish men indicates a change in the epidemiology of the disease. *Circulation.* 2011;124:1118-1123.
2. Nordon IM, Hinchliffe RJ, Loftus IM, Thompson MM. Pathophysiology and epidemiology of abdominal aortic aneurysms. *Nat Rev Cardiol.* 2011;8:92-102.
3. Lederle FA, Johnson GR, Wilson SE, et al. The aneurysm detection and management study screening program: validation cohort and final results. Aneurysm Detection and Management Veterans Affairs Cooperative Study Investigators. *Arch Intern Med.* 2000;160:1425-1430.

Alternative Ankle-Brachial Index Method Identifies Additional At-Risk Individuals

Nead KT, Cooke JP, Olin JW, et al (Stanford Univ School of Medicine, CA; Mount Sinai School of Medicine, NY)

J Am Coll Cardiol 62:553-559, 2013

Objectives.—The aim of this study was to determine whether use of an alternative ankle-brachial index (ABI) calculation method improves mortality risk prediction compared with traditional methods.

Background.—The ABI is used to diagnose peripheral arterial disease (PAD) and to identify those at risk for cardiovascular events. Traditionally, the ABI is calculated with the higher of the dorsalis pedis and posterior tibial ankle arteries. Studies directly comparing calculation methods are limited.

Methods.—The ABI was calculated at baseline in 1,413 study participants undergoing non-emergent coronary angiography subsequently followed for all-cause and cardiovascular mortality. There were 224 individuals assigned to the traditional-PAD group (ABI <0.90) with the traditional ABI method. Of those remaining, an alternative ABI method using the lower of the 2 ankle pressures assigned 282 patients to the alternative-PAD group. The 862 individuals not assigned to PAD by either method were the no-PAD group.

Results.—There were 163 mortalities during a median follow-up of 5.0 years. Adjusted Cox regression models showed that the alternative-PAD group had an increased risk for all-cause (hazard ratio [HR]: 1.49; 95% confidence interval: 1.01 to 2.19) and cardiovascular mortality (HR: 3.21; 95% confidence interval: 1.53 to 6.37) versus the no-PAD group. Additionally, in the no-PAD group, there was an 11% (HR: 1.11; 95% confidence interval: 1.05 to 1.17) increased risk of all-cause mortality/1-mm Hg increased difference between the left and right brachial systolic pressures.

Conclusions.—The implementation of an alternative ABI method and use of the brachial difference identifies individuals at an increased risk for mortality who are currently missed with traditional ABI methods. Current ABI protocols might need to be evaluated.

▶ The authors propose reconsideration of the known value of ankle-brachial index (ABI) evaluation in patients with coronary artery disease. It is broadly understood that a reduced ABI consistent with peripheral arterial disease (PAD) is a powerful indicator of increased cardiovascular mortality, especially among patients with concomitant coronary artery disease (CAD). As such, this study confirms this clinical pillar. The proposal to use the higher brachial pressure and the lowest ankle pressure obviously stacks the deck to detect more patients as abnormal, and indeed this captured an additional—and shocking—24% of patients as PAD using the alternative calculation (see Fig 2 in the original article). These alternative-PAD patients then were identified to have a hazard ratio for cardiovascular mortality that approximates the traditional PAD groups. Ultimately, it is incumbent on any physician to interpret an ordered study with caution. In the arena of CAD, it is also incumbent on them to consider a deep dive on a reported ABI. Perhaps the conventional wisdom, or at least clinical reassurance, that one's cardiovascular risk is less advanced if PAD has not set in should be questioned. In particular, differences in distal extremity pressures are now known indicators of mortality, and maximizing modern medical management for these patients is true "best medical therapy."

J. Black, MD

Modifiable risk factor burden and the prevalence of peripheral artery disease in different vascular territories

Berger JS, Hochman J, Lobach I, et al (New York Univ School of Medicine)

J Vasc Surg 58:673-681.e1, 2013

Background.—The precise relationship between risk factor burden and prevalence of peripheral artery disease (PAD) in different vascular territories (PAD, carotid artery stenosis [CAS], and abdominal aortic aneurysms [AAAs]) is unclear.

Methods.—We investigated the association of modifiable risk factors (hypertension, hypercholesterolemia, smoking, diabetes, and sedentary lifestyle) with any and type-specific peripheral vascular disease (PVD) among 3.3 million patients in the U.S., aged 40 to 99, who underwent screening bilateral ankle brachial indices, carotid duplex ultrasound, and abdominal aortic ultrasound in the Life Line Screening program between 2004 and 2008. Multivariate logistic regression analysis was used to estimate the odds of disease in different risk factor categories. Population-attributable risk was calculated to estimate the proportion of disease that could be potentially ascribed to modifiable risk factors.

Results.—Among 3,319,993 participants, prevalence of any PVD was 7.51% (95% confidence interval [CI], 7.50%-7.53%). PAD was present in 3.56% (95% CI, 3.54%-3.58%), CAS in 3.94% (95% CI, 3.92%-3.96%), and AAAs in 0.88% (95% CI, 0.86%-0.89%). The multivariate-adjusted prevalence with the presence of 0, 1, 2, 3, 4, and 5 modifiable risk factors was 2.76, 4.63, 7.12, 10.73, 16.00, and 22.08 ($P < .0001$ for trend) for any PVD; 1.18, 2.09, 3.28, 5.14, 8.32, and 12.43 ($P < .0001$ for trend) for PAD; 1.41, 2.36, 3.72, 5.73, 8.48, and 11.58 ($P < .0001$ for trend) for CAS; and 0.31, 0.54, 0.85, 1.28, 1.82, and 2.39 ($P < .0001$ for trend) for AAAs, respectively. These associations were similar for men and women. For every additional modifiable risk factor that was present, the multivariate-adjusted odds of having vascular disease increased significantly (any PVD [odds ratio (OR), 1.58; 95% CI, 1.58-1.59]; PAD [OR, 1.62; 95% CI, 1.62-1.63]; CAS [OR, 1.57; 95% CI, 1.56-1.57]; and AAA [OR, 1.51; 95% CI, 1.50-1.53]).

Conclusions.—This very large contemporary database demonstrates that risk factor burden is associated with an increased prevalence of PVD, and there is a graded association between the number of risk factors present and the prevalence of PAD, CAS, and AAAs (Tables 1 and 2).

▶ This analysis of the Life Line Screening program data set provides valuable insight into prevalence of peripheral vascular disease and associated risk factors. As the authors point out, the participants are a nonrandom sample subject to selection bias related to volunteerism and/or socioeconomic status (the latter being related to the out-of-pocket expense associated with participation). More than 100 000 participants were excluded because they did not undergo screening for all 3 of the disease manifestations used to define peripheral vascular disease (PVD): peripheral arterial disease (PAD), carotid artery stenosis (CAS), and abdominal aortic aneurysm (AAA). It is therefore likely that selective screening in this subgroup of participants may reflect selection bias related to specific risk profiles (such as family history of previous abnormal testing prompting participants to seek only a specific screen) or socioeconomic status related to the increased cost associated with complete evaluation. Despite these considerations, it is interesting to note that cardiovascular disease prevalence in this study was generally similar to that noted in the National Health and Nutrition Examination Survey[1] (Table 1).

TABLE 1.—Baseline Characteristics of Study Participants Included in the Analysis

Characteristic	Study Participants (n = 3,696,778)
Age, years, ± SD	64.1 ± 10.2
Female sex, %	62.5
Race or ethnic group, %	
White	85.8
Black	3.0
Hispanic	2.37
Asian	1.93
Native American	2.76
Other	0.62
Body mass index, kg/m^2, ± SD	27.4 ± 6.07
Obesity,[a] %	27.6
Cigarette smoking status, %	
Never smoked	59.65
Former smoker	30.78
Current smoker	23.48
Hypertension, %	47.0
Hyperlipidemia, %	53.3
Diabetes mellitus, %	10.8
Sedentary lifestyle, %	58.2
Family history of cardiovascular disease, %	23.0

SD, Standard deviation.
[a]Obesity is defined by a body mass index >30 kg/m^2.

TABLE 2.—Prevalence and 95% CI of PVD Disease by Sex and Race

	Prevalence of any PVD (95% CI)	Prevalence of PAD (95% CI)	Prevalence of CAS (95% CI)	Prevalence of AAA (95% CI)
All subjects	7.51 (7.50-7.53)	3.56 (3.54-3.58)	3.94 (3.92-3.96)	0.88 (0.86-0.89)
Men				
Race/ethnicity				
White	8.47 (8.41-8.52)	3.04 (3.00-3.07)	4.61 (4.57-4.65)	1.99 (1.97-2.02)
Black	8.20 (7.9-8.5)	5.43 (5.19-5.69)	2.57 (2.40-2.75)	1.02 (0.92-1.14)
Asian	4.61 (4.34-4.89)	1.79 (1.62-1.96)	2.50 (2.31-2.71)	0.80 (0.69-0.92)
Hispanic	4.74 (4.5-5.0)	1.95 (1.8-2.39)	2.56 (2.38-2.75)	0.75 (0.66-0.86)
Native American	13.81 (13.4-14.22)	5.67 (5.4-5.9)	7.56 (7.25-7.88)	2.9 (2.7-3.11)
Other	7.23 (6.66-7.85)	3.06 (2.69-3.48)	3.68 (3.27-4.14)	1.37 (1.13-1.67)
Women				
Race/ethnicity				
White	6.82 (6.78-6.85)	3.61 (3.59-3.64)	3.6 (3.58-3.63)	0.29 (0.29-0.30)
Black	8.91 (8.7-9.11)	6.79 (6.6-6.96)	2.56 (2.45-2.68)	0.28 (0.24-0.32)
Asian	4.1 (3.9-4.3)	2.37 (2.23-2.51)	1.86 (1.74-1.99)	0.09 (0.07-0.12)
Hispanic	4.25 (4.08-4.42)	2.39 (2.26-2.52)	2.04 (1.92-2.16)	0.10 (0.07-0.13)
Native American	11.42 (11.18-11.66)	6.35 (6.18-6.54)	5.90 (5.72-6.08)	0.56 (0.51-0.62)
Other	7.67 (7.24-8.13)	4.63 (4.29-4.98)	3.42 (3.113-3.74)	0.44 (0.34-0.57)

AAA, Abdominal aortic aneurysm; *CAS*, carotid artery stenosis; *CI*, confidence interval; *PAD*, peripheral artery disease; *PVD*, peripheral vascular disease.

The analysis provides valuable data related to vascular disease and vascular disease risk factor prevalence. It is interesting to note that only 10% of participants (with a mean age of 64 years) had 0 risk factors. Several gender- and race-specific differences in disease prevalence were identified. Prevalence of

AAA and CAS were both higher in men, but women had a higher prevalence of PAD. Prevalence of any PVD was highest among Native American men, who also had the highest prevalence of CAS and AAA. PAD, however, was most common in black women (Table 2). Race–gender interactions for PVD risk were not evaluated but have been suggested by others.[2]

Hypertension, hypercholesterolemia, smoking, diabetes, and sedentary lifestyle were regarded as "modifiable" risk factors, but this designation may be overzealous. Although the authors discuss the potential impact of decreasing an individual's number of risk factors, hypertension, diabetes, and hypercholesterolemia are chronic diseases that are generally treated without being cured. Although hypertension and diabetes can be controlled with varying degrees of success through medical management (and therefore might be considered modifiable in that regard), these risk factors were identified in the current study through the fact that they were currently being treated with medications; the assumption that risk associated with these conditions can be further reduced may therefore be somewhat ambitious. Nonetheless, as the authors point out, sedentary lifestyle and smoking are both modifiable (and indeed curable), although for the latter risk factor, former smoking status imparts risk comparable to that of current smoking (suggesting that modification may have limited impact).

M. Corriere, MD, MS

References

1. Roger VL, Go AS, Lloyd-Jones DM, et al. Heart disease and stroke statistics—2012 update: a report from the American Heart Association. *Circulation*. 2012;125: e2-220.
2. Nguyen LL, Hevelone N, Rogers SO, et al. Disparity in outcomes of surgical revascularization for limb salvage: race and gender are synergistic determinants of vein graft failure and limb loss. *Circulation*. 2009;119:123-130.

The BASIL survival prediction model in patients with peripheral arterial disease undergoing revascularization in a university hospital setting and comparison with the FINNVASC and modified PREVENT scores

Moxey PW, Brownrigg J, Kumar SS, et al (St George's Vascular Inst, London, UK)

J Vasc Surg 57:1-8, 2013

Background.—Critical limb ischemia carries a significant risk of morbidity and mortality. The development of scores to predict risk can aid clinical decision making. The Bypass versus Angioplasty in Severe Ischaemia of the Leg (BASIL) trial investigators developed a model to predict death, which has not been previously validated.

Methods.—Data were collected in a prospectively maintained database on all patients who underwent angioplasty or arterial bypass for peripheral artery disease in a university hospital between January 2008 and June 2010. The main outcome measures were all-cause mortality and amputation-free survival at 3, 6, 12, and 24 months after the index intervention. The BASIL survival predictor, Finland National Vascular (FINNVASC) registry, and Edifoligide for the Prevention of Infrainguinal Vein Graft Failure (PREVENT) models were applied and receiver-operating characteristic (ROC) curve analysis was used to evaluate their predictive power.

Results.—Data on 342 patients were collected. Patients with isolated iliac disease or claudication were excluded. The 6-, 12-, and 24-month all-cause mortality rates were 11.6%, 17.9%, and 26.8%, respectively. The area under the ROC curve (95% confidence interval) using the BASIL score to predict mortality at 6, 12, and 24 months was 0.700 (0.60-0.80; $P < .001$), 0.651 (0.56-0.74; $P < .003$), and 0.681 (0.59-0.74; $P < .001$), respectively. ROC curve analysis indicated that the performance of the BASIL score in this cohort was comparable to other validated predictive scores.

Conclusions.—The BASIL survival prediction model can moderately predict short-term and medium-term mortality in patients with limb ischemia and may be a useful adjunct to decision making in everyday clinical practice.

▶ As society grapples with the continually rising costs of health care, third-party payers, government, or private industry will seek to determine the "value" of any given treatment option. Models to predict survival and other outcomes will become more and more common and influential because the "value" of a given health care treatment will in some part be predicated on the predicted outcomes with or without the given treatment. As government assumes or increasingly regulates payments for health care, concerns about spending will demand greater proof of "value" from any proposed treatment.

This article attempts to develop a survival prediction model from the Bypass versus Angioplasty in Severe Ischaemia of the Leg (BASIL) trial. The authors describe the impetus for constructing this model as the observation from the BASIL trial that patients who did not survive past 2 years gained little benefit from the more complicated and more expensive treatment option of bypass. Those who did survive past 2 years did benefit more from bypass than angioplasty. The authors suggest that patients who will not survive 2 years "could be better treated with angioplasty." Hence the need for a survival prediction model. Although prediction models might be of some use to the clinician in forming judgments about a particular patient, their utility is clearly dependent on their accuracy. As the authors concede and as Dr Joseph Mills clearly points out in his excellent commentary, this model must be used with great caution. When the area under the receiver operating characteristic curve of a model is less than 0.7, the model must be used with caution. This model only touches this threshold with its 6-month survival predictions and falls short at 12 and 24 months. Two other models used in the article for comparison fared even more poorly. Unfortunately, this model does not seem to offer a clear advantage to the physician in forming his or her clinical judgment about a particular case.

P. White, MD, FACS

Incidence of chronic venous disease in the Edinburgh Vein Study

Robertson L, Lee AJ, Evans CJ, et al (Univ of Edinburgh, UK; Univ of Aberdeen, UK; et al)

J Vasc Surg Venous Lymphat Disord 1:59-67, 2013

Background.—Epidemiologic research in chronic venous disease has focused on prevalence and associated risk factors. Evidence on the risks and incidence that this condition will develop is limited. The aim of this study was to measure the incidence of new varicose veins and chronic venous insufficiency (CVI) in an adult population and to investigate risk factors associated with the development of these conditions.

Methods.—The Edinburgh Vein Study is a cohort study of a random sample of the general population. Invitations were sent to 1456 men and women at baseline to participate in a 13-year follow-up examination. Each participant completed a questionnaire on lifestyle and medical history and underwent an examination that included clinical classification of venous disease.

Results.—After a mean follow-up of 13.4 (standard deviation, 0.4) years, 880 of 1456 individuals participated (60.4% response). The overall incidence (95% confidence interval [CI]) of C_2 varicose veins was 18.2% (15.2%-21.6%), giving an annual incidence rate of 1.4% (1.1%-1.7%), with incidence rates similar in men and women: the 13-year age-adjusted incidence of varicose veins was 15.2% (10.4%-20.0%) in men and 17.4% (13.1%-21.7%) in women ($P = .97$). The 13-year incidence of varicose veins increased consistently with age from 9.8% in those aged 18 to 34 years to 25.7% in those aged 55 to 64 years ($P < .001$). The 13-year incidence (95% CI) of CVI was 9.2% (7.0%-11.9%), and the annual incidence rate was 0.7% (0.5%-0.9%). The incidence of CVI was similar in men and women and increased consistently with age ($P < .001$). Participants with a family history of venous disease were more likely to develop C_2 varicose veins (odds ratio, 1.75; 95% CI, 1.12-2.71). Obesity was associated with the development of CVI: the 13-year incidence (95% CI) was 6.1% (3.7%-9.6%) in those who were of normal weight and 23.6% (14.2%-37.0%) in obese participants, with an age-adjusted odds ratio of 3.58 (1.70-7.56).

Conclusions.—The Edinburgh Vein Study is one of a few cohort studies to report the incidence of varicose veins and CVI in the general population. The incidence of varicose veins and CVI did not differ significantly by sex and was strongly associated with increasing age. The risk of developing varicose veins was increased in those with a family history, and the risk of CVI was increased in those with higher body mass index.

▶ Most studies evaluating the epidemiology of varicose veins and chronic venous disease are cross-sectional; there are few longitudinal studies.[1] The Edinburgh Vein Study is a prospective population-based cohort with a random sample of 1566 men and women, aged 18 to 64 years, who were randomly selected from the general population from practices in Edinburgh, Scotland, and examined between 1994 and 1996. The Edinburgh Vein Study evaluated the prevalence of venous disease, associated risk factors, extent of varicose veins, and reflux patterns.[2,3] Most epidemiologic research has focused on the prevalence of varicose veins and venous ulceration. Prevalence is useful in estimating the total burden of disease in a population at any given time but is limited in that it does not provide information on the risk of acquiring new varicose veins and venous insufficiency. In this follow-up study from the Edinburgh Vein Study, the authors sought to determine the incidence of new varicose veins, chronic venous insufficiency defined as skin changes and ulceration, and the associated risk factors in an adult population. The study population was reassessed 13 years later to determine the incidence and risk factors.

An important aspect in this study was the standardization in the evaluation of varicose veins and that all patients who followed up were examined for new varicose veins by an experienced examiner; therefore, there was no self-reporting by the subjects, eliminating confounders. Importantly, the study also minimized variations in measurements by the 4 observers to improve the accuracy of the results, with excellent agreement and k scores for interobserver and intraobserver variability. Of 1456 subjects eligible for the follow-up study, 880 were examined, giving a response rate of 60.4%. At mean follow-up of 13.4 years, the overall incidence of varicose vein development was 18.2%, with an annual incidence rate of 1.2%, which is much in line with what was found in the Framingham study (annual incidence of 2.6% for women and 1.9% for men) and the Bonn Vein Study II (annual incidence of varicose veins 2.07%). The overall incidence of more advanced disease (edema and skin changes) was 9.2%, with an annual incidence rate of 0.7%. This was lower than that found for the Bonn Vein Study, which had an annual incidence of 1.97%. The 13-year incidence of CEAP clinical class C3, C4, and C5 to C6 chronic venous insufficiency was 5.3% (3.7%–7.5%), 3.3% (2.1%–5.2%), and 0.5% (0.2%–1.6%), respectively. Importantly, the overall incidence of C2 varicose veins was not significantly different between women and men (18.6% vs 17.7%, respectively, $P = .97$), which is consistent with what was found in the Bonn Vein Study II. In addition, there was no difference in the incidence of chronic venous insufficiency between women and men (8.1% vs 10.6%, respectively, $P = .25$). The incidence of varicose veins increased with age for both women and men, and the age-adjusted incidence of varicose veins for women and men was similar (17.4% vs 15.2%, respectively). Risk factors that were significantly associated with varicose veins after adjusting for age were family history of varicose veins or ulcer. After adjusting for age and sex, risk factors not associated with varicose veins were obesity, sex, pregnancies, hormone replacement therapy, smoking, oral contraceptive use, and mobility at work. However, for advanced disease (C3–C6), and after adjusting for age and sex, a significant factor for developing advanced disease was obesity (body mass index ≥30; risk was 3.6-fold higher in obese participants), but unlike for varicose veins, a family history of venous disease did not increase risk. This would suggest genetic influences for varicose veins and environmental influences for advanced disease.

This important study teaches us several facts: (1) both varicose veins (C2) and advanced venous disease (C3–C6) increase significantly with age but do not differ by sex; (2) varicose veins are significantly associated with family history of venous disease, but advanced disease does not seem to be related; and (3) obesity is a significant risk factor for advanced venous disease. Further work in this area is required to determine the answers to the following: (1) How can advanced forms of chronic venous disease be prevented? (2) Does early intervention of varicose veins benefit by limiting progression of advanced venous disease? and (3) What genetic influences are responsible for development of varicose veins?

J. D. Raffetto, MD

References

1. Brand FN, Dannenberg AL, Abbott RD, Kannel WB. The epidemiology of varicose veins: the Framingham Study. *Am J Prev Med.* 1988;4:96-101.
2. Ruckley CV, Evans CJ, Allan PL, Lee AJ, Fowkes FG. Chronic venous insufficiency: clinical and duplex correlations. The Edinburgh Vein Study of venous disorders in the general population. *J Vasc Surg.* 2002;36:520-525.
3. Evans CJ, Fowkes FG, Ruckley CV, Lee AJ. Prevalence of varicose veins and chronic venous insufficiency in men and women in the general population: Edinburgh Vein Study. *J Epidemiol Community Health.* 1999;53:149-153.

3 Vascular Laboratory and Imaging

Editor's Choice: Five-year Outcomes in Men Screened for Abdominal Aortic Aneurysm at 65 Years of Age: A Population-based Cohort Study

Svensjö S, Björck M, Wanhainen A (Uppsala Univ, Sweden)

Eur J Vasc Endovasc Surg 47:37-44, 2014

Objective.—Acquiring contemporary data on prevalence and natural history of abdominal aortic aneurysms (AAA) is essential in the effort to optimise modern screening programmes. The primary aim of this study was to determine the fate of a 65-year-old male population 5 years following an invitation to an aortic ultrasound (US) examination.

Methods.—In this population-based cohort-study, men were invited to US examination at age 65, and were re-invited at age 70. Mortality, AAA repair, and risk factors were recorded. An AAA was defined as a diameter ≥30 mm, and a sub-aneurysmal aorta as 25–29 mm.

Results.—In 2006–2007, 3,268 65-year-old men were invited, and 2,736 (83.7%) were examined. After 5 years, 24 had completed AAA repair (6 died within 0–4 years), an additional 239 had died, and 194 had moved. Thus, 2,811 70-year-old men were re-invited, and 2,247 (79.9%) were examined. The AAA prevalence increased from 1.5% at 65 to 2.4% (95% CI: 1.8 to 3.0) at 70, and of sub-aneurysmal aortas from 1.7% at 65 to 2.6% (2.0 to 3.3), at 70. Of 2,041 with <25 mm at 65, 0.7% had an AAA at 70. Of 40 with a sub-aneurysmal aorta at 65, 52.5% progressed to AAA at 70. In a Cox regression analysis, sub-aneurysmal aorta at 65 (hazard ratio [HR] 59.78) and smoking (HR 2.78) were independent risk factors for AAA formation. Among 44 with AAA at 65, 22 completed AAA repair with no 30-day mortality.

Conclusion.—AAA screening in a contemporary setting was safe at 5 years, with a single AAA rupture observed among non-attenders. Men with a screening detected AAA had a high repair rate and high non-AAA related mortality. AAA-formation was common among men with sub-aneurysmal dilatation, indicating a possible need for surveillance of this group (Fig 4).

► So if I have an aortic ultrasound at age 65 and my aortic size is normal, am I good to go? Do I ever need to be screened again in my lifetime? The authors of this study sought to answer this question. Evidence from randomized controlled

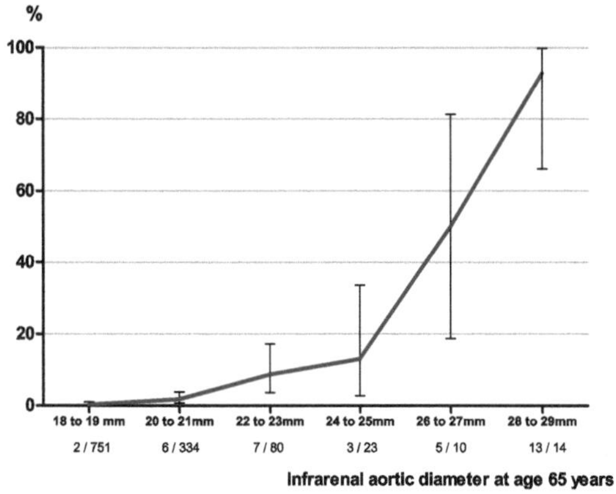

FIGURE 4.—Risk of progression to AAA. Error bars indicate 95% confidence intervals. (Reprinted from Svensjö S, Björck M, Wanhainen A. Editor's choice: five-year outcomes in men screened for abdominal aortic aneurysm at 65 years of age: a population-based cohort study. *Eur J Vasc Endovasc Surg*. 2014;47:37-44, Copyright 2014, with permission from European Society for Vascular Surgery.)

trials and observational studies demonstrate that screening elderly men for abdominal aortic aneurysm (AAA) reduces long-term mortality for ruptured AAA. The most widespread strategy, screening men once at age 65, is partially or even fully implemented in many countries. This first report, from an ongoing population-based cohort study started in 2006 in Uppsala, Sweden, describes the fate of a 65 year-old male population 5 years after an invitation to an aortic ultrasound examination.

A large cohort of men were screened and divided into groups based on aortic size. An AAA was defined as an aorta > 30 mm and subaneurysmal aorta as 25 to 29 mm. Risk of progression was then calculated (Fig 4) after a follow-up examination 5 years later. For those patients with normal-sized aortas, < 1% had an AAA 5 years later. Of those with a subaneurysmal aorta, a whopping 52% progressed to develop an aneurysm within 5 years. This article teaches us that perhaps not all screening can be reduced to a simple positive or negative result and that those patients with aortic diameters between 25 and 30 mm should be followed up at least 5 years after the initial screen and probably for life.

B. W. Starnes, MD

Foot CT perfusion in patients with peripheral arterial occlusive disease (PAOD): A feasibility study

Iezzi R, Santoro M, Dattesi R, et al ("A. Gemelli" Hosp — Catholic Univ, Rome, Italy)

Eur J Radiol 82:e455-e464, 2013

Purpose.—To prospectively assess the technical feasibility and reproducibility of quantitative foot perfusion multidetector-row computed tomography (MDCT) in patients with peripheral occlusive artery disease (PAOD)

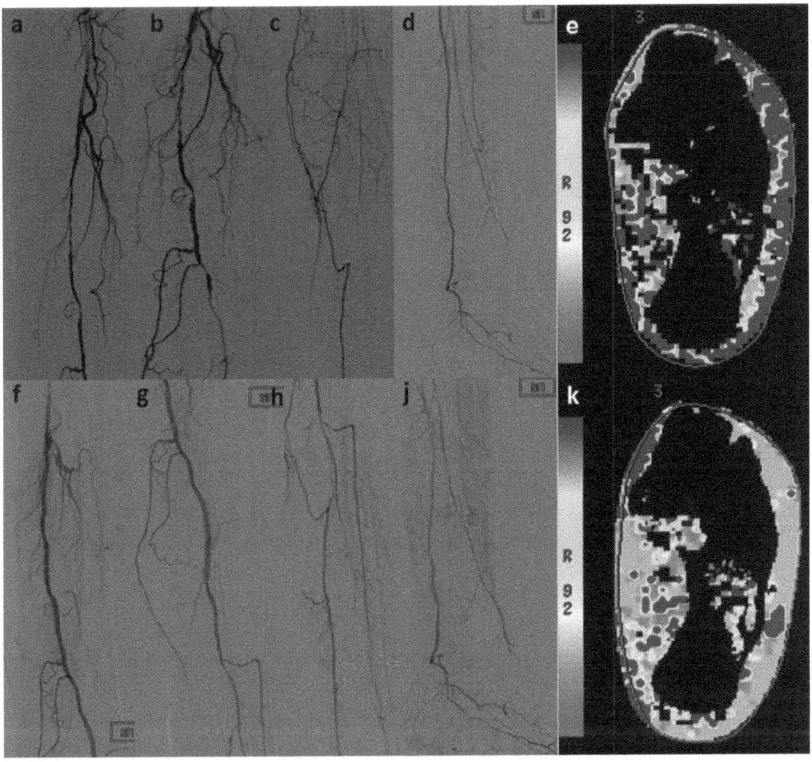

FIGURE 10.—DSA images before (a)—(d) and after (f)—(j) femoro-popliteal revascularization in 74-year man with PAOD. The perfusion map shows a significant MTT decrease before(e) and after (k) endovascular treatment. (Reprinted from Iezzi R, Santoro M, Dattesi R, et al. Foot CT perfusion in patients with peripheral arterial occlusive disease (PAOD): a feasibility study. *Eur J Radiol.* 2013;82:e455-e464, Copyright 2013 with permission from Elsevier.)

and to evaluate perfusion parameters changes after endovascular treatment.

Materials and Methods.—Institutional review board approval and informed patient consent were obtained. 10 patients older than 65 years (mean 74.1 years, range 66—95 years) with PAOD and who were referred to our department for single-limb endovascular treatment were enrolled prospectively. All patients underwent foot CT perfusion examinations before and within 72 h after endovascular treatment. A 64-row CT light-speed VCT scanner (GE Medical Systems) was used with acquisition of eight contiguous 5-mm reconstructed sections (60-s acquisition time; 40 mL Iomeprol 400 mgI/mL, @4 mL/s). Data were analyzed by two blinded readers using commercially available software to calculate perfusion parameters. Inter-observer and intra-observer agreement of perfusion CT analysis was assessed using Bland—Altman analyses and intra-class correlation coefficient (ICC). Changes in perfusion parameters after endovascular treatment were assessed using Wilcoxon's test.

Results.—Good inter-observer and intra-observer agreement was obtained in all patients. Good agreement was obtained for perfusion parameters for the untreated foot and in repeated studies. By comparing perfusion parameters in the treated foot, a significantly shorter mean transit time (MTT) was obtained.

Conclusions.—Foot CT perfusion is a feasible and reproducible technique. A significant decrease of MTT between pre- and post-revascularization suggests improved flow in the below-the-knee arteries (Fig 10).

▶ This prospective study explores the feasibility, reproducibility, and interobserver reliability of foot computed tomography (CT) perfusion in patients with peripheral arterial occlusive disease (PAD). Ten participants with PAD were enrolled to have foot CT perfusion studies before and within 72 hours after endovascular treatment, but 3 were excluded from analysis because of motion artifact, calcification, and lack of vessels suitable for evaluation. Among perfusion parameters evaluated (blood volume, blood flow, mean transit time, and permeability surface), only mean transit time changed significantly after revascularization, suggesting that it may be the most sensitive of these measures. Given that one of the radiologists interpreting the results was a resident with limited vascular experience, the reported intraclass correlations likely represent relatively conservative estimates (but indicated excellent agreement nonetheless).

Assessment of foot microcirculation using CT perfusion may have specific relevance for treatment decisions in diabetic patients, particularly those with foot wounds that are not primarily ischemic (including neuropathic ulcers). Given the feasibility, reliability, and reproducibility of foot CT perfusion demonstrated in this analysis, the logical next step to determine clinical utility would be an assessment of this technique's ability to predict wound healing or other clinical endpoints. Given that the method requires contrast administration and has limitations related to calcification and motion artifact, specific advantages over transcutaneous oxygen tension (the available alternative for assessing microvascular perfusion) would need to be identified for it to become a routine tool for clinical care.

M. Corriere

A Mismatch Between Aortic Pulse Pressure and Pulse Wave Velocity Predicts Advanced Peripheral Arterial Disease

Brand M, Woodiwiss AJ, Michel F, et al (Univ of the Witwatersrand, Johannesburg, South Africa)

Eur J Vasc Endovasc Surg 46:338-346, 2013

Objectives.—To determine whether increases in central aortic pulse pressure (PPc), but decreases in carotid–femoral pulse wave velocity (PWV) predict the presence of advanced peripheral arterial disease (PAD).

Methods.—Applanation tonometry and vascular ultrasound were employed to assess carotid–femoral PWV, PPc, and carotid intima media

TABLE 2.—Comparison of Multivariate Adjusted Measures of Large Artery Structure and Function Between Participants with Chronic Critical Lower Limb Ischaemia (CLI) and Healthy Participants from a Community Sample

Large Artery Structure and Function	Controls	CLI	*p* Value[a]
Age- and sex-matched controls vs CLI			
Carotid–femoral pulse wave velocity (m/s)	8.62 ± 3.41 (*n* = 194)	5.72 ± 3.65 (*n* = 136)	<.0001
Aortic augmentation index (%)	29.3 ± 10.6 (*n* = 194)	32.4 ± 11.5 (*n* = 136)	<.05
Aortic pulse pressure (mmHg)	39.8 ± 14.4 (*n* = 194)	49.1 ± 15.4 (*n* = 136)	<.0001
Carotid intima–media thickness (mm)	0.69 ± 0.18 (*n* = 88)	0.80 ± 0.17 (*n* = 136)	.0001
Women from age- and sex-matched controls vs women with CLI			
Carotid–femoral pulse wave velocity (m/s)	8.19 ± 2.79 (*n* = 70)	4.74 ± 3.07 (*n* = 41)	<.0001
Aortic augmentation index (%)	33.4 ± 8.2 (*n* = 70)	33.7 ± 9.3 (*n* = 41)	.89
Aortic pulse pressure (mmHg)	41.9 ± 12.3 (*n* = 70)	48.7 ± 14.4 (*n* = 41)	<.05
Carotid intima–media thickness (mm)	0.68 ± 0.13 (*n* = 33)	0.80 ± 0.13 (*n* = 41)	<.001
Men from age- and sex-matched controls vs men with CLI			
Carotid–femoral pulse wave velocity (m/s)	8.77 ± 3.76 (*n* = 124)	6.27 ± 3.99 (*n* = 95)	<.0001
Aortic augmentation index (%)	27.3 ± 11.5 (*n* = 124)	32.4 ± 12.5 (*n* = 95)	<.01
Aortic pulse pressure (mmHg)	37.7 ± 14.0 (*n* = 124)	49.5 ± 14.8 (*n* = 95)	<.0001
Carotid intima–media thickness (mm)	0.69 ± 0.20 (*n* = 55)	0.81 ± 0.19 (*n* = 95)	<.005
Community sample vs CLI			
Carotid–femoral pulse wave velocity (m/s)	6.66 ± 2.15 (*n* = 1030)	4.25 ± 2.68 (*n* = 136)	<.0001
Aortic augmentation index (%)	26.5 ± 9.3 (*n* = 1030)	30.1 ± 11.6 (*n* = 136)	<.001
Aortic pulse pressure (mmHg)	35.2 ± 11.3 (*n* = 1030)	42.8 ± 14.0 (*n* = 136)	<.0001
Carotid intima–media thickness (mm)	0.65 ± 0.14 (*n* = 429)	0.73 ± 0.16 (*n* = 136)	<.0001

Note. Data are mean ± SD. Adjustments are for age, sex (in all participants), pulse rate, body height, mean arterial pressure, body weight, presence of hypertension, diabetes mellitus, and smoking.

[a]Probability values were further adjusted for non-independence of family members.

thickness (IMT) in 136 patients of African ancestry with chronic critical lower limb ischaemia (CLI) and in 1,030 randomly selected healthy adults of African ancestry, 194 of whom were age- and sex matched (controls).

Results.—With adjustments for confounders, compared with age- and sex-matched controls, participants with CLI had an increased carotid IMT ($p = .0001$) and PPc ($p < .0001$), but a markedly reduced PWV (m/second) (CLI = 5.7 ± 3.7, controls = 8.6 ± 3.4, $p < .0001$). PWV was correlated with PPc in controls ($r = .52$, $p < .0001$), but not in CLI ($r = -.06$). A PPc/PWV mismatch index showed increased values in participants with CLI over the full adult age range assessed. With carotid IMT, PPc, or aortic augmentation index in the same regression model, an increase in the PPc/PWV mismatch index was independently associated with CLI ($p < .0001$) and a PPc/PWV value upper 95% confidence interval in the community sample predicted CLI (odds ratio = 32 [6–169], $p < .0001$). PPc/PWV predicted CLI with a similar level of performance and accuracy and a greater specificity (98%) than that of IMT (82%).

TABLE 3.—Independent Relationships Between Factors Associated with Chronic Critical Lower Limb Ischaemia (CLI) with Central Aortic Pulse Pressure (PPc)/Carotid–femoral Pulse Wave Velocity (PWV) Mismatch Index, PPc, Carotid Intimaemedia Thickness (IMT), or Central Aortic Augmentation Index (AIx) in the Same Regression Models ($n = 136$ with CLI vs 194 Age- and Sex-Matched Controls with Arterial Function Parameters and 88 Age- and Sex-Matched Controls with IMT)

CLI versus	β-coeff. ± SEM[a]	*p* Value[b]	β-coeff. ± SEM[a]	*p* Value[b]	β-coeff. ± SEM[a]	*p* Value[b]
PPc/PWV	.18 ± .04	<.0001	.15 ± .04	.0005	.23 ± .04	<.0001
PPc	.14 ± .05	<.01	–	–	–	–
Carotid IMT	–	–	.19 ± .05	<.0001	–	–
AIx	–	–	–	–	.08 ± .05	.13
Age	.06 ± .05	.17	.04 ± .05	.40	.10 ± .04	<.05
Regular smoking	.20 ± .05	<.0001	.25 ± .06	<.0001	.20 ± .05	<.0001
Regular alcohol	.09 ± .04	.05	.14 ± .06	<.05	.09 ± .04	<.05
Diabetes mellitus	.10 ± .04	<.05	.17 ± .05	<.005	.10 ± .04	<.05
Pulse rate	.52 ± .04	<.0001	.43 ± .05	<.0001	.52 ± .05	<.0001
Mean arterial pressure	−.20 ± .04	<.0001	−.06 ± .05	.23	−.16 ± .04	.0001
Body height	.17 ± .06	<.005	.10 ± .06	.11	.17 ± .06	<.005
Female gender	.12 ± .05	<.05	.15 ± .07	<.05	.12 ± .05	<.05
Body weight	.08 ± .05	.07	.09 ± .05	.07	.09 ± .05	<.05

[a]Standardized β-coefficient. Also included in the regression models was the presence of hypertension which was not significantly associated with CLI.

[b]Probability values were further adjusted for non-independence of family members.

Conclusion.—In CLI, while PPc increases, carotid–femoral PWV is markedly reduced. A PPc/PWV mismatch may be a new risk marker for advanced PAD (Tables 2 and 3).

▶ This analysis explores associations between critical limb ischemia (CLI) and noninvasive measures of large artery structure and function. Comparisons between participants with CLI and healthy participants matched for both age and sex revealed significant differences in carotid-femoral pulse wave velocity (PWV), central aortic pulse pressure (PPc), and aortic augmentation index (although differences for this last measure were not significant for all subgroup comparisons; Table 2). Associations between these parameters and CLI remained significant in multivariable models adjusting for demographic, anthropometric, and clinical risk factors (including smoking, diabetes, and hypertension) as well as for the more familiar carotid intima-media thickness (Table 3). PWV could not be measured in >10% of community participants because of extreme obesity, reflecting a technical limitation of this measure that resulted in exclusion of a subgroup of patients that would be expected to have a high prevalence of both hypertension and type II diabetes.

Although the authors identify the need for novel tools capable of predicting CLI (which is not always on a continuum preceded by claudication symptoms), advantages of these more complex measures over the simpler ankle-brachial index will need to be demonstrated to justify their widespread use. The sensitivity, specificity, and predictive value of these measures for CLI were included in the analysis, but their utility as screening tests is a somewhat artificial consideration given that CLI is symptomatic by definition. It is also worth noting that this case-control study identified an association between increased PPc/PWV mismatch and baseline CLI but did not evaluate predictive value of these parameters for future development of CLI (as perhaps implied by the title). Although the utility of PPc and PWV for clinical management therefore remains to be defined, this exploratory analysis still provides insight into the pathophysiology of peripheral arterial disease and suggests that these measures may be capable of characterizing specific clinical disease phenotypes. Given that all patients in this study were of black African descent, it will also be interesting to see if future investigations uncover race- or gender-specific associations that might inform individualized treatment strategies.

M. Corriere, MD, MS

ACCF/ACR/AIUM/ASE/IAC/SCAI/SCVS/SIR/SVM/SVS/SVU 2013 Appropriate Use Criteria for Peripheral Vascular Ultrasound and Physiological Testing Part II: Testing for Venous Disease and Evaluation of Hemodialysis Access: A Report of the American College of Cardiology Foundation Appropriate Use Criteria Task Force

Gornik HL, Gerhard-Herman MD, Misra S, et al

J Am Coll Cardiol 62:649-665, 2013

The American College of Cardiology Foundation (ACCF), in partnership with key specialty and subspecialty societies, conducted a review of common clinical scenarios where noninvasive vascular testing (venous ultrasound and physiological testing) is frequently considered. The indications (clinical scenarios) were derived from common applications or anticipated uses, as well as from current clinical practice guidelines and results of studies examining the implementation of the original appropriate use criteria (AUC). The 116 indications in this document were developed by a diverse writing group and scored by a separate independent technical panel on a scale of 1 to 9, to designate appropriate use (A) (median 7 to 9), maybe appropriate use (M) (median 4 to 6), and rarely appropriate use (R) (median 1 to 3) (Tables 1-8).

▶ Providers are increasingly being challenged to use fewer resources without compromising quality. Our natural tendency is to take advantage of imaging to maximize diagnostic accuracy and decrease the chance of errors, making responsible stewardship difficult at times. Expansion of available noninvasive imaging technologies has been accompanied by corresponding increases in utilization, reflecting the conflict that often exists between technology and value.

This report, authored by members of the American College of Cardiology Foundation Appropriate Use Criteria Task Force plus representatives from a broad range of stakeholder medical societies, assesses appropriate use criteria for 116 venous disease and hemodialysis access physiologic testing indications. Panelists independently rated testing indications before and after panel meetings in which blinded scores were discussed, and the final scores were used to categorize indications as appropriate, maybe appropriate, or rarely

TABLE 1.—Venous Duplex of the Upper Extremities for Patency and Thrombosis

	Indication	Appropriate Use Rating
Limb Swelling		
1.	• Unilateral–acute	A (9)
2.	• Unilateral–chronic, persistent	A (7)
3.	• Bilateral–acute • Suspected central venous obstruction	A (8)
4.	• Bilateral–chronic, persistent • No alternative diagnosis identified (e.g., no CHF or anasarca from hypoalbuminemia) • Suspected central venous obstruction	A (7)
Limb Pain (Without Swelling)		
5.	• Nonarticular pain in the upper extremity (no indwelling upper extremity venous catheter)	M (5)
6.	• Nonarticular pain in the upper extremity with indwelling upper extremity venous catheter	A (7)
7.	• Tender, palpable cord in the upper extremity	A (8)
Shortness of Breath		
8.	• Suspected pulmonary embolus (no indwelling upper extremity venous catheter)	M (4)
9.	• Suspected pulmonary embolus with indwelling upper extremity venous catheter	M (6)
10.	• Diagnosed pulmonary embolus (no indwelling upper extremity venous catheter)	M (4)
11.	• Diagnosed pulmonary embolus with indwelling upper extremity venous catheter	M (6)
Fever		
12.	• Fever of unknown origin (no indwelling upper extremity venous catheter)	R (2)
13.	• Fever with indwelling upper extremity venous catheter	M (4)
Known Upper Extremity Venous Thrombosis		
14.	• New upper extremity pain or swelling while on anticoagulation	A (7)
15.	• New upper extremity pain or swelling, not on anticoagulation (i.e., contraindication to anticoagulation)	A (7)
16.	• Before anticipated discontinuation of anticoagulation treatment	M (5)
17.	• Shortness of breath in a patient with known upper extremity DVT	R (3)
18.	• Surveillance after diagnosis of upper extremity superficial phlebitis • Not on anticoagulation, phlebitis location ≤5 cm from deep vein junction	M (6)
19.	• Surveillance after diagnosis of upper extremity superficial phlebitis • Not on anticoagulation, phlebitis location ≥5 cm from deep vein junction	M (4)
Vein Mapping Prior to Bypass Surgery (Coronary or Peripheral)		
20.	• In the absence of adequate leg vein for harvest	A (8)
21.	• In the presence of adequate leg vein for harvest	M (4)
Screening Examination for Upper Extremity DVT*		
22.	• Prior to pacemaker or implantable cardiac defibrillator placement	R (3)
23.	• Prolonged ICU stay (e.g., >4 days) • No indwelling upper extremity venous catheter	R (2)
24.	• Prolonged ICU stay (e.g., >4 days) with indwelling upper extremity venous catheter	R (3)
25.	• Monitoring indwelling upper extremity venous catheter that is functional	R (2)
26.	• In those with high risk: acquired, inherited, or hypercoagulable state	R (2)
27.	• Positive D-dimer test in a hospital inpatient	R (1)

A = appropriate; CHF = congestive heart failure; DVT = deep vein thrombosis; ICU = intensive care unit; M = maybe appropriate; R = rarely appropriate.

*Screening examination performed in the absence of upper extremity pain or swelling.

TABLE 2.—Venous Duplex of the Lower Extremities for Patency and Thrombosis

	Indication	Appropriate Use Rating
Limb Swelling		
28.	• Unilateral—acute	A (9)
29.	• Unilateral—chronic, persistent	A (7)
30.	• Bilateral—acute	A (8)
31.	• Bilateral—chronic, persistent • No alternative diagnosis identified (e.g., no CHF or anasarca from hypoalbuminemia)	M (6)
Limb Pain (Without Swelling)		
32.	• Nonarticular pain in the lower extremity (e.g., calf or thigh)	A (7)
33.	• Knee pain	M (4)
34.	• Tender, palpable cord in the lower extremity	A (8)
Shortness of Breath		
35.	• Suspected pulmonary embolus	A (8)
36.	• Diagnosed pulmonary embolus	A (7)
Fever		
37.	• Fever of unknown origin (no indwelling lower extremity venous catheter)	M (5)
38.	• Fever with indwelling lower extremity venous catheter	M (5)
Known Lower Extremity Venous Thrombosis		
39.	• Surveillance of calf vein thrombosis for proximal propagation in patient with contraindication to anticoagulation (within 2 weeks of diagnosis)	A (7)
40.	• New lower extremity pain or swelling while on anticoagulation	A (7)
41.	• New lower extremity pain or swelling, not on anticoagulation (i.e., contraindication to anticoagulation)	A (8)
42.	• Before anticipated discontinuation of anticoagulation treatment	M (5)
43.	• Shortness of breath in a patient with known lower extremity DVT	M (5)
44.	• Surveillance after diagnosis of lower extremity superficial phlebitis • Not on anticoagulation, phlebitis location ≤5 cm from deep vein junction	A (7)
45.	• Surveillance after diagnosis of lower extremity superficial phlebitis • Not on anticoagulation, phlebitis location ≥5 cm from deep vein junction	M (5)
Vein Mapping Prior to Bypass Surgery (Coronary or Peripheral)		
46.	• In the absence of prior lower extremity vein harvest or ablation procedure	A (8)
47.	• In the presence of prior lower extremity vein harvest or ablation procedure	A (8)
Screening Examination for Lower Extremity DVT*		
48.	• After orthopedic surgery	R (3)
49.	• Prolonged ICU stay (e.g., >4 days)	R (3)
50.	• In those with high risk: acquired, inherited, or hypercoagulable state	R (3)
51.	• Positive D-dimer test in a hospital inpatient	R (2)
Post-Endovenous (Great or Small) Saphenous Ablation		
52.	• Lower extremity swelling or pain	A (8)
53.	• Routine post-procedural follow-up, no lower extremity pain or swelling Within 10 days post-procedure	A (7)
Other Symptoms or Signs of Vascular Disease		
54.	• Physiological testing positive for venous obstruction	A (7)
55.	• Patent foramen ovale with suspected paradoxical embolism for patient without lower extremity pain or swelling obstruction	A (7)

A = appropriate; DVT = deep vein thrombosis; ICU = intensive care unit; M = maybe appropriate; R = rarely appropriate.
*Screening examination performed in the absence of lower extremity pain or swelling.

appropriate care based on median scores. Although the authors state their objective is to improve patient care and health outcomes in a cost-effective manner, the criteria seem to more directly target the process of payer authorization than clinical decision making or outcomes. Providers approaching a clinical scenario with the mindset of confirming or ruling out a specific diagnosis may

TABLE 3.—Duplex Evaluation for Venous Incompetency

	Indication	Appropriate Use Rating
Venous Insufficiency (Venous Duplex With Provocative Maneuvers for Incompetency)		
56.	• Active venous ulcer	A (9)
57.	• Healed venous ulcer	A (7)
58.	• Spider veins (telangiectasias)	R (3)
59.	• Varicose veins, entirely asymptomatic	M (5)
60.	• Varicose veins with lower extremity pain or heaviness	A (7)
61.	• Visible varicose veins with chronic lower extremity swelling or skin changes of chronic venous insufficiency (e.g., hyperpigmentation, lipodermatosclerosis)	A (7)
62.	• Skin changes of chronic venous insufficiency without visible varicose veins (e.g., hyperpigmentation, lipodermatosclerosis)	A (7)
63.	• Lower extremity pain or heaviness without signs of venous disease	M (5)
64.	• Mapping prior to venous ablation procedure	A (8)
65.	• Prior endovenous (great or small) saphenous ablation procedure with new or worsening varicose veins in the ipsilateral limb	A (8)
66.	• Prior endovenous (great or small) saphenous ablation procedure with no residual symptoms	R (3)

A = appropriate; M = maybe appropriate; R = rarely appropriate.

TABLE 4.—Venous Physiological Testing (Plethysmography) With Provocative Maneuvers to Assess for Patency and/or Incompetency

	Indication	Appropriate Use Rating
Limb Pain, Swelling, or Other Signs of Venous Disease		
67.	• Active venous ulcer	A (7)
68.	• Varicose veins, entirely asymptomatic	M (5)
69.	• Varicose veins with lower extremity pain or heaviness	A (7)
70.	• Varicose veins with chronic lower extremity swelling or skin changes of chronic venous insufficiency (e.g., hyperpigmentation or lipodermatosclerosis)	A (7)
71.	• Skin changes of chronic venous insufficiency without visible varicose veins (e.g., hyperpigmentation or lipodermatosclerosis)	A (7)
72.	• Lower extremity pain or heaviness without signs of venous disease	M (6)
73.	• Limb swelling: unilateral—acute	
	• Suspected acute venous thrombosis	R (3)
Shortness of Breath		
74.	• Suspected pulmonary embolus	R (2)

A = appropriate; M = maybe appropriate; R = rarely appropriate.

be more interested in test sensitivity, specificity, or predictive value rather than whether it is considered appropriate versus maybe or rarely appropriate. Nonetheless, these criteria provide a standardized algorithm for redirecting providers with limited familiarity with physiologic testing to the most appropriate study for the clinical scenario in question. The criteria may also be useful from a health system or vascular laboratory perspective as a means of decreasing waste while maximizing efficiency and reimbursement while reducing waste and costs

TABLE 5.—Duplex of the IVC and Iliac Veins for Patency and Thrombosis

	Indication	Appropriate Use Rating
	Prior to IVC Filter Placement	
75.	• Prior to IVC filter placement • For procedural access planning	M (6)
	Evaluation for Suspected Deep Vein Thrombosis	
76.	• Lower extremity swelling–unilateral or bilateral–as a "stand-alone test" without a venous duplex of the lower extremities	R (3)
77.	• Lower extremity swelling–unilateral or bilateral–combined routinely with a venous duplex of the lower extremities	M (4)
78.	• Lower extremity swelling–unilateral or bilateral–performed selectively –when the lower extremity venous duplex is normal	M (6)
79.	• Lower extremity swelling–unilateral or bilateral–performed selectively –when the lower extremity venous duplex is positive for acute proximal DVT	A (7)
80.	• Selectively–when the flow pattern in 1 or both common femoral veins is abnormal	A (8)
	Evaluation for Suspected Pulmonary Embolus	
81.	• Pulmonary symptoms (suspected pulmonary embolus)–as a "stand-alone test" without a venous duplex of the lower extremities	R (2)
82.	• Pulmonary symptoms (suspected pulmonary embolus)–combined routinely with a venous duplex of the lower extremities	M (4)
	Evaluation of Other Symptoms or Signs of Abdominal Vascular Disease	
83.	• Abdominal pain	R (3)
84	• Abdominal bruit	R (3)
85.	• Fever of unknown origins	R (3)

A = appropriate; DVT = deep vein thrombosis; IVC = inferior vena cava; M = maybe appropriate; R = rarely appropriate.

TABLE 6.—Duplex of the Hepatoportal System (Portal Vein, Hepatic Veins, Splenic Vein, Superior Mesenteric Vein, Inferior Vena Cava) for Patency, Thrombosis, and Flow Direction*

	Indication	Appropriate Use Rating
	Evaluation of Hepatic Dysfunction or Portal Hypertension	
86.	• Abnormal liver function tests • No alternative diagnosis identified (e.g., medication related or infectious hepatitis)	M (6)
87.	• Cirrhosis with or without ascites	A (7)
88.	• Jaundice • As an initial diagnostic test	R (3)
89.	• Jaundice • No alternative diagnosis identified after initial evaluation (e.g., no biliary obstruction)	M (6)
90.	• Hepatomegaly and/or splenomegaly	A (7)
91.	• Portal hypertension	A (7)
	Surveillance Following Portal Decompression Procedure	
92.	• Follow-up of a TIPS	A (8)
	Evaluation of Other Symptoms or Signs of Abdominal Vascular Disease	
93.	• Abdominal pain	M (4)
94.	• Fever of unknown origin	R (3)
	Evaluation of Cardiac and/or Pulmonary Symptoms	
95.	• Pulmonary symptoms (suspected pulmonary embolus)	R (3)
96.	• Cor pulmonale	R (3)

A = appropriate; TIPS = transjugular intrahepatic portosystemic shunt; M = maybe appropriate; R = rarely appropriate.
*Testing indications refer to evaluation of native hepatoportal venous system only (i.e., hepatic transplant sites and arterial system excluded).

TABLE 7.—Duplex of the Renal Veins for Patency and Thrombosis*

Indication		Appropriate Use Rating
Evaluation for Suspected Renal Vein Thrombosis—Potential Signs and/or Symptoms		
97.	• Gross hematuria	R (3)
98.	• Acute renal failure	M (5)
99.	• Acute flank pain	M (5)
Evaluation of Cardiac and/or Pulmonary Symptoms		
100.	• Pulmonary symptoms (suspected pulmonary embolus)	R (3)
Evaluation of Other Symptoms or Signs of Abdominal Vascular Disease		
101.	• Drug-resistant hypertension (suspected renal artery stenosis)	R (3)
102.	• Microscopic hematuria (prior to urological evaluation)	R (2)
103.	• Fever of unknown origin	R (2)
104.	• Epigastric bruit	R (2)

A = appropriate; DVT = deep vein thrombosis; IVC = inferior vena cava; M = maybe appropriate; R = rarely appropriate.

*Testing indications refer to evaluation of native renal veins only for patency (i.e., renal transplant sites and renal arteries excluded).

TABLE 8.—Pre-Operative Planning and Post-Operative Assessment of a Vascular Access Site*

Indication		Appropriate Use Rating
Assessment Prior to Access Site Placement*		
105.	• Pre-operative mapping study (upper extremity arterial and venous duplex) ≥3 months prior to access placement	R (3)
106.	• Pre-operative mapping study (upper extremity arterial and venous duplex) <3 months prior to access placement	A (8)
"Failure to Mature"		
107.	• "Failure to mature" on basis of physical examination 0–6 weeks after placement	M (6)
108.	• "Failure to mature" on basis of physical examination >6 weeks after placement	A (8)
Symptoms and Signs of Disease†		
109.	• Signs of access site malfunction during dialysis (e.g., low blood flows, kt/V, recirculation times, or increased venous pressure)	A (8)
110.	• Mass associated with an AVF/AVG	A (8)
111.	• Loss of palpable thrill of AVF/AVG	A (8)
112.	• Arm swelling	A (8)
113.	• Hand pain, pallor, and/or digital ulceration (i.e., evaluation for suspected arterial steal syndrome)	A (8)
114.	• Cool extremity	
	• Without pain, pallor, or ulceration	R (3)
115.	• Difficult cannulation by multiple personnel on multiple attempts	A (8)
Asymptomaticy†		
116.	• Routine surveillance of a functioning AVF or AVG	R (3)

A = appropriate; AVF = autogenous arteriovenous fistula (including venous transpositions); AVG = prosthetic arteriovenous graft; M = maybe appropriate; R = rarely appropriate.

*Ultrasound assessment prior to creation of dialysis access (AVF or AVG) typically includes a combined arterial and venous duplex examination that is performed to determine the adequacy of superficial veins (patency, size, and length of conduit), patency of central venous outflow, and adequacy of adequate arterial inflow. Determination of central venous patency is particularly important for patients with a history of prior central venous catheter(s).

†In a mature AVF or AVG that is being accessed for hemodialysis.

related to inappropriate testing. The authors acknowledge that the criteria are not substitutes for clinical judgment and experience, but despite this qualification, they may have the unintended consequence of creating authorization barriers in complex or unusual circumstances where they may not apply.

M. Corriere, MD, MS

Computed tomography angiography-based evaluation of great saphenous vein conduit for lower extremity bypass

deFreitas DJ, Love TP, Kasirajan K, et al (Atlanta VA Med Ctr, GA; Emory Univ School of Medicine, Atlanta, GA; et al)

J Vasc Surg 57:50-55, 2013

Objective.—Lower extremity computed tomography angiography (CTA) is frequently used for anatomic assessment of lower extremity peripheral arterial disease. When lower extremity bypass is planned, duplex ultrasound (DUS) is routinely obtained to evaluate the great saphenous vein (GSV) for use as conduit. Although GSV can be visualized on CTA images, diameter assessment is not routinely included in formal study interpretation. We hypothesized that CTA images could be used to measure GSV diameters and that CTA-based diameters would correlate with measurements obtained using DUS.

Methods.—Consecutive patients undergoing lower extremity arterial bypass who were evaluated preoperatively with both CTA and DUS vein mapping were identified at a single hospital. Minimum above- and below-knee GSV diameters were measured from electronically archived CTA images by two independent observers. CTAs were performed using standard arterial phase protocol without additional venous phase imaging. Between-observer reproducibility of CTA-based diameter measurements was evaluated using intraclass correlation coefficients. Correlation between CTA and DUS-based GSV diameters was evaluated with Spearman correlation coefficients. CTA diameter cut-points for identification of adequate GSV bypass conduit, defined as DUS-based minimum GSV diameter ≥3 mm, were determined using receiver-operating characteristic curves.

Results.—Sixty-three lower extremities were evaluated in 36 patients. In the absence of previous surgical removal, GSV was visible on all CTAs reviewed. No instances of GSV thrombosis were identified on DUS. Minimum DUS-based above-knee GSV diameter was 2.9 ± 0.1 mm (range, 1.4-4.6 mm), and mean below-knee diameter was 2.6 ± 0.1 mm (range, 1.3-4.0 mm). When GSV was visible and exceeded the minimum diameter threshold for CTA measurement, correlation between CTA- and DUS-based diameters was both positive and highly significant ($\rho = 0.595$; $P < .0001$). CTA-based diameters also had excellent reliability between observers (r [95% CI]: 0.88 [0.85-0.91]). For identification of adequate bypass conduit using CTA, above-knee GSV diameter ≥3.9 mm was 67% sensitive and 73% specific; below-knee GSV diameter ≥3.0 mm was 75% sensitive and 84% specific.

Conclusions.—CTA-based GSV diameter measurements have good reproducibility and highly significant correlation with DUS-based diameters. CTA-based GSV diameter is a specific but relatively insensitive indicator of adequate bypass conduit. When CTA-based diameters indicate inadequate GSV bypass conduit, confirmatory DUS vein mapping is warranted. Confirmatory DUS vein mapping may be unnecessary when adequate vein diameter is identified on CTA.

▶ It is clear that the development of new computed tomographic (CT) angiography imaging is changing our practice. I would estimate that vascular surgeons practicing these days use more computer-assisted imaging and design to help their patients than ever before. As such, new applications for these technologies are a natural progression. In this article, the group from Emory attempt to answer the provocative question of whether CT angiograms obtained to assess the aorta and its runoff may be used simultaneously to assess whether such patients have adequate vein conduit to perform distal bypass. Overall, the study is well designed and statistically robust. All lower extremity venous duplex exams were performed in the supine position to make the tests comparable. In short, they found good reliability between the tests as long as the greater saphenous vein diameter was ≥3.9 mm for the above knee segment or ≥3.0 mm for the below knee segment. In these cases, duplex ultrasound vein mapping may be unnecessary. To be sure, it is not that cumbersome to perform a quick intraoperative duplex examination of the greater saphenous vein mapping in patients with questionable or small vein size. Certainly if preoperative duplex ultrasound vein mapping were not performed, this would be preferable to prosthetic below knee or tibial bypass.

D. L. Gillespie, MD, RVT, FACS

Computed tomography angiography-based evaluation of great saphenous vein conduit for lower extremity bypass

deFreitas DJ, Love TP, Kasirajan K, et al (Emory Univ School of Medicine, Atlanta, GA; et al)

J Vasc Surg 57:50-55, 2013

Objective.—Lower extremity computed tomography angiography (CTA) is frequently used for anatomic assessment of lower extremity peripheral arterial disease. When lower extremity bypass is planned, duplex ultrasound (DUS) is routinely obtained to evaluate the great saphenous vein (GSV) for use as conduit. Although GSV can be visualized on CTA images, diameter assessment is not routinely included in formal study interpretation. We hypothesized that CTA images could be used to measure GSV diameters and that CTA-based diameters would correlate with measurements obtained using DUS.

Methods.—Consecutive patients undergoing lower extremity arterial bypass who were evaluated preoperatively with both CTA and DUS vein mapping were identified at a single hospital. Minimum above- and below-knee GSV diameters were measured from electronically archived CTA images by two independent observers. CTAs were performed using standard arterial phase protocol without additional venous phase imaging. Between-observer reproducibility of CTA-based diameter measurements was evaluated using intraclass correlation coefficients. Correlation between CTA and DUS-based GSV diameters was evaluated with Spearman correlation coefficients. CTA diameter cut-points for identification of adequate GSV bypass conduit, defined as DUS-based minimum GSV diameter ≥3 mm, were determined using receiver-operating characteristic curves.

Results.—Sixty-three lower extremities were evaluated in 36 patients. In the absence of previous surgical removal, GSV was visible on all CTAs reviewed. No instances of GSV thrombosis were identified on DUS. Minimum DUS-based above-knee GSV diameter was 2.9 ± 0.1 mm (range, 1.4-4.6 mm), and mean below-knee diameter was 2.6 ± 0.1 mm (range, 1.3-4.0 mm). When GSV was visible and exceeded the minimum diameter threshold for CTA measurement, correlation between CTA- and DUS-based diameters was both positive and highly significant ($\rho = 0.595$; $P < .0001$). CTA-based diameters also had excellent reliability between observers (r [95% CI]: 0.88 [0.85-0.91]). For identification of adequate bypass conduit using CTA, above-knee GSV diameter ≥3.9 mm was 67% sensitive and 73% specific; below-knee GSV diameter ≥3.0 mm was 75% sensitive and 84% specific.

Conclusions.—CTA-based GSV diameter measurements have good reproducibility and highly significant correlation with DUS-based diameters. CTA-based GSV diameter is a specific but relatively insensitive indicator of adequate bypass conduit. When CTA-based diameters indicate inadequate GSV bypass conduit, confirmatory DUS vein mapping is warranted. Confirmatory DUS vein mapping may be unnecessary when adequate vein diameter is identified on CTA (Fig 2).

► Color flow duplex ultrasound scan is used in many studies involving the vasculature, including during vein mapping of the great saphenous vein (GSV), small saphenous vein, and upper extremity cephalic and basilica veins in preparation for bypass surgery. In this retrospective study, the authors hypothesized that computed tomographic angiography (CTA) images could be used for GSV assessment for use as a bypass conduit, and that CTA-based diameter measurements are correlated with those obtained using duplex ultrasonography (DUS). This study included 36 patients with a total of 63 lower extremities evaluated with both CTA and DUS. Of the 63 lower extremities studied with DUS vein mapping, the GSV could be visualized and measured at all intended above-knee anatomic locations in 59 limbs (93.7%) and all intended below-knee anatomic locations in 51 limbs (81.0%). CTA-based GSV assessments were possible in 54 of 59 (91.5%) above-knee and 43 of 51 below-knee (84.3%) anatomic locations where DUS measurements were obtained. When GSV was visible and exceeded the minimum diameter threshold of CTA measurement, correlation

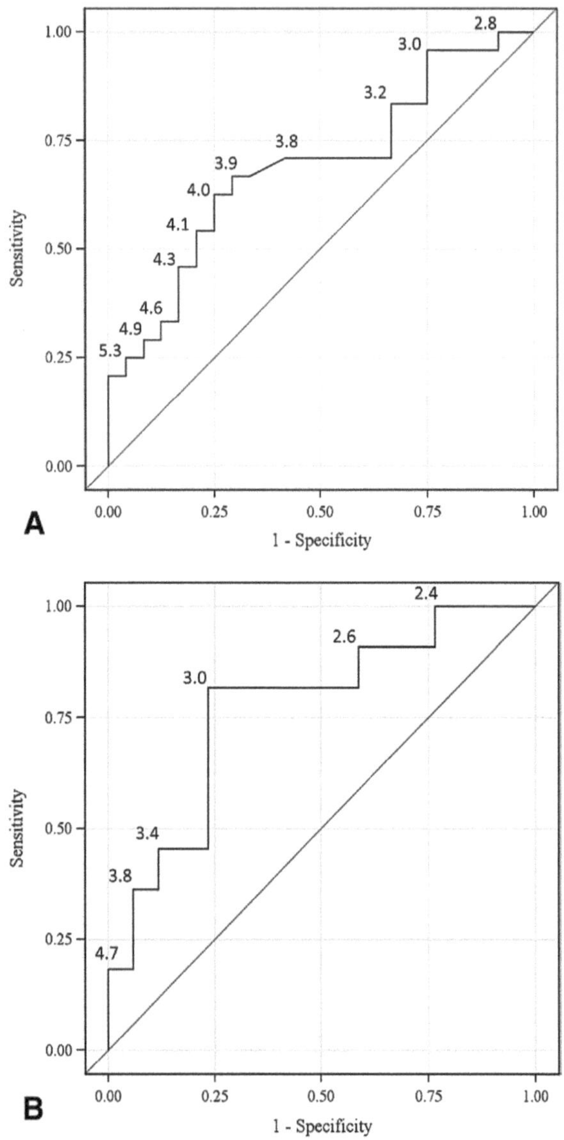

FIGURE 2.—Receiver-operating characteristic curves: computed tomography angiography (CTA)-based minimum great saphenous vein (GSV) diameter as indicator of adequate bypass conduit. Above-knee (**A**) and below-knee (**B**) CTA-based diameter cutpoints in millimeters are indicated along the curve. Adequate conduit defined as diameter ≥3.0 mm by duplex ultrasound (DUS). (Reprinted from the Journal of Vascular Surgery. Defreitas DJ, Love TP, Kasirajan K, et al. Computed tomography angiography-based evaluation of great saphenous vein conduit for lower extremity bypass. *J Vasc Surg*. 2013;57:50-55, Copyright 2013, with permission from The Society for Vascular Surgery.)

between CTA- and DUS-based diameters was both positive and highly significant. By receiver operator characteristic, the CTA determined that adequate GSV diameter above the knee was 3.9 mm and below the knee was 3.0 mm (Fig 2). For identification of adequate lower extremity bypass conduit, CTA-based categorical assessment of above-knee GSV had a sensitivity of 67% and a specificity of 73%. Below the knee, CTA-based assessment of GSV had a sensitivity of 75% and a specificity of 84%. These data would indicate that if GSV diameters as determined by CTA appear adequate, DUS may not be necessary to confirm; however, if GSV diameters as determined by CTA appear inadequate, confirmation with DUS may be necessary. An advantage of US, in addition to not posing radiation risks, is its ability to assess vein morphology, compressibility, duplication, branches and perforators, and evidence of previous superficial thrombophlebitis. Because CTA-based GSV diameters are measured from arterial phase images with veins in a noncontrasted state, the limitations are the inability to assess patency or detect thrombus because of lack of venous phase images. Another important consideration is that the resolution may be limited with CTA, and the role of DUS vein mapping becomes particularly important when vein diameter is borderline, or technical factors, such as inflammation, edema, or paucity of surrounding adipose tissue, impair visualization with CTA. Because the nature of this study was retrospective, prospective validation will be necessary to endorse CTA as an imaging modality for GSV diameters as a suitable bypass conduit for lower extremity ischemia.

J. D. Raffetto, MD

A Prospective Randomized Trial of Ultrasound- vs Landmark-Guided Central Venous Access in the Pediatric Population

Bruzoni M, Slater BJ, Wall J, et al (Lucile Packard Children's Hosp - Stanford Univ Med Ctr, Palo Alto, CA; et al)

J Am Coll Surg 216:939-943, 2013

Background.—The purpose of this prospective randomized study was to compare landmark- to ultrasound-guided central venous access when performed by pediatric surgeons. The American College of Surgeons advocates for use of ultrasound in central venous catheter placement; however, this is not universally embraced by pediatric surgeons. Complication risk correlates positively with number of venous cannulation attempts.

Study Design.—With IRB approval, a randomized prospective study of children under 18 years of age undergoing tunneled central venous catheter placement was performed. Patient accrual was based on power analysis. Exclusion criteria included known nonpatency of a central vein or coagulopathy. After randomization, the patients were assigned to either ultrasound-guided internal jugular vein access or landmark-guided subclavian/internal jugular vein access. The primary outcomes measure was number of attempts at venous cannulation. Secondary outcomes measures included: access times, number of arterial punctures, and other complications. Continuous variables were compared using 2-tailed Student's *t*-test. Discrete variables were analyzed with chi-square. Significance was defined as $p < 0.05$.

Results.—There were 150 patients enrolled between April 2008 and September 2011. There was no difference when comparing demographic data. Success at first attempt was achieved in 65% of patients in the ultrasound group vs 45% in the landmark group ($p = 0.021$). Success within 3 attempts was achieved in 95% of ultrasound group vs 74% of landmark group ($p = 0.0001$).

Conclusions.—Ultrasound reduced the number of cannulation attempts necessary for venous access. This indicates a potential to reduce complications when ultrasound is used by pediatric surgeons.

▶ Is it now common in surgical training programs to utilize ultrasound imaging in the placement of central lines? I certainly hope so, with the data showing that the use of an ultrasound scan is "associated with an increased success rate, decreased operating time, reduced number of cannulation attempts, and a decreased number of carotid artery punctures." This study is very specific in that it looks at the utility of this imaging modality in central venous catheterization performed by pediatric surgeons or pediatric surgery fellows. The patients were within a wide range of ages (0–18 years); thus, many were adult size. The surgeons all completed training as well as 20 proctored cases before enrolling patients in the study. Interestingly, all patients underwent subclavian vein puncture attempts, and no internal jugular veins were used. As would be expected from prior studies, those allocated to ultrasound guidance did much better in first-time attempts and within 3 attempts.

Although the discussion emphasizes the challenging nature of central venous catheterization in the pediatric population, the cohort was broad in age and weight of participants. I would be interested to see results by age and size distribution. The weight range was from 4 kg to 106 kg or between 8.8 and 233 pounds! Definitely not small children! Only the average size is given, not the median. The limitations section does include some comments about line placement in infants and toddlers. Perhaps this is the group in whom the focus should lie to improve outcomes. The main message from this study is good—use ultrasound imaging to improve 1st time subclavian vein cannulation rates for central line placement. However, the authors really should look at a truly pediatric population to validate their claims.

R. L. Bush, MD, JD, MPH

4 Perioperative Considerations

Unplanned readmissions after vascular surgery

Gupta PK, Fernandes-Taylor S, Ramanan B, et al (Univ of Wisconsin Hosp and Clinics, Madison; Creighton Univ, Omaha, NE)

J Vasc Surg 59:473-482, 2014

Objective.—Existing literature on readmission after vascular surgery is limited. The upcoming reduction in Medicare reimbursement for institutions with high readmission rates mandates an accurate understanding of this issue. In this study, we characterize the frequency and causes of 30-day unplanned readmissions after elective vascular surgery.

Methods.—Patients who underwent elective carotid endarterectomy (CEA), endovascular aortic repair (EVAR), open abdominal aortic aneurysm (oAAA) repair, or infrainguinal bypass grafting (BPG) were identified from the American College of Surgeons (ACS) National Surgical Quality Improvement Program (NSQIP) 2011 database (n = 11,246). Multivariable logistic regression was used to determine variables that contributed to 30-day unplanned readmissions for each surgery type.

Results.—The unadjusted unplanned readmission rates after the four vascular procedures ranged from 6.5% for CEA to 15.7% for BPG. In multivariable analyses, patient comorbidities were associated with unplanned readmission after BPG and CEA ($P < .05$), whereas postoperative complications were more consistently associated with unplanned readmission after EVAR and oAAA repair ($P < .05$). For all procedures, complications leading to readmission developed more frequently after discharge. Thirty-day mortality was significantly higher in readmitted patients after BPG (1.9% vs 0.3%), EVAR (3.9% vs 0.1%), and CEA (2.2% vs 0.2%; $P < .001$ for each), but not after oAAA repair.

Conclusions.—Select comorbidities and postoperative complications contribute to unplanned readmissions after vascular surgery. The characteristics of readmitted patients vary with the type of procedure. Interventions designed to mitigate these factors have the potential to reduce unplanned readmissions but likely need to vary with the type of vascular treatment.

► The objective of this study was to characterize 30-day unplanned readmission rates for 4 common vascular procedures: open abdominal aortic aneurysm (oAAA) repair, endovascular abdominal aortic aneurysm repair (EVAR), infrainguinal bypass grafting (BPG), and carotid endarterectomy (CEA), and analyze preoperative and postoperative factors associated with unplanned readmissions after these vascular procedures. Their primary outcome of interest was an unplanned readmission 30 days after discharge after a qualifying surgical procedure, defined as any unplanned inpatient stay at the same or different institution. The association between 30-day readmission and subsequent 30-day mortality was also evaluated. Data were extracted from the 2011 American College of Surgeons National Surgical Quality Improvement Program (NSQIP) Participant Use Data File. They found overall (planned and unplanned) readmission rates of 16.4%, 8.2%, 8.1%, and 8.0% after BPG, EVAR, oAAA repair, and CEA, respectively. These results are significantly less than prior reports gleaned primarily from Medicare databases. The higher rate of readmission seen in the Medicare population may be related to the inclusion of planned readmissions in the Medicare analyses and a higher burden of morbidity among older Medicare patients, as analysis of NSQIP data included a significant number of patients age less than 65 years. Once again, multivariate analyses showed that discharge to a skilled nursing or rehabilitation facility was associated with readmission after EVAR and CEA but not BPG and oAAA repair. An interesting study finding was that complications eventually leading to readmission more often developed after discharge than during the index admission. The preoperative comorbidities or postoperative complications that predisposed to unplanned readmission were different for all 4 vascular procedures studied. This implies that factors predisposing patients to readmission vary depending on the surgical procedure and raises the possibility that interventions to reduce readmissions may be different for each intervention.

M. T. Watkins, MD

Impact of postoperative nadir hemoglobin and blood transfusion on outcomes after operations for atherosclerotic vascular disease

Kougias P, Orcutt S, Pak T, et al (Michael E. DeBakey VA Med Ctr, Houston, TX; Baylor College of Medicine, Houston, TX)

J Vasc Surg 57:1331-1337, 2013

Objective.—Controversy surrounds the topic of transfusion policy after noncardiac operations. This study assessed the combined impact of postoperative nadir hemoglobin (nHb) levels and blood transfusion on adverse events after open surgical intervention in patients who undergo operative intervention for atherosclerotic vascular disease.

Methods.—Consecutive patients who underwent peripheral arterial disease (PAD)-related operations were balanced on baseline characteristics by inverse weighting on propensity score calculated as their probability to have nHb greater than 10 gm/dL on the basis of operation type, demographics, and comorbidities, including the revised cardiac risk index. A multivariate generalized estimating equation analysis was performed to investigate associations between nHb, transfusion, and a composite outcome of perioperative death and myocardial infarction. Logistic and Cox proportional hazards regressions were used to assess the impact of nHb and transfusion on respiratory and wound complications; and a composite end point (CE) of death, myocardial infarction during a 2-year follow-up. Level of statistical significance was set at alpha of 0.0125 to adjust for the increased probability of type I error attributable to multiple comparisons.

Results.—The analysis cohort included 880 patients (1074 operations). After adjusting for nHb level, the number of units transfused was not associated with the perioperative occurrence of the CE (odds ratio [OR], 1.13; $P = .025$). Adjusted for the number of units transfused, nHb had no impact on the perioperative CE (OR, 0.62; $P = .22$). An interaction term between transfusion and nHb level remained nonsignificant ($P = .312$), indicating that the impact of blood transfusion was the same regardless of the nHb level. Perioperative respiratory complications were more likely in patients receiving transfusions (OR, 1.22; $P = .009$), and perioperative wound infections were less common in patients with nHb > 10 gm/dL (OR, 0.65; $P = .01$). During an average follow-up of 24 months, transfused patients were more likely to develop the CE (hazard ratio [HR], 1.15, $P = .009$), whereas nHb level did not impact the long-term adverse event rate (HR, 0.78; $P = .373$). The above associations persisted even after adjusting the Cox regression model for the occurrence of perioperative cardiac events.

Conclusions.—Although nHb less than 10 gm/dL is not associated with death or ACS after PAD-related operations, maintaining nHb greater than 10 gm/dL appears to decrease the risk of wound infection. Blood transfusion is associated with increased risk of perioperative respiratory complications. Until a randomized trial settles this issue definitively, a restrictive transfusion strategy is justified in patients undergoing operations for atherosclerotic vascular disease.

▶ Triggers for blood transfusion have been subjected to rigorous randomized controlled trials suggesting safety for combined end points of cardiovascular and mortality outcomes. Unfortunately, post hoc analyses have introduced specific patient subsets that may or may not benefit from more liberal transfusion strategies. Vascular patients and their anticipated concomitant coronary artery disease are a prime example of the exceptions being called on for more not less red blood cell mass. This study from Kougias and colleagues provides cautious reassurance that hemoglobin levels under 10 g/dL are safely tolerated. Ultimately, I was eager to hear a hint for those patients with a hemoglobin approaching 8 g/dL, yet the data are not provided. So for now, we are left with the best data on the subject, which is still the randomized controlled trials with patient populations much more heterogeneous than our patients with peripheral arterial disease and the unlikely prospect that multicenter randomized trials are on the horizon.

J. Black, MD

5 Grafts and Graft Complications

Vacuum-assisted wound closure versus alginate for the treatment of deep perivascular wound infections in the groin after vascular surgery

Monsen C, Wann-Hansson C, Wictorsson C, et al (Skåne Univ Hosp, Malmö, Sweden; Malmö Univ, Sweden)

J Vasc Surg 59:145-151, 2014

Background.—Vacuum-assisted wound closure (VAC) therapy may heal wounds faster than conventional dressings after surgical debridement of perivascular groin infections after vascular surgery.

Methods.—Patients with deep infected wounds (Szilagyi grade III) were surgically revised and left open for secondary healing, then randomized to either VAC or alginate (Sorbalgon) therapy, between February 2007 and November 2011. To test the hypothesis, it was calculated that 42 patients needed to be included (90% power, 5% level of significance). It was decided to perform an interim analysis after inclusion of 20 patients.

Results.—Among 66 patients undergoing groin revision, 20 patients were included in this study. Patients were randomized to VAC (n = 10) or alginate (n = 10). The two groups were comparable in patient and wound characteristics. Time to full skin epithelialization was significantly shorter in the VAC group (median, 57 days) compared with the alginate group (median, 104 days; $P = .026$). The number of positive wound cultures of bacteria and C-reactive protein values decreased equally in both groups between surgical revision and day 21. One femur amputation was performed in each group as a consequence of the groin infection, one patient died during the in-hospital stay in the alginate group, and none died in the VAC group.

Conclusions.—VAC achieves faster healing than alginate therapy after wound debridement for deep perivascular wound infections in the groin after vascular surgery. This finding does not allow further inclusion of patients from an ethical point of view, and this study was, therefore, stopped prematurely.

▶ This report takes on a challenging surgical problem: management of deep perivascular wound infection in the groin after vascular surgery. The authors are to be congratulated for attempting to study this problem in a methodical and scientific manner; however, the super selectivity of the patients studied and thus reported becomes rapidly apparent. The comparison of a vacuum-assisted wound closure

(VAC) to local therapy with absorptive dressing seems appropriate, but there is no mention of the relative cost of each therapy. Nowhere in the article is the denominator—that is, the total number of patients who had vascular procedures involving cutdowns during the study—described. Thus the incidence of deep perivascular wound infection in the groin at this tertiary center is not reported. Only 20 of 66 potential patients were eventually randomized to the study protocol in this study. This report considers the treatment outcomes for patients who have had primarily groin explorations consisting of limited open and endovascular procedures. There appear to be 4 prosthetic bypass patients in each treatment group based on data in the table. One might assume that some of the other procedures performed might include a patch, but whether this is indeed the case is unclear. Although the time to wound healing was significantly shorter in the VAC-treated patients, the small number of patients in the study prevented the authors from making a significant conclusion about the incidence of failed therapy, even though there was 5-fold difference in failed therapy between the 2 groups. It seems to me that there is plenty of opportunity for this problem to be analyzed, allowing for definitive recommendations.

M. T. Watkins, MD

A 14-year Experience with Aortic Endograft Infection: Management and Results

Lyons OTA, Patel AS, Saha P, et al (Guy's and St Thomas' NHS Foundation Trust, London, UK)

Eur J Vasc Endovasc Surg 46:306-313, 2013

Objectives.—The management of thoracic and abdominal aortic endograft infection is complex and associated with high mortality. Cases are rare: a recent systematic review identified 117 reported cases; the largest reported series comprises 12 infected endografts.

Methods.—We report 22 consecutive patients with infected abdominal or thoracic aortic endovascular devices implanted from 1998 to 2012. Management included extension with new devices, aneurysm sac drainage of pus/irrigation with antibiotics, endograft explantation, and axillo-(bi) femoral reconstruction.

Results.—Twenty-two patients (16 men) were identified. Median age was 71 years (range, 43–88 years). Index devices were infra-renal endovascular repair ($n = 13$), and thoracic endovascular repair ($n = 9$) all for aneurysmal or pseudoaneurysmal disease. Seven (32%) had prior aortic surgery. Follow-up was complete in all cases; in survivors follow-up was a median of 29 (range, 12–45) months. The mortality from explantation of ten infrarenal devices was 1/10 (10%) on-table and a further 2/10 (20%) within 30 days. Device retention led to disease progression and death in all patients with infected endografts. Sac drainage/irrigation provided only temporary control of sepsis. Device extension can treat rupture, but additional devices became infected.

Conclusion.—Abdominal endograft explantation is high risk but may be curative. Appropriate selection of patients for infected endograft explantation remains a major challenge.

▶ Infection is a rare complication of endovascular treatment, and there is no good evidence to guide management. Without device removal, aortic endograft infection is uniformly fatal, but abdominal endograft explantation carries a 30-day mortality of 30%. Traditionally, endograft infection has been managed by removal of all foreign material with debridement of infected tissue by arterial reconstruction, either in situ using biological conduit or extra-anatomically using prosthetic graft, followed by prolonged antibiotic therapy.

No endograft is intended to be removable, and bare proximal stents in some stent graft designs may become imbedded in the aortic wall, complicating explantation. This series is probably the largest consecutive series of infected endografts and of explanted devices. The major risk factors for device infection included a period of sepsis after implantation in 50%, primarily infected aortic pathology to begin with in 50%, reintervention in 27%, and fistula in 23% of patients. In this series, patients with an index device deployed in primarily infected pathology were more likely to present with infection within 3 months of deployment.

One of the most important messages of this series was that all patients with a documented aortic endograft infection who did not have their endografts explanted died of aortic disease progression. Other important lessons were as follows:

1 Mortality from management of thoracic aortic endograft infection without explantation is reported at 70%, but in this series with longer and more complete follow-up, the mortality was 100%.
2 Extension with more devices was used in salvage situations to prevent immediate death from rupture. Although temporary control was often achieved, this routinely failed in the relatively short term.
3 Drainage of pus and irrigation of the sac improved systemic sepsis but did not prevent progression to death.

The authors' conclusions, as stated, are worth reprinting here:

"Explantation of infected abdominal endografts carries a high early mortality and morbidity, and appropriate selection of patients for such a high risk procedure remains a major challenge, but explantation can result in cure of aortic graft infection. Conservative (non-operative) management with retention of the infected aortic endograft inevitably results in death from disease progression, usually within two years of presentation with infection."

B. W. Starnes, MD

Conservative management of persistent aortocaval fistula after endovascular aortic repair

van de Luijtgaarden KM, Bastos Gonçalves F, Rouwet EV, et al (Erasmus Univ Med Ctr, Rotterdam, The Netherlands)

J Vasc Surg 58:1080-1083, 2013

Endovascular repair is a valid alternative for patients with abdominal aortic aneurysms. However, in patients with concomitant aortocaval fistulas, type II endoleaks may result in a persistent communication between the aneurysm sac and the inferior vena cava. In these patients, prompt closure of the persistent fistula has been advocated. We present a patient with an abdominal aortic aneurysm, with aortocaval fistula, who was managed

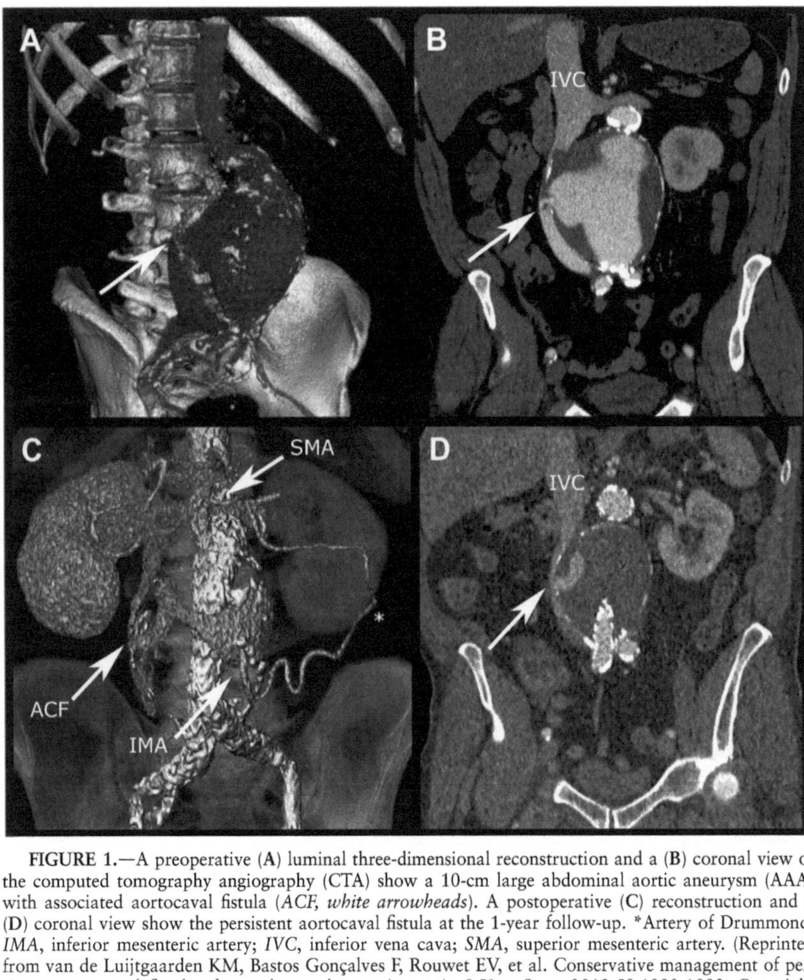

FIGURE 1.—A preoperative (**A**) luminal three-dimensional reconstruction and a (**B**) coronal view of the computed tomography angiography (CTA) show a 10-cm large abdominal aortic aneurysm (AAA) with associated aortocaval fistula (*ACF, white arrowheads*). A postoperative (**C**) reconstruction and a (**D**) coronal view show the persistent aortocaval fistula at the 1-year follow-up. *Artery of Drummond; *IMA*, inferior mesenteric artery; *IVC*, inferior vena cava; *SMA*, superior mesenteric artery. (Reprinted from van de Luijtgaarden KM, Bastos Gonçalves F, Rouwet EV, et al. Conservative management of persistent aortocaval fistula after endovascular aortic repair. *J Vasc Surg*. 2013;58:1080-1083, Copyright 2013, with permission from The Society for Vascular Surgery.)

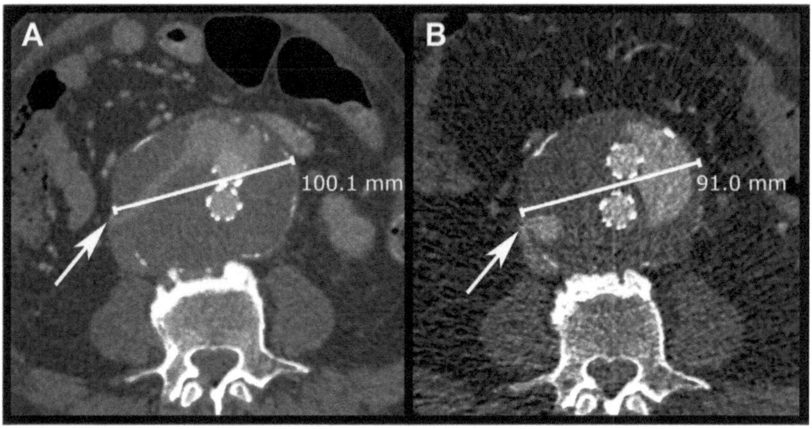

FIGURE 2.—Postoperative computed tomography angiography (CTA) at (**A**) 6 weeks and at the (**B**) 1-year follow-up shows a 10-mm decrease in diameter. Notice the large type II endoleak associated with a persistent aortocaval fistula (*white arrowheads*). (Reprinted from van de Luijtgaarden KM, Bastos Gonçalves F, Rouwet EV, et al. Conservative management of persistent aortocaval fistula after endovascular aortic repair. *J Vasc Surg*. 2013;58:1080-1083, Copyright 2013, with permission from The Society for Vascular Surgery.)

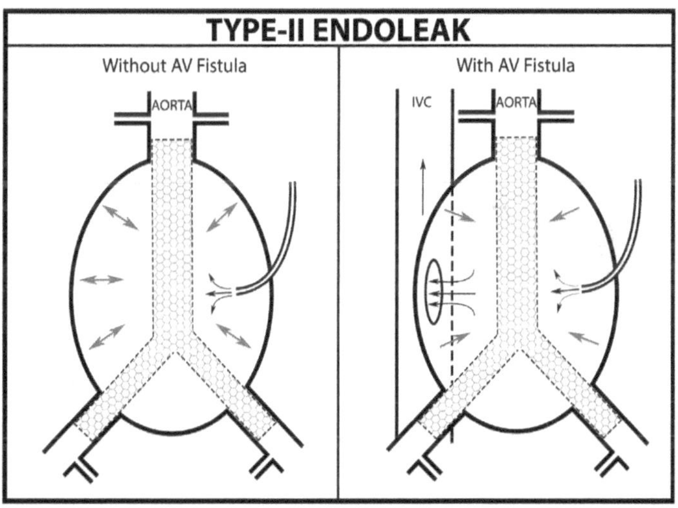

FIGURE 3.—Different dynamics are shown in the aneurysm sac between a type II endoleak (left) without and (right) with an arteriovenous (*AV*) fistula. *IVC*, Inferior vena cava. (Reprinted from van de Luijtgaarden KM, Bastos Gonçalves F, Rouwet EV, et al. Conservative management of persistent aortocaval fistula after endovascular aortic repair. *J Vasc Surg*. 2013;58:1080-1083, Copyright 2013, with permission from The Society for Vascular Surgery.)

endovascularly. Aneurysm sac shrinkage was observed despite persistent aortocaval communication due to type II endoleak. This case demonstrates that conservative management of type II endoleaks associated with persistent aortocaval fistulas is possible and may result in favorable aneurysm sac remodelling (Figs 1-3).

▶ Described herein is a case of conservative management of a persistent aortocaval fistula after endovascular aneurysm repair (EVAR). The patient had dramatic sac-size reduction of 10 mm on follow-up at 1 year (Figs 1 and 2). This fistula stayed patent because of a type 2 endoleak, effectively acting as a sump with low resistance, emanating from the inferior mesenteric artery.

This case report brings up some interesting points. Persistent arteriovenous fistulas (AVF) after EVAR have been reported, but the natural history of this complication remains unknown; moreover, there is no clear evidence in current literature supporting a strategy of treatment over observation alone. In the presence of persistent caval communication, type 2 endoleaks are subject to different flow and pressure dynamics caused by the connection with the low-pressure venous system. The connection causes a pressure gradient, resulting in a decrease of intrasac pressure (Fig 3). Owing to the low-pressure nature of this communication, this special type of type 2 endoleak has a low probability of aneurysm sac growth. This may stimulate a young mind out there somewhere to try and reproduce this physiology in all EVAR patients with endoleak to achieve the same result described here.

It should be noted, however, that close observation, including periodic cardiac evaluation, is mandatory in this setting. Secondary intervention may be reserved for patients with persistent aortocaval fistulas combined with aneurysm sac enlargement or systemic manifestations.

B. W. Starnes, MD

6 Aortic Aneurysm

Debate: Whether young, good-risk patients should be treated with endovascular abdominal aortic aneurysm repair

Vallabhaneni R, Farber MA, Schneider F, et al (Univ of North Carolina, Chapel Hill; Univ of Poitiers, France)

J Vasc Surg 58:1709-1715, 2013

As endovascular abdominal aortic aneurysm repair has become increasingly prominent in our vascular surgery practices, the discussion regarding long-term durability continues. The initial randomized trials that enrolled patients almost 10 years ago revealed a short-term survival advantage with endovascular abdominal aortic aneurysm repair at the expense of a higher reintervention rate and loss of that initial survival advantage in the longer term. Continuing and healthy debate over the practical importance of these findings has resulted in somewhat differing practice patterns on either side of the Atlantic. This debate explores the issues surrounding whether younger, good-risk patients with a long life expectancy should be treated with endovascular repair.

▶ This is a knock-down, drag-out between Chapel Hill, North Carolina, USA, and Poitiers, France, with the Americans defending the position of endovascular aneurysm repair (EVAR) for young patients and the French defending open repair as first-line therapy. I must say that I side with the Americans on this one.

It should be noted that the first 2 studies examining this issue in young patients (one reviewed yet again in this edition of the YEAR BOOK), began enrollment nearly a decade ago. Since that time, additional device advances, technique improvement, and understanding in management of patients has occurred.

I tend to smile when anyone describes to me the young, "healthy" patient with a 5.5-cm abdominal aortic aneurysm (AAA). These patients are not healthy! If they were, they wouldn't have an aneurysm. Sure, there are unfortunate young patients with connective tissue disorders but the fact still remains that the majority of these patients have significant histories of tobacco abuse and other risk factors for vascular disease. A recently published report from the Nottingham group looked at midterm survival in young patients treated with EVAR and open surgical repair.[1] When patients treated at their institution since 1995 were analyzed, nearly 40% of patients who were treated with open repair or EVAR died less than 6 years after their surgery; however, most of these patients did not die of aneurysmal disease. Patients with aneurysmal aortas may not have the same life expectancy as patients in the general population, and this may be a risk factor for early mortality.

The French state very simply in their conclusions that there is no evidence in the literature to support EVAR as first-line therapy in young patients. I think this is shortsighted and disregards the opinion of the patient when presented with modern data.

B. W. Starnes, MD

Reference

1. Altaf N, Abisi S, Yong Y, et al. Mid-term results of endovascular aortic aneurysm repair in the young. *Eur J Vasc Endovasc Surg.* 2013;46:315-319.

The Shortfall in Long-term Survival of Patients with Repaired Thoracic or Abdominal Aortic Aneurysms: Retrospective Case–Control Analysis of Hospital Episode Statistics

Karthikesalingam A, Bahia SS, Patterson BO, et al (St George's Hosp, London, UK)

Eur J Vasc Endovasc Surg 46:533-541, 2013

Objective.—To report the contemporary life expectancy of patients undergoing abdominal (AAA) or thoracic aortic aneurysm (TAA) repair in England, relative to a healthy control population.

Methods.—A retrospective observational case–control study was carried out of Hospital Episode Statistics (HES) data, an administrative dataset covering the entire English National Health Service. Patients undergoing elective repair of an abdominal or thoracic aortic aneurysm in an English NHS hospital between April 2006 and March 2011 were included. Outcome measures were 5-year all-cause mortality (in- and out-of-hospital) and adverse cardiovascular events (myocardial infarction, stroke, emergency amputation or limb revascularisation).

Results.—19,505 AAA and 730 TAA repairs were identified, with 75,260 and 2,721 control participants, respectively, and 27.5 (1.0–60.0) months' median (range) follow-up. Five-year survival was 67.4% for AAA against 81.1% for control participants, and 65.3% for TAA against 89.1% for control participants ($p < .001$). Freedom from adverse cardiovascular events was 86.1% for AAA against 93% for control participants and 89.1% for TAA against 94.4% for control participants ($p < .001$).

Conclusion.—Long-term survival remains poor after aneurysm repair and adverse cardiovascular events are common relative to the wider population. Further research is required to characterise and optimise cardiovascular risk prevention in patients with aortic aneurysms (Fig 5).

▶ It has previously been reported that long-term survival of patients undergoing abdominal aortic aneurysm (AAA) repair was considerably worse than age and gender-matched controls. This is thought to be related to the higher cardiovascular burden of disease in this patient population. The epidemiology of AAA has

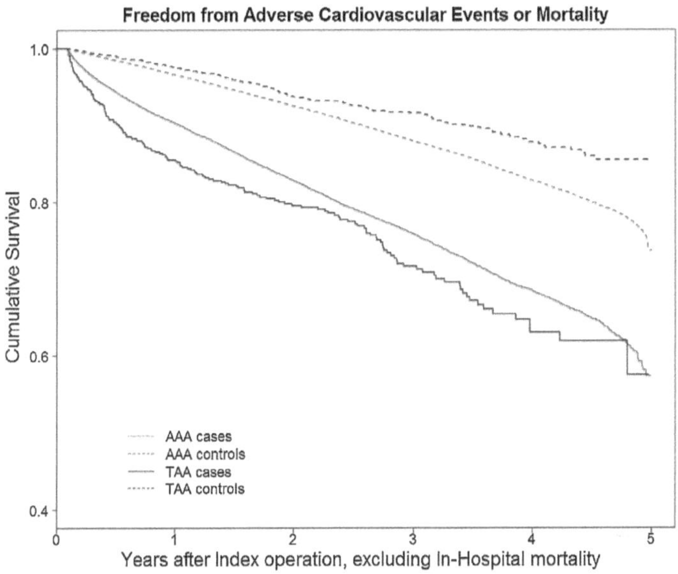

FIGURE 5.—Freedom from adverse cardiovascular events or mortality. (Reprinted from Karthikesalingam A, Bahia SS, Patterson BO, et al. The shortfall in long-term survival of patients with repaired thoracic or abdominal aortic aneurysms: retrospective case–control analysis of hospital episode statistics. *Eur J Vasc Endovasc Surg*. 2013;46:533-541, Copyright 2013, with permission from European Society for Vascular Surgery.)

been improved by modern trends in smoking behavior, public health measures, and improvements in cardiovascular risk management. It is reasonable to say, therefore, that there exists a potential opportunity for focused medical therapy to improve life expectancy. To accomplish this, we must first reappraise the life expectancy of these patients and compare it with the general population, thus clarifying whether modern medical therapy and the effects of recent health policy have reduced the shortfall in long-term survival that has been observed after AAA repair.

These authors have nicely analyzed a large contemporary dataset in the United Kingdom, and although the prevalence of AAA has fallen with improvements in public health, patients surviving AAA or thoracic aortic repair continue to demonstrate considerable morbidity and mortality compared with age- and gender-matched controls (Fig 5).

Currently there is a paucity of data defining whether these comorbidities are modifiable or whether this represents an end-stage process. Future studies may use these benchmark data for comparison.

B. W. Starnes, MD

Outcomes After Open Repair for Ruptured Abdominal Aortic Aneurysms in Patients with Friendly Versus Hostile Aortoiliac Anatomy

van Beek SC, On behalf of the Amsterdam Acute Aneurysm Trial Collaborators (Univ of Amsterdam, The Netherlands; Onze Lieve Vrouwe Gasthuis, Amsterdam, The Netherlands; et al)

Eur J Vasc Endovasc Surg 47:380-387, 2014

Objectives.—In patients with a ruptured abdominal aortic aneurysm (RAAA), anatomic suitability for endovascular aneurysm repair (EVAR) depends on aortic neck and iliac artery characteristics. If the aortoiliac anatomy is unsuitable for EVAR ("hostile anatomy"), open repair (OR) is the next option. We hypothesized that the death rate for OR is higher in patients with hostile anatomy than in patients with friendly anatomy.

Methods.—We conducted an observational cohort study in 279 consecutive patients with an RAAA treated with OR between 2004 and 2011. The primary endpoint was 30-day or in-hospital death. Aortoiliac anatomy (friendly vs. hostile) was determined prospectively by the vascular surgeon and the interventional radiologist treating the patient. A multivariable logistic regression analysis was done to assess the risk of dying in patients with hostile anatomy after adjustment for age, sex, comorbidity, and hemodynamic stability.

Results.—Aortoiliac anatomy was friendly in 71 patients and hostile in 208 patients. Death rate was 38% (95% confidence interval (CI): 28 to 50%) in patients with friendly anatomy and 30% (95% CI: 24 to 37%) in patients with hostile anatomy ($p = .23$). After multivariable adjustment, the risk of dying was not higher in patients with hostile anatomy (adjusted odds ratio 0.744, 95% CI 0.394 to 1.404).

Conclusion.—The death rate after open repair for an RAAA is comparable in patients with friendly and hostile aortoiliac anatomy (Fig 2, Table 1).

▶ In any ruptured abdominal aortic aneurysm (rAAA) scenario, if anatomy is unsuitable for endovascular aneurysm repair (EVAR; "hostile anatomy"), open surgical repair is the next best option. As the number of patients treated with EVAR increases, fewer patients with "friendly anatomy" are being treated with open repair. This leaves patients with more challenging anatomy for open repair (Table 1).

The authors interestingly found no difference in outcome based on friendly or hostile aortic anatomy (Fig 2). The reasons for this are probably not what you think. In the Netherlands, there are now only 3 hospitals that care for patients with rAAA (Academic Medical Center, University of Amsterdam; Onze Lieve Vrouwe Gasthuis; and VU University Medical Center). All of these units are in Amsterdam, and this has been a recent change with centralization of care for rAAA. It will be interesting (and important/controversial) in years to come to see if this strategy should be applied in the United States. This article is the

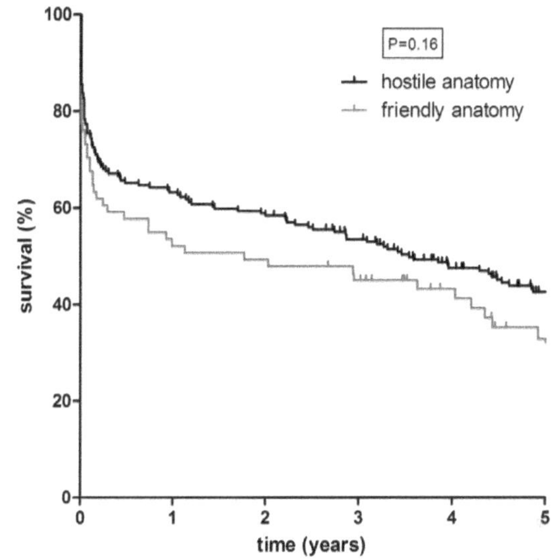

friendly anatomy	patients at risk	71	37	35	31	22	14
	death	0	34	36	39	40	45
	censored	0	0	0	1	9	12
hostile anatomy	patients at risk	208	130	120	105	82	63
	death	0	76	86	96	107	115
	censored	0	2	2	7	19	30

FIGURE 2.—Survival analysis of patients with friendly and hostile aortoiliac anatomy for EVAR. (Reprinted from van Beek SC, On behalf of the Amsterdam Acute Aneurysm Trial Collaborators. Outcomes after open repair for ruptured abdominal aortic aneurysms in patients with friendly versus hostile aortoiliac anatomy. *Eur J Vasc Endovasc Surg*. 2014;47:380-387, Copyright 2014, with permission from European Society for Vascular Surgery.)

TABLE 1.—Criteria for Friendly and Hostile Aortoiliac Anatomy Based on the Instructions for use of An Aorto-Uni-Iliac Endograft

Suitable infrarenal anchoring segment
- A minimum length of the infrarenal segment of at least 10–15 mm
- An infrarenal diameter of 20–32 mm
- No obstructing calcifications, tortuosity, or thrombus

Suitable iliac anchoring segment
- An ipsilateral iliac diameter of 8–18 mm
- A contralateral iliac diameter of 10–20 mm
- At least one iliac artery should be able to accommodate an endograft
- No obstructing calcifications, tortuosity, or thrombus

EVAR = endovascular aneurysm repair.

first to show that with regionalization of care, outcomes improve, most likely related to factors such as streamlined protocols, case volume, and experience.

B. W. Starnes, MD

Survival Following Ruptured Abdominal Aortic Aneurysm Before and During the IMPROVE Trial: A Single-Centre Series

Ambler GK, Twine CP, Shak J, et al (Cambridge Univ Hosps NHS Foundation Trust, UK)

Eur J Vasc Endovasc Surg 47:388-393, 2014

Objectives.—The first large-scale randomised trial (Immediate Management of the Patient with Rupture: Open Versus Endovascular repair [IMPROVE]) for endovascular repair of ruptured abdominal aortic aneurysm (rEVAR) has recently finished recruiting patients. The aim of this study was to examine the impact on survival after rEVAR when the IMPROVE protocol was initiated in a high volume abdominal aortic aneurysm (AAA) centre previously performing rEVAR.

Methods.—One hundred and sixty-nine patients requiring emergency infrarenal AAA repair from January 2006 to April 2013 were included. Eighty-four patients were treated before (38 rEVAR, 46 open) and 85 (31 rEVAR, 54 open) were treated during the trial period. A retrospective analysis was performed.

Results.—Before the trial, there was a significant survival benefit for rEVAR over open repair (90-day mortality 13% vs. 30%, $p = .04$, difference remained significant up to 2 years postoperatively). This survival benefit was lost after starting randomisation (90-day mortality 35% vs. 33%, $p = .93$). There was an increase in overall 30-day mortality from 15% to 31% ($p = .02$), while there was no change for open repair ($p = .438$). There was a significant decrease in general anaesthetic use ($p = .002$) for patients treated during the trial. Randomised patients had shorter hospital and intensive treatment unit stays ($p = .006$ and $p = .03$ respectively).

Conclusions.—The change in survival seen during the IMROVE trial highlights the need for randomised rather than cohort data to eliminate selection bias. These results from a single centre reinforce those recently reported in IMPROVE (Fig 2).

▶ I still have a hard time wrapping this study around my simple little brain. This single center, as part of the Immediate Management of the Patient with Rupture: Open Versus Endovascular repair (IMPROVE) trial on ruptured abdominal aortic aneurysms (rAAA), noticed a significant deterioration in their mortality statistics *after* entering the trial (Fig 2)! The unit already had a rupture protocol in place and was using endovascular aneurysm repair (EVAR) for rAAA quite successfully before the trial; but after starting randomization, the survival benefit of EVAR for rAAA over open surgical repair was lost.

The most probable explanation is that this effect was due to bias from selecting patients with more suitable anatomy for EVAR before IMPROVE. This

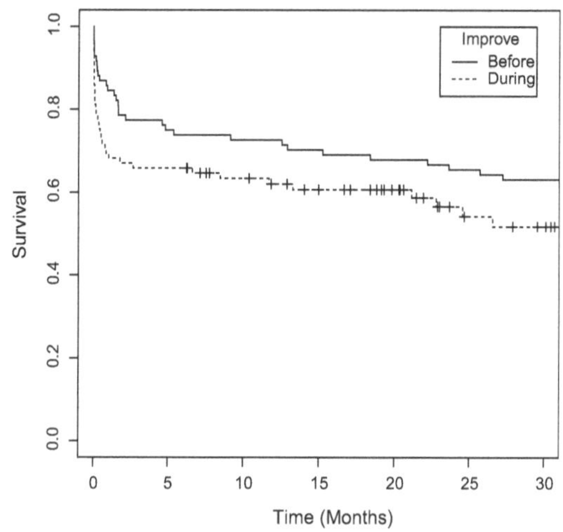

FIGURE 2.—Comparative survival of ruptured abdominal aortic aneurysm repair before and during the IMPROVE trial. The solid line shows survival pre-IMPROVE, the dashed line shows survival during the trial period. (Reprinted from Ambler GK, Twine CP, Shak J, et al. Survival following ruptured abdominal aortic aneurysm before and during the IMPROVE trial: a single-centre series. *Eur J Vasc Endovasc Surg*. 2014;47:388-393, Copyright 2014, with permission from European Society for Vascular Surgery.)

suggests that looking at all patients with rAAA, when truly randomized, there is no difference in mortality. I'm fine with that and will continue to manage patients with rAAA with EVAR when I can because I know it is better (I've proved it to myself in my institution[1]). We thought our open mortality would rise after implementation of a rupture protocol because more of the patients undergoing open repair would have complex anatomy, but we saw that the pre- and postprotocol mortality for open repair remained exactly the same.

We must be careful here because the patients randomized into the EVAR group had shorter, more angulated necks, which is associated with worse outcomes after EVAR, and EVAR-suitable patients may have better outcomes with open repair than those with unsuitable anatomy. I think we all know that what will come out of all this is that EVAR is superior in the setting of rAAA for those patients with suitable anatomy.

B. W. Starnes, MD

Reference

1. Starnes BW, Quiroga E, Hutter C, et al. Management of ruptured abdominal aortic aneurysm in the endovascular era. *J Vasc Surg*. 2010;51:9-17.

Statin therapy is associated with improved survival after endovascular and open aneurysm repair

de Bruin JL, for the DREAM Study Group (Vrije Universiteit Medical Center, Amsterdam, The Netherlands; et al)

J Vasc Surg 59:39-44.e1, 2014

Background.—The relationship between numerous risk factors and perioperative mortality after cardiovascular surgery has been studied extensively. While improved perioperative survival and fewer cardiovascular events have been related to statin therapy, its effect on long-term survival after aneurysm repair remains to be elucidated. The aim of this study is to determine the effect of statin therapy on long-term survival after open and endovascular aneurysm repair and to identify other cardiovascular and patient-related risk factors in this respect.

Methods.—A post-hoc analysis of a randomized trial comparing open and endovascular abdominal aortic aneurysm repair was performed. In this multicenter trial, 351 patients were randomly assigned to undergo either open abdominal aortic aneurysm repair or endovascular repair. Patients who were on lipid-lowering medication at their inclusion in the trial (n = 135) were compared with those who were not (n = 216).

Results.—During 6 years of follow-up, 118 (33.6%) patients died after randomization. Statin therapy, baseline characteristics, Society for Vascular Surgery/International Society for Cardiovascular Surgery risk factors, aneurysm size, reinterventions, antiplatelet or anticoagulant agents, and β-blockers were used to identify prognostic factors influencing survival. After identification of significant factors in a Kaplan-Meier analysis, a multivariable Cox regression analysis was applied. Statin therapy at inclusion in the trial was independently associated with better overall survival after open or endovascular aneurysm repair (hazard ratio [HR], 0.5; 95% confidence interval [CI], 0.3-0.8; $P = .004$). Statins were especially associated with fewer cardiovascular deaths (HR, 0.4; 95% CI, 0.2-0.9; $P = .025$). Several risk factors were associated with poor survival after open and endovascular aneurysm repair: age >70 (HR, 3.4; 95% CI, 2.2-5.0; $P < .001$), a history of cardiac disease at baseline (HR, 1.9; 95% CI, 1.3-2.8; $P = .001$), and moderate/severe tobacco use (HR, 1.7; 95% CI, 1.2-2.5; $P = .004$). Gender, aneurysm size, the need for reintervention, pulmonary disease, renal disease, carotid disease, hypertension, diabetes mellitus, antiplatelet or anticoagulant agents, and β-blockers were not significantly associated with impaired long-term survival ($P > .05$).

Conclusions.—Despite the limitations of a post-hoc analysis of a prospectively maintained trial, we conclude that statin therapy at the beginning of the trial is independently associated with improved long-term survival after open or endovascular aneurysm repair, while age above

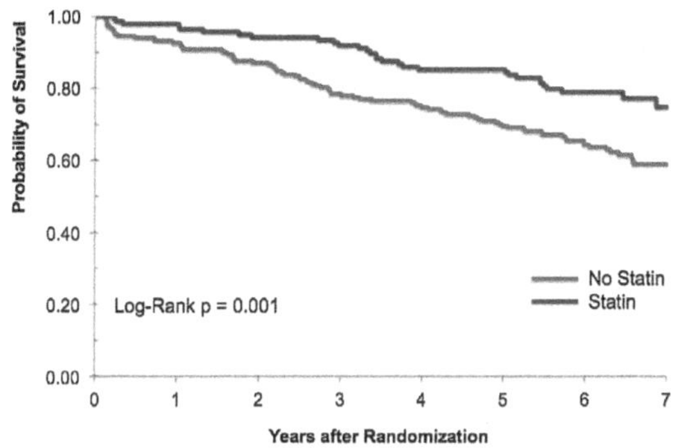

Number at Risk								
No Statin	216	200	188	168	160	149	98	38
Statin	135	131	127	124	115	113	60	24

FIGURE 1.—Kaplan-Meier estimates of survival between patients with or without statins. The standard error of both survival estimates does not exceed 10%; the maximum standard errors are 5.5% and 4.5%, respectively, at the end of both curves. (Reprinted from de Bruin JL, for the DREAM Study Group. Statin therapy is associated with improved survival after endovascular and open aneurysm repair. *J Vasc Surg*. 59:39-44.e1, 2014, Copyright 2014, with permission from the Society for Vascular Surgery.)

70 years, a history of cardiovascular disease, and tobacco use are associated with decreased long-term survival (Fig 1).

▶ This prospective study showed statin therapy to be independently associated with better long-term survival after open or endovascular aneurysm repair. In the univariate risk-factor analysis, the absence of statin therapy was significantly associated with poor survival (Fig 1). Statin therapy was associated with better long-term survival after open or endovascular repair (hazard ratio [HR], 0.5; 95% confidence interval [CI], 0.3–0.8; $P = .004$).

Cardiovascular deaths in the endovascular aneurysm repair group appear to contribute to a catch-up mortality phenomenon during the first 2 postoperative years. Consequently, long-term survival is equal for both types of aneurysm repair, with cardiovascular and cancer as main causes of death. Convergence of all-cause mortality or catch-up mortality between endovascular and open aneurysm repair in the DREAM and EVAR-1 trials is mostly explained by higher rates of cardiovascular deaths in the endovascular repair groups during the first 2 years. Improving the cardiovascular risk profile with intensive vascular counseling and optimal cardioprotective medication can play a key role in sustaining the beneficial effect of endovascular aneurysm repair postoperatively.

Statin therapy at the beginning of this trial was independently associated with improved long-term survival after open or endovascular repair. These findings support the view that statin treatment is an essential element of risk management in patients undergoing aortic aneurysm treatment.

B. W. Starnes, MD

Fenestrated endograft for recurrent paravisceral aortic pseudoaneurysm after thoracoabdominal aortic aneurysm open repair

Gargiulo M, Gallitto E, Freyrie A, et al (Univ of Bologna, Italy)
J Vasc Surg 58:790-793, 2013

Paravisceral aortic pseudoaneurysm is an uncommon late graft-related complication after thoracoabdominal aortic aneurysm open repair. The redo surgery and hybrid procedures are the treatments of choice, with significant perioperative morbidity and mortality rates. We report a total endovascular repair of a 56-mm paravisceral aortic pseudoaneurysm in a 65-year-old patient with a history of type V thoracoabdominal aortic aneurysm open repair and redo open procedure for a distal anastomotic pseudoaneurysm. The lesion was successfully treated with a custom-made four-fenestration endograft. At 18 months, the patient was asymptomatic without liver, renal, or pancreatic problems. Computed tomography

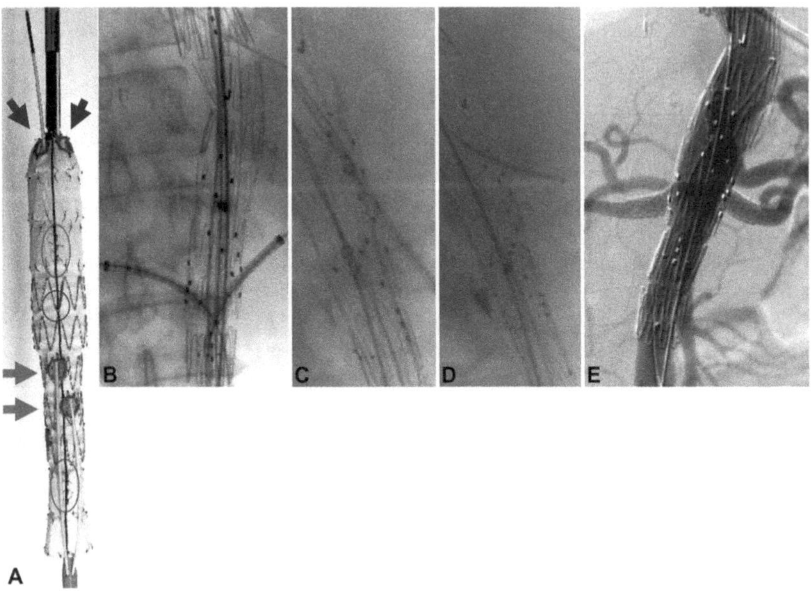

FIGURE 2.—**A,** An anterior view of the endograft shows the proximal reinforced scallops with the two preloaded catheters for the celiac trunk and superior mesenteric artery fenestrations. **B,** A posterior view of the endograft shows the double reducing tie system. **C,** Anterior view shows the endograft is completely opened. **D,** An intraoperative angiographic image shows the left renal artery cannulation using a C2 Cook Catheter and a 0.035-inch floppy guidewire. **E,** Cannulation of the superior mesenteric artery is shown with the top cap still in place: a 10F Cook-Flexor introducer was inserted from the axillary artery through the dedicated scallop, and a 7F Cook-Flexor introducer was advanced in the right renal artery from the left femoral access. (Reprinted from Gargiulo M, Gallitto E, Freyrie A, et al. Fenestrated endograft for recurrent paravisceral aortic pseudoaneurysm after thoracoabdominal aortic aneurysm open repair. *J Vasc Surg*. 2013;58:790-793, Copyright 2013, with permission from The Society for Vascular Surgery.)

angiography demonstrated the absence of endoleaks, the antegrade perfusion of visceral vessels, and the absence of stent graft fractures (Fig 2).

▶ This case report emphasizes specific important technical considerations for managing a complication of open repair of a thoracoabdominal aortic aneurysm with a fenestrated endovascular approach. We as vascular surgeons are finding new ways to treat complex aortic pathology with simplified, minimally invasive techniques.

One of the requirements for successful fenestrated endografting is perfect alignment of fenestrations with the intended target vessels. This can be facilitated by selection of the target vessels from within the stent graft before full deployment of the graft and further by the placement of diameter-reducing ties to lower the profile of the device and create " offset," or a space between the graft and the target vessel. This novel technique uses a device with preloaded catheters through 2 additional fenestrations in the top portion of the graft. This allows the diameter-reducing ties to remain in place and, more important, the top cap to stay undeployed during cannulation of the fenestrated graft from above. The only expertise required is the simple advancement of a guidewire from below, through the preloaded catheters and snared from a transaxillary or brachial access (Fig 2). Sheaths are advanced into the graft from above and used to select the visceral fenestrations and secure access within the superior mesenteric artery. We will continue to see these sorts of ingenious advancements in endograft design in the near future. I like to tell our residents that if we are not careful that, like LASIK eye surgery, we will soon see these procedures being done in the local shopping mall.

B. W. Starnes, MD

A systematic review and meta-analysis of the association between markers of hemostasis and abdominal aortic aneurysm presence and size

Sidloff DA, Stather PW, Choke E, et al (Univ of Leicester, UK)

J Vasc Surg 59:528-535.e4, 2014

Objective.—The purpose of this study was to summarize the current evidence of the association between markers of hemostasis and both the presence and size of abdominal aortic aneurysms (AAAs).

Methods.—A systematic review and meta-analysis was performed according to Preferred Reporting Items for Systematic reviews and Meta-Analyses guidelines by use of the search terms "aneurysm AND abdominal AND aortic AND coagulation" NOT "thoracic." Outcome data including concentration of hemostatic marker, number of patients, and significance level were recorded.

Results.—A total of 22 nonrandomized studies were included in the analysis, with a total of 9862 patients. Fibrinogen mean difference (MD) (0.43 g/L; 95% confidence interval [CI], 0.28-0.58 g/L; $P \leq .00001$), D-dimer MD (325.82 ng/mL; 95% CI, 199.74-451.89 ng/mL; $P \leq .00001$),

Study or Subgroup	AAA Mean	AAA SD	AAA Total	Control Mean	Control SD	Control Total	Weight	Mean Difference IV, Random, 95% CI
Aramato 1994	8,400	10,800	41	2,100	2,700	30	0.1%	6300.00 [2855.88, 9744.12]
Fowkes 2006	441.5	423.8	89	93	74.81	98	12.8%	348.50 [259.22, 437.78]
Golledge 2010	342.9	530	337	112.4	102.07	923	13.4%	230.50 [173.53, 287.47]
Ihara 2003	858	1,253	22	125.7	46.1	26	4.1%	732.30 [208.41, 1256.19]
Jelenska 2004	778	311	20	362	242	22	11.0%	416.00 [246.28, 585.72]
Lee 1996	142	92.96	40	83	45.5	200	13.6%	59.00 [29.51, 88.49]
Nomura 2003	420	256	17	104	46	72	12.2%	316.00 [193.84, 438.16]
Parry 2010	346.7	307.1	75	120.2	66.1	90	13.2%	226.50 [155.67, 297.33]
Serino 2002	421	400	18	238	180	10	9.8%	183.00 [-32.85, 398.85]
Wallinder 2009	625	723.7	40	86	102.2	41	9.5%	539.00 [312.56, 765.44]
Yamazumi 1998	7,700	6,700	36	1,000	1,200	25	0.3%	6700.00 [4461.39, 8938.61]
Total (95% CI)			**735**			**1537**	**100.0%**	**326.10 [199.67, 452.54]**

Heterogeneity: Tau² = 30326.05; Chi² = 145.46, df = 10 (P < 0.00001); I² = 93%
Test for overall effect: Z = 5.06 (P < 0.00001)

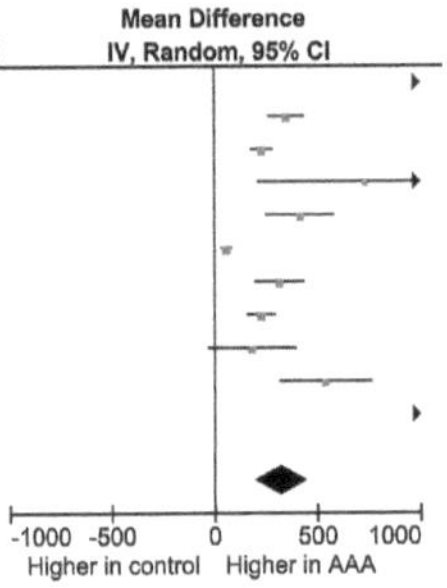

FIGURE 3.—Forest plot compares mean plasma concentration of D-dimer between studies. A random-effects model was used for meta-analysis. *AAA*, Abdominal aortic aneurysm; *CI*, confidence interval; *SD*, standard deviation. (Reprinted from Sidloff DA, Stather PW, Choke E, et al. A systematic review and meta-analysis of the association between markers of hemostasis and abdominal aortic aneurysm presence and size. *J Vasc Surg*. 2014;59:528-535.e4, Copyright 2014, with permission from the Society for Vascular Surgery.)

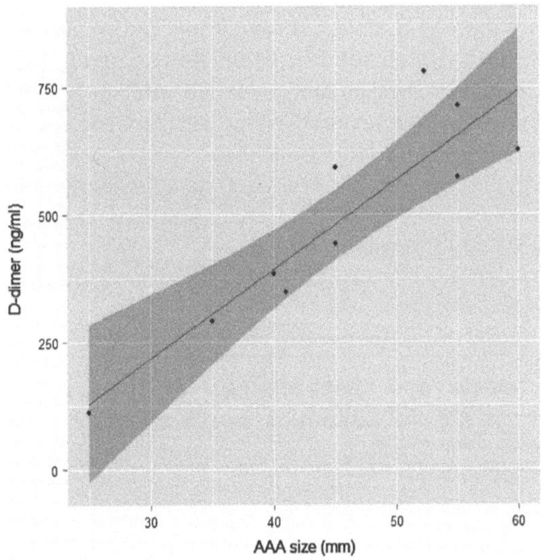

FIGURE 4.—Meta-regression demonstrates the association between abdominal aortic aneurysm (*AAA*) diameter and D-dimer concentration. (Reprinted from Sidloff DA, Stather PW, Choke E, et al. A systematic review and meta-analysis of the association between markers of hemostasis and abdominal aortic aneurysm presence and size. *J Vasc Surg*. 2014;59:528-535.e4, Copyright 2014, with permission from the Society for Vascular Surgery.)

and thrombin-antithrombin III complex MD (5.58 g/L; 95% CI, 3.34-7.83 g/L; $P \leq .0001$) were significantly elevated in the presence of AAAs. Tissue plasminogen activator, prothrombin fragments F1DF2, and platelet count were not shown to be significantly different between patients with and those without AAAs. Meta-regression of studies reporting plasma D-dimer concentration and aneurysm diameter suggests a strong and significant association ($r^2 = 0.94$; $P \leq .0001$).

Conclusions.—This study suggests that the presence of AAAs is associated with increased fibrin turnover, fibrinolysis, and thrombin generation, as shown by increased levels of fibrinogen, D-dimer, and thrombin-antithrombin III complex. This is clinically relevant because markers of hemostasis are independent risk factors for cardiovascular events, highlighting the necessity of addressing all modifiable cardiovascular risk factors in patients with AAAs. Furthermore, the finding that plasma D-dimer concentration appears to have a linear relationship with aneurysm diameter may be useful as a future biomarker of AAAs (Figs 3 and 4).

▶ This is one of the coolest papers I read for the YEAR BOOK this year. It is a systematic review and meta-analysis comparing hemostatic markers in patients with and without abdominal aortic aneurysm (AAA) and represents the largest of its kind to date. These authors have found a significant association between the presence of AAA and plasma levels of fibrinogen, D-dimer, and thrombin-antithrombin III complex, suggesting that AAAs are associated with increased fibrin turnover, fibrinolysis, and thrombin generation. Several studies have already shown that circulating markers of hemostasis are elevated in patients with aortic dilatation and that they are independently associated with cardiovascular events.[1]

Pooled analysis of the data (Fig 3) shows that patients with AAAs have a significantly higher plasma concentration of D-dimer (325.82 ng/mL; 95% confidence interval 199.74–451.89 ng/mL; $P < .00001$). There was a significant heterogeneity between studies ($I^2 = 80\%$) and accordingly, a random-effects model was used. Five studies reported on the association of AAA size with plasma concentration of D-dimer, all finding a positive association with the largest correlation coefficient value equaling 0.644. Meta-regression of studies reporting AAA diameter and D-dimer concentration (Fig 4) reveals a highly significant, strongly positive association between aneurysm diameter and D-dimer concentration.

Imagine being able to draw a blood sample and determine aneurysm size! Although it is unlikely that these biomarkers will replace ultrasound as a first-line diagnostic tool for the presence of AAAs, one possible strategy to reduce the cost of negative screening is to use a 2-stage approach with the use of a cheaper, high-sensitivity diagnostic test such as D-dimer, followed by a high-specificity test such as ultrasound.

Future studies of the use of hemostatic markers in identifying patients with AAAs should match patients for both age and smoking habits and should exclude patients with peripheral vascular disease. Further analysis of the use of hemostatic markers to predict aneurysm presence and size is necessary to determine any potential role in new diagnostic/prognostic pathways for patients with AAAs.

B. W. Starnes, MD

Reference

1. Ernst E, Koenig W. Fibrinogen and cardiovascular risk. *Vasc Med.* 1997;2:115-125.

Endovascular repair for ruptured abdominal aortic aneurysm confers an early survival benefit over open repair

Antoniou GA, Georgiadis GS, Antoniou SA, et al (Hellenic Red Cross Hosp, Athens, Greece; Democritus Univ of Thrace, Alexandroupolis, Greece; Univ of Crete, Greece; et al)

J Vasc Surg 58:1091-1105, 2013

Background.—Despite the intuitive advantages of endovascular repair (EVAR) of ruptured abdominal aortic aneurysms (AAAs), uncertainty remains about the optimal management in the absence of convincing high-quality evidence. Our objective was to undertake a comprehensive literature review and perform a meta-analysis of outcome data of treatment modalities for ruptured AAAs.

Methods.—Systematic searches were conducted of electronic information sources to identify studies comparing perioperative outcomes of EVAR and open repair for AAA rupture. Summary estimates of odds ratios (ORs) or standardized mean difference and 95% confidence intervals (CIs) were obtained with a random-effects model. Meta-regression models were formed to explore potential heterogeneity as a result of changes in practice over time.

Results.—We selected 41 studies for analysis. The entire meta-analysis population comprised 59,941 patients (8201 EVAR patients and 51,740 open repair patients). EVAR was associated with a significantly lower

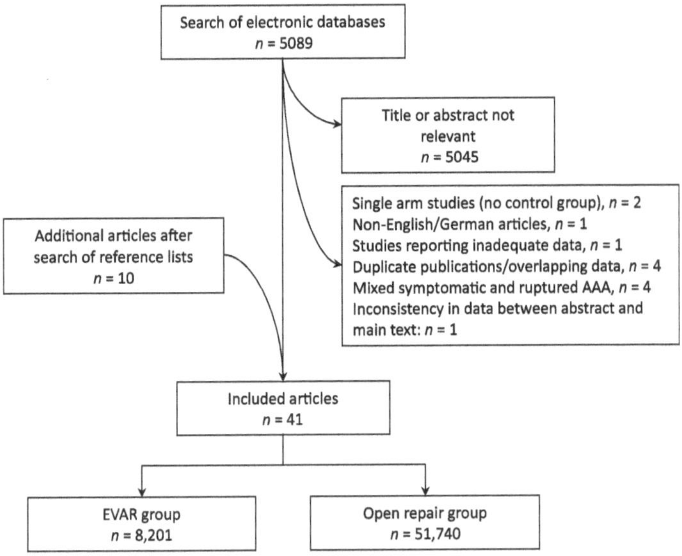

FIGURE 1.—Flow chart shows the strategy used for the literature search. *AAA*, Abdominal aortic aneurysm. (Reprinted from Antoniou GA, Georgiadis GS, Antoniou SA, et al. Endovascular repair for ruptured abdominal aortic aneurysm confers an early survival benefit over open repair. *J Vasc Surg*. 2013;58:1091-1105, with permission from The Society for Vascular Surgery.)

	EVAR		Open repair			Odds Ratio	
Study or Subgroup	**Events**	**Total**	**Events**	**Total**	**Weight**	**M-H, Random, 95% CI**	**Year**
Yilmaz	4	17	12	29	0.8%	0.44 [0.11, 1.67]	2002
Reichart	1	6	4	13	0.2%	0.45 [0.04, 5.21]	2003
Resch	4	14	8	23	0.7%	0.75 [0.18, 3.17]	2003
Lee 2	1	13	1	4	0.2%	0.25 [0.01, 5.26]	2004
Brandt	0	11	2	13	0.1%	0.20 [0.01, 4.64]	2005
Larzon	2	15	12	26	0.5%	0.18 [0.03, 0.96]	2005
Alsac	4	17	10	20	0.7%	0.31 [0.07, 1.28]	2005
Vaddineni	2	9	4	15	0.4%	0.79 [0.11, 5.49]	2005
Greco	114	290	2627	5508	9.5%	0.71 [0.56, 0.90]	2006
Hinchliffe	8	15	9	17	0.7%	1.02 [0.25, 4.08]	2006
Coppi	10	33	42	91	1.7%	0.51 [0.22, 1.19]	2006
Dalainas	8	20	5	8	0.5%	0.40 [0.07, 2.16]	2006
Peppelenbosch	17	49	20	51	1.9%	0.82 [0.36, 1.86]	2006
Acosta	19	56	48	106	2.6%	0.62 [0.32, 1.22]	2007
Sharif	17	52	38	74	2.2%	0.46 [0.22, 0.96]	2007
Ockert	9	29	9	29	1.1%	1.00 [0.33, 3.04]	2007
Anain	5	30	4	10	0.5%	0.30 [0.06, 1.47]	2007
Wibmer	4	16	9	31	0.7%	0.81 [0.21, 3.21]	2008
Lee 1	6	17	15	20	0.7%	0.18 [0.04, 0.75]	2008
Vun	0	7	16	38	0.2%	0.09 [0.00, 1.71]	2009
Verhoeven	9	45	31	114	1.8%	0.67 [0.29, 1.55]	2009
Vogel	37	82	324	618	4.6%	0.75 [0.47, 1.19]	2009
Visser	15	58	57	143	2.6%	0.53 [0.27, 1.04]	2009
Giles 2	29	121	160	446	4.7%	0.56 [0.36, 0.89]	2009
Veith	6	45	1	12	0.3%	1.69 [0.18, 15.59]	2009
Giles 1	758	2323	10804	26106	14.2%	0.69 [0.63, 0.75]	2009
Davenport	22	99	122	328	3.9%	0.48 [0.29, 0.81]	2010
Bosch	5	25	15	33	0.9%	0.30 [0.09, 0.99]	2010
Starnes	5	27	13	24	0.8%	0.19 [0.05, 0.68]	2010
Lyons	2	18	6	19	0.4%	0.27 [0.05, 1.57]	2010
Chagpar	5	32	59	135	1.3%	0.24 [0.09, 0.66]	2010
Holt	108	335	1935	4079	9.6%	0.53 [0.42, 0.67]	2010
Sarac	10	32	41	128	1.8%	0.96 [0.42, 2.22]	2011
Mandawat	11	64	74	207	2.4%	0.37 [0.18, 0.76]	2012
Noorani	6	52	14	50	1.2%	0.34 [0.12, 0.96]	2012
Ioannidis	14	20	10	23	0.8%	3.03 [0.86, 10.72]	2012
Mayer	31	198	61	163	4.2%	0.31 [0.19, 0.51]	2012
Saqib	8	37	25	111	1.6%	0.95 [0.39, 2.34]	2012
Nedeau	3	19	27	55	0.8%	0.19 [0.05, 0.74]	2012
Reimerink	16	57	17	59	1.9%	0.96 [0.43, 2.16]	2013
Park	1039	3786	5227	12761	14.5%	0.54 [0.50, 0.59]	2013
Total (95% CI)		**8201**		**51740**	**100.0%**	**0.56 [0.50, 0.64]**	
Total events	2374		21918				

Heterogeneity: $Tau^2 = 0.02$; $Chi^2 = 62.70$, df = 40 (P = 0.01); $I^2 = 36\%$

Test for overall effect: Z = 9.39 (P < 0.00001)

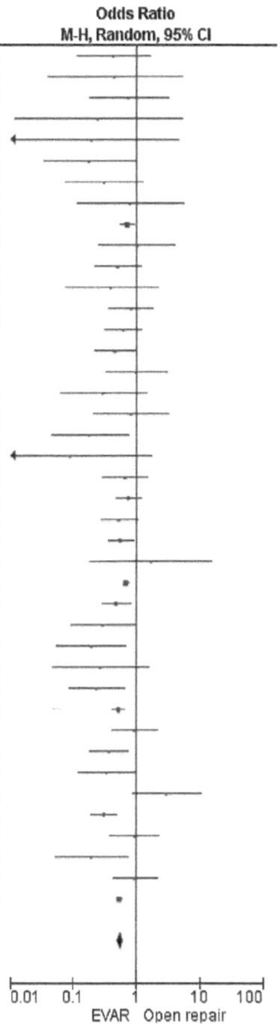

FIGURE 2.—Forest plot shows comparison of in-hospital mortality among the studies in the meta-analysis. *CI*, Confidence interval; *EVAR*, endovascular aneurysm repair; *M-H*, Mantel-Haenszel. (Reprinted from Antoniou GA, Georgiadis GS, Antoniou SA, et al. Endovascular repair for ruptured abdominal aortic aneurysm confers an early survival benefit over open repair. *J Vasc Surg*. 2013;58:1091-1105, with permission from The Society for Vascular Surgery.)

incidence of in-hospital mortality (OR, 0.56; 95% CI, 0.50-0.64; $P < .01$; meta-analysis of risk-adjusted observational studies and randomized controlled trials: OR, 0.58; 95% CI, 0.46-0.73; $P < .01$). EVAR patients had a significantly decreased risk of developing respiratory complications (OR, 0.59; 95% CI, 0.49-0.69; $P < .01$) and acute renal failure (OR, 0.65; 95% CI, 0.55-0.78; $P < .01$) and a trend toward a reduced incidence of cardiac complications (OR, −0.02; 95% CI, −0.03 to 0.00; $P = .05$) and mesenteric ischemia (OR, 0.66; 95% CI, 0.44-1.00; $P = .05$). Patients treated with EVAR had significantly less requirements of intraoperative blood transfusion (standardized mean difference, −0.88; 95% CI, −1.06 to −0.70; $P < .01$). Random-effects meta-regression revealed no statistical evidence for an association between death and year of publication ($P = .19$).

Conclusions.—Our analysis provides evidence to motivate the adoption of an EVAR-first policy in a nonelective setting and the establishment of standardized protocols for the management ruptured AAAs (Figs 1 and 2).

▶ The objective of this study was to undertake a comprehensive literature review and define the effect of endovascular repair (EVAR) on the management of ruptured abdominal aortic aneurysms (AAA) by conducting an analysis of perioperative outcomes of such a treatment strategy compared with conventional open repair. This is the most comprehensive meta-analysis to date, with the population comprising 59 941 patients across 41 studies (Fig 1).

In-hospital mortality occurred in 30% of patients treated with EVAR and in 42% of the patients who underwent open repair (odds ratio, 0.56; 95% confidence interval, 0.50–0.64; $P < .01$; Fig 2). These are very narrow confidence intervals and thus quite convincing.

The combined outcome estimate of mortality was not substantially affected when the primary analysis was repeated again after excluding each single study at a time. Sensitivity analyses and subgroup meta-regression comparing outcome measures in hospital-based and population-based reports consistently showed survival superiority of EVAR over open repair of ruptured AAA.

Hopefully, these data will help motivate the widespread adoption of EVAR for ruptured AAA. We don't need a randomized trial!

B. W. Starnes, MD

What is the Best Option for Elective Repair of an Abdominal Aortic Aneurysm in a Young Fit Patient?

Sandford RM, Choke E, Bown MJ, et al (Univ Hosps of Leicester, UK)
Eur J Vasc Endovasc Surg 47:13-18, 2014

Objective.—The lower procedural risk associated with endovascular aneurysm repair (EVAR) compared with open aneurysm repair (OAR) is well known. Younger patients are likely to represent a group at low perioperative risk. The long-term durability and late complications following EVAR may have more significance when considering the optimal treatment for young patients with a longer life expectancy. This study examined perioperative and long-term outcomes of young patients undergoing aneurysm repair by either open surgical or endovascular means.

Methods.—A retrospective review of a prospectively collated database was performed. Patients undergoing elective aneurysm repair at the age of 65 years or younger between January 2000 and September 2010 were included. All EVAR patients were followed up in a nurse-led clinic. Data regarding long-term outcomes for patients undergoing open repair were gathered from case note review.

Results.—There were 99 patients who underwent open repair and 59 patients who underwent endovascular repair. Groups were well matched in terms of demographics and co-morbidities. 30-day mortality was 1%

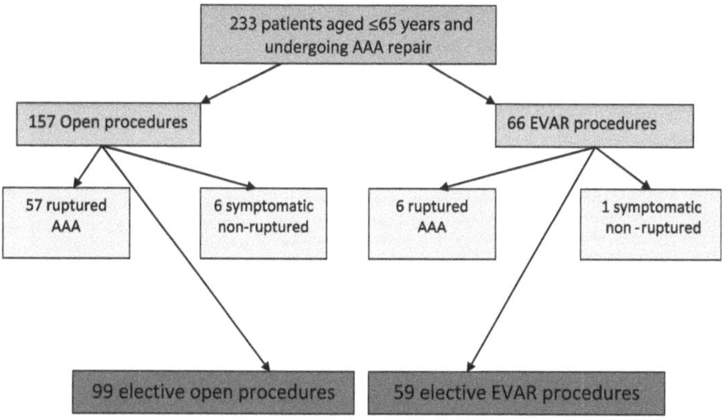

FIGURE 1.—Patients undergoing abdominal aortic aneurysm (AAA) repair between January 2000 and September 2010. (Reprinted from Sandford RM, Choke E, Bown MJ, et al. What is the best option for elective repair of an abdominal aortic aneurysm in a young fit patient? *Eur J Vasc Endovasc Surg*. 2014;47:13-18, Copyright 2014, with permission from the European Society for Vascular Surgery.)

after open repair. There were no perioperative deaths after endovascular repair. Overall, 30-day complication rates were 15% after open repair and 12% after EVAR. The nature of complications differed between the two groups with the EVAR group experiencing endoleaks and the OAR group demonstrating more cardiorespiratory complications. Mean follow-up was 75.5 months and there was a 14% reintervention rate after EVAR compared with 7% after OAR.

Conclusion.—Young patients are likely to have a lower procedural risk for EVAR and OAR than described in published figures. Although mortality and complication rates in these two groups were similar, the nature of complications occurring following open surgery were often more significant than those occurring after EVAR. There remains a risk of late reintervention following either form of repair (Fig 1).

▶ How many publications do we need to see attempting to sway opinion to one side or the other for open surgical versus endovascular repair for abdominal aortic aneurysm (AAA) in the young, fit patient? Ultimately, the decision will be made by the patient with appropriate counseling and informed consent.

This is yet another attempt to question whether young patients are better served with EVAR or open repair of AAA in the elective setting. The authors confirmed in their analysis that young patients had lower periprocedural risk for EVAR and open repair than in previously published reports.

Criticisms of this study were that it was small and from a moderate-volume center. Only 30% of patients aged less than 65 years were treated with EVAR (Fig 1). Although the early complication rates between groups were similar, the nature of those complications varied between groups, with the predominant endovascular complication being endoleak, a proportion of which were type 2 and considered benign. Among the open surgical group, complications were generally of a more significant nature, including hemorrhage, acute coronary syndromes, and limb and mesenteric ischemia.

Both this study, and a recent publication examining midterm outcomes after EVAR,[1] reiterate the often unreported risk of long-term reinterventions after open repair of AAA.

B. W. Starnes, MD

Reference

1. Altaf N, Abisi S, Yong Y, Saunders JH, Braithwaite BD, MacSweeney ST. Mid-term results of endovascular aortic aneurysm repair in the young. *Eur J Vasc Endovasc Surg*. 2013;46:315-319.

Development of a risk index for prediction of mortality after open aortic aneurysm repair

Ramanan B, Gupta PK, Sundaram A, et al (Creighton Univ, Omaha, NE; Univ of Wisconsin Hosp & Clinics, Madison; et al)

J Vasc Surg 58:871-878, 2013

Objective.—Open infrarenal abdominal aortic aneurysm (oAAA) repair is associated with significant morbidity and mortality. Although there has been a shift toward endovascular repair, many patients continue to undergo an open repair due to anatomic considerations. Tools currently existing for estimation of periprocedural risk in patients undergoing open aortic surgery have certain limitations. The objective of this study was to develop a risk index to estimate the risk of 30-day perioperative mortality after elective oAAA repair.

Methods.—Patients who underwent elective oAAA repair (n = 2845) were identified from the American College of Surgeons' 2007 to 2009 National Surgical Quality Improvement Program (NSQIP), a prospective database maintained at >250 centers. Univariable and multivariable analyses were performed to evaluate risk factors associated with 30-day mortality after oAAA repair and a risk index was developed.

Results.—The 30-day mortality after oAAA repair was 3.3%. Multivariable analysis identified six preoperative predictors of mortality, and a risk index was created by assigning weighted points to each predictor using the β-coefficients from the regression analysis. The predictors included dyspnea (at rest: 8 points; on moderate exertion: 2 points; none: 0 points), history of peripheral arterial disease requiring revascularization or amputation (3 points), age >65 years (3 points), preoperative creatinine >1.5 mg/dL (2 points), female gender (2 points), and platelets <150,000/mm^3 or >350,000/mm^3 (2 points). Patients were classified as low (<7%), intermediate (7%-15%), and high (>15%) risk for 30-day mortality based on a total point score of <8, 8 to 11, and >11, respectively. There were 2508 patients (88.2%) patients in the low-risk category, 278

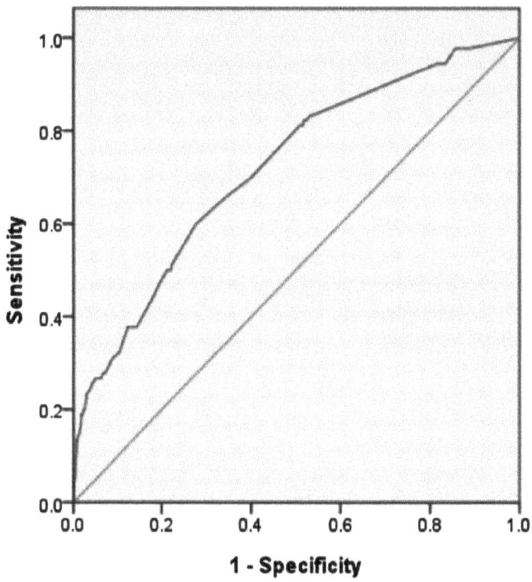

FIGURE.—Receiver-operating characteristic curve. (Reprinted from Ramanan B, Gupta PK, Sundaram A. et al. Development of a risk index for prediction of mortality after open aortic aneurysm repair. *J Vasc Surg*. 2013;58:871-878, Copyright 2013, with permission from The Society for Vascular Surgery.)

(9.8%) in the intermediate-risk category, and 59 (2.1%) in the high-risk category.

Conclusions.—This risk index has excellent predictive ability for mortality after oAAA repair and awaits validation in subsequent studies. It is anticipated to aid patients and surgeons in informed patient consent, preoperative risk assessment, and optimization (Fig).

▶ For any given procedure, including open aortic surgery, the process of informed consent requires a fairly thorough explanation of the risks and benefits of the procedure to the patient and the patient's family. The risks presented by vascular surgeons for patients undergoing abdominal aortic surgery are based on anecdotal experience or on currently available risk estimation tools.

This study found age older than 65 years, dyspnea, female gender, abnormal platelet count, history of peripheral arterial disease requiring revascularization or amputation, and abnormal creatinine level (>1.5 mg/dL) were associated with perioperative mortality after elective open AAA repair. These risk factors have also been found to be components of previous risk estimation tools.

Overall mortality in the well-known GAS (Glasgow Aneurysm Score) study[1] was 20% (8.6% for nonruptured aneurysms). Thirty-day mortality in the current series was 3.3%. This raises the question of applicability of the GAS when perioperative mortality rates have decreased from 8.6% to 3.3% in the current series. The risk index in this study, which provides an estimate of perioperative mortality in an individual patient, has a much higher C-statistic than the GAS at 0.72 (Fig). I foresee this risk index, like many others being reported, as an important tool in the modern informed consent process. Obviously, this risk index needs to be validated in future studies.

B. W. Starnes, MD

Reference

1. Samy AK, Murray G, MacBain G. Glasgow aneurysm score. *Cardiovasc Surg.* 1994;2:41-44.

Family history of aortic disease predicts disease patterns and progression and is a significant influence on management strategies for patients and their relatives

Brown CR, Greenberg RK, Wong S, et al (Cleveland Clinic, OH)
J Vasc Surg 58:573-581, 2013

Background.—While a positive family history (FH) is a known risk factor for developing an aneurysm, its association with the extent of disease has not been established. We evaluated the influence of a FH of aortic disease with respect to the pattern and distribution of aortic aneurysms in a given patient.

Methods and Results.—From November 1999 to November 2011, 1263 patients were enrolled in physician-sponsored endovascular device trials to treat aortic aneurysms. Of the 555 patients who were alive and returning for follow-up, we obtained 426 (77%) family histories. Three-dimensional imaging studies were used to identify the presence of aneurysms; 36% (155/426) of patients had a FH of aortic aneurysms and 5% (21/155) had isolated intracranial aneurysms. A logistic regression model was used to compare aortic morphology between patients with a positive or negative FH for aneurysms. Patients with a positive FH of aortic aneurysms were younger at their initial aneurysm (63 vs 70 years; $P < .0001$), more frequently had proximal aortic involvement (root: odds ratio [OR], 5.4; $P < .0001$; ascending: OR, 2.9; $P < .001$; thoracic: OR, 2.2; $P = .01$) with over 50% of FH patients ultimately developing suprarenal aortic involvement ($P = .0001$) and had a greater incidence of bilateral iliac artery aneurysm (OR, 1.8; $P = .03$).

Conclusions.—FH is an important tool that provides insight into the expected behavior of the untreated aorta and has significant implications for the development of treatment strategies. These findings should be used to guide patient's management with regard to treatment, follow-up paradigms, genetic testing, and screening of other family members (Fig 2).

▶ This is the first of 2 reports on familial abdominal aortic aneurysm that I chose for the Year Book this year. Over the last several decades, the role of genetics in aortic aneurysmal disease and dissection has become increasingly appreciated. Current knowledge dictates that between 15% and 30% of patients with an aortic aneurysm or dissection will have a positive family history. Based on

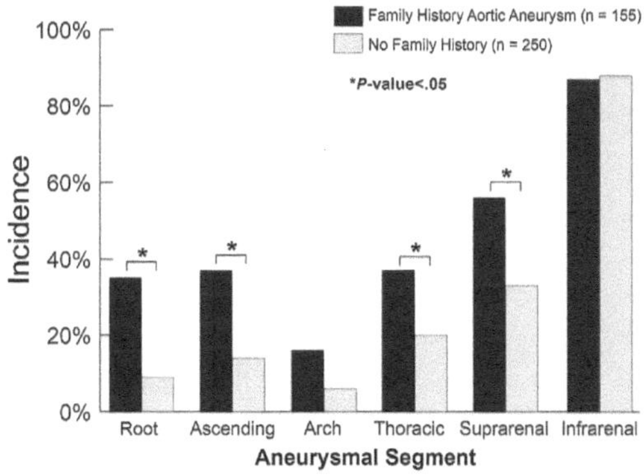

FIGURE 2.—Incidence of patients with aneurysmal segments in the aorta based on family history (FH) of aortic disease. The *asterisk* represents statistically significant differences based on adjusted *P* values. (Reprinted from Brown CR, Greenberg RK, Wong S, et al. Family history of aortic disease predicts disease patterns and progression and is a significant influence on management strategies for patients and their relatives. *J Vasc Surg*. 2013;58:573-581, with permission from The Society for Vascular Surgery.)

their clinical experience, these authors postulated that patients with a positive family history have more extensive aortic aneurysms and entirely different pattern of disease than patients without a positive family history.

Of 1263 patients enrolled in 1 of 3 investigational device exemptions, 555 were both alive and returning for follow-up. A total of 426 family pedigrees were ascertained (77%), and, of those, 176 or 41% had a positive family history for aneurysm. Deceased patients reported by relatives to have had sudden death of unknown etiology were considered to potentially have had an aneurysm.

These findings are important. Patients with a positive family history of aortic aneurysm were younger at initial presentation compared with those with no family history. These data indicate that the presence of a family history of aortic aneurysmal disease influences the pattern and anatomic distribution of aneurysms in the proband's aorta and iliofemoral arteries. The presence of positive family history significantly increased the likelihood of aneurysmal disease development in the aortic root ($P < .0001$), ascending aorta ($P < .0001$), descending thoracic aorta ($P = .01$), and suprarenal aorta ($P = .0001$) (Fig 2).

These findings suggest that obtaining an accurate family history for patients with aortic disease is a much more powerful tool than simple screening.

B. W. Starnes, MD

Calcification as a Risk Factor for Rupture of Abdominal Aortic Aneurysm

Buijs RVC, Willems TP, Tio RA, et al (Univ of Groningen, The Netherlands)

Eur J Vasc Endovasc Surg 46:542-548, 2013

Objectives.—Abdominal aortic aneurysm (AAA) is a major cause of death in developed countries. The AAA diameter is still the only validated prognostic measure for rupture, and therapeutic interventions are initiated

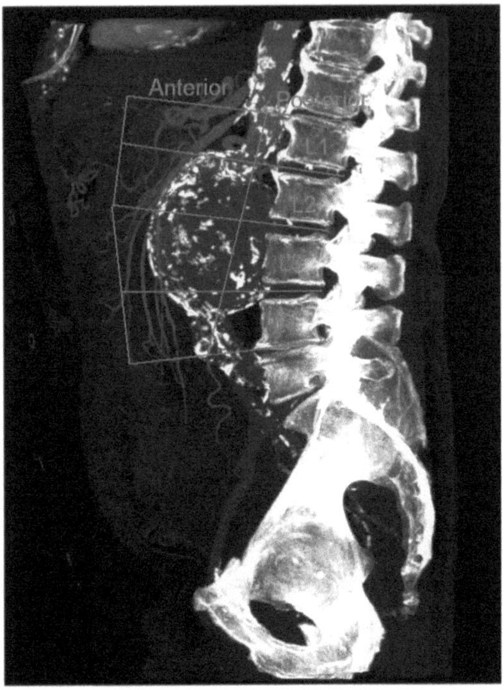

FIGURE 3.—A sagittal maximum intensity projection image from a thoracic computed tomography scan in an abdominal aortic aneurysm (AAA) patient with visualization of the measurement protocol according to the Abdominal Aortic Calcification-8 score. Each lumbar vertebra up to number four has been numbered. A crude midline is drawn to show the anterior and posterior side of the AAA. The calcifications alongside the most ventral and dorsal wall are counted as either present or absent. (Reprinted from Buijs RVC, Willems TP, Tio RA, et al. Calcification as a risk factor for rupture of abdominal aortic aneurysm. *Eur J Vasc Endovasc Surg*. 2013;46:542-548, Copyright 2013, with permission from the European Society for Vascular Surgery.)

accordingly. This still leads to unnecessary interventions in some cases or unidentified impending ruptures. Vascular calcification has been validated abundantly as a risk factor in the cardiovascular field and may strengthen the rupture risk assessment of the AAA. With this study we aim to assess the correlation between AAA calcification and rupture risk in a retrospective unmatched case-control population.

Methods.—A database of 334 AAA patients was evaluated. Three groups were formed: elective (eAAA; $n = 233$), ruptured (rAAA; $n = 73$) and symptomatic non-ruptured (sAAA; $n = 28$) AAA patients. The Abdominal Aortic Calcification-8 score (AAC-8) was used to measure the severity of vascular calcification.

Results.—The AAA diameter (61 ± 12 mm vs. 74 ± 21 mm; $p < .001$) and AAC-8 score (3.4 ± 2 points vs. 4.9 ± 2.3 points; $p < .001$) of the eAAA and the combined rAAA and sAAA groups, respectively, were significantly different after univariate analysis. Multivariate analysis showed that larger AAA diameter (odds ratio [OR]: 1.048/mm increase; 95% confidence interval [CI]: 1.042–1.082; $p < .001$) and a higher AAC-8 score

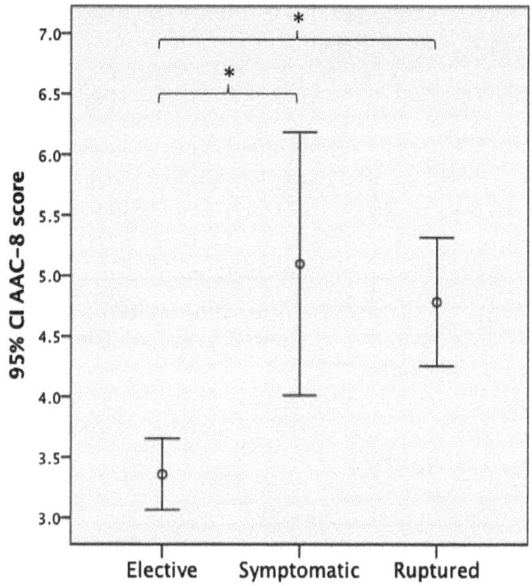

FIGURE 5.—95% Confidence interval (CI) of the mean bar graph of the Abdominal Aortic Calcification-8 (AAC-8) score for elective, ruptured, and symptomatic abdominal aortic aneurysms (AAAs). *Note.* *$p < .05$. (Reprinted from Buijs RVC, Willems TP, Tio RA, et al. Calcification as a risk factor for rupture of abdominal aortic aneurysm. *Eur J Vasc Endovasc Surg*. 2013;46:542-548, Copyright 2013, with permission from the European Society for Vascular Surgery.)

(OR: 1.34/point increase; 95% CI: 1.19–1.53; $p < .001$) were significantly associated with development into a sAAA or rAAA. Peripheral artery disease was significantly correlated to eventual elective treatment (OR: 0.39; 95% CI: .15–1; $p = .049$).

Conclusion.—This study suggests a trend of an increased degree of calcification in symptomatic or even ruptured AAA patients compared with elective AAA patients (Figs 3 and 5).

▶ Risk stratification for abdominal aortic aneurysm (AAA) in its current state is based solely on the maximum diameter of the aorta. Calcification has been shown to be a sign of a degenerative inflammatory process involved in the arterial wall but has received little attention in relation to AAA. This study shows a clear association between aortic wall calcification and rupture.

To reliably image all calcifications in a 3-dimensional plane, a maximum-intensity projection was created from a sagittal perspective (Fig 3 in the original article). Calcification was measured by independent radiologists using the AAC-8 Score,[1] which essentially assigns points based on calcium burden in the anterior and posterior aortic walls between L1 and L4. Agreement for inter-rater reliability of the AAC-8 Score was good (Kappa = 0.69; $P < .001$).

Three hundred thirty-four computed tomography scans were evaluated and divided into 3 groups (elective, symptomatic, and ruptured; Fig 5 in the original article). This study is interesting in that the degree of calcification has value not only as an addendum to diameter but could also be associated with the development of symptoms in AAA patients.

B. W. Starnes, MD

Reference

1. Schousboe JT, Wilson KE, Kiel DP. Detection of abdominal aortic calcification with lateral spine imaging using DXA. *J Clin Densitom.* 2006;9:302-308.

A Novel Strategy to Translate the Biomechanical Rupture Risk of Abdominal Aortic Aneurysms to their Equivalent Diameter Risk: Method and Retrospective Validation

Gasser TC, Nchimi A, Swedenborg J, et al (Royal Inst of Technology (KTH), Stockholm, Sweden; Univ Hosp of Liège, Belgium; Karolinska Univ Hosp and Inst, Stockholm, Sweden; et al)

Eur J Vasc Endovasc Surg 47:288-295, 2014

Objective.—To translate the individual abdominal aortic aneurysm (AAA) patient's biomechanical rupture risk profile to risk-equivalent diameters, and to retrospectively test their predictability in ruptured and non-ruptured aneurysms.

Methods.—Biomechanical parameters of ruptured and non-ruptured AAAs were retrospectively evaluated in a multicenter study. General patient data and high resolution computer tomography angiography (CTA) images from 203 non-ruptured and 40 ruptured aneurysmal infrarenal aortas. Three-dimensional AAA geometries were semi-automatically derived from CTA images. Finite element (FE) models were used to predict peak wall stress (PWS) and peak wall rupture index (PWRI) according to the individual anatomy, gender, blood pressure, intra-luminal thrombus (ILT) morphology, and relative aneurysm expansion. Average PWS diameter and PWRI diameter responses were evaluated, which allowed for the PWS equivalent and PWRI equivalent diameters for any individual aneurysm to be defined.

Results.—PWS increased linearly and PWRI exponentially with respect to maximum AAA diameter. A size-adjusted analysis showed that PWS equivalent and PWRI equivalent diameters were increased by 7.5 mm ($p = .013$) and 14.0 mm ($p < .001$) in ruptured cases when compared to non-ruptured controls, respectively. In non-ruptured cases the PWRI equivalent diameters were increased by 13.2 mm ($p < .001$) in females when compared with males.

Conclusions.—Biomechanical parameters like PWS and PWRI allow for a highly individualized analysis by integrating factors that influence the risk of AAA rupture like geometry (degree of asymmetry, ILT morphology, etc.) and patient characteristics (gender, family history, blood pressure, etc.). PWRI and the reported annual risk of rupture increase similarly with the diameter. PWRI equivalent diameter expresses the PWRI through the

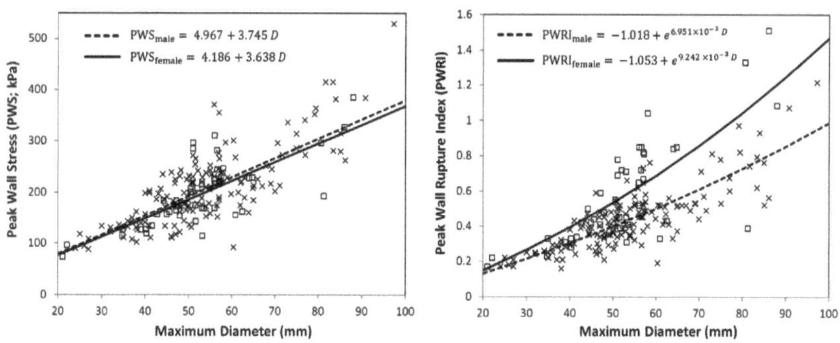

FIGURE 2.—Development of peak wall stress (PWS) and peak wall rupture index (PWRI) with respect to the maximum diameter of nonruptured abdominal aortic aneurysms (AAAs). Squares denote female and crosses male patients. Solid lines (female) and dashed lines (male) denote regression curves. (Reprinted from Gasser TC, Nchimi A, Swedenborg J, et al. A novel strategy to translate the biomechanical rupture risk of abdominal aortic aneurysms to their equivalent diameter risk: method and retrospective validation. *Eur J Vasc Endovasc Surg*. 2014;47:288-295, Copyright 2014, with permission from European Society for Vascular Surgery.)

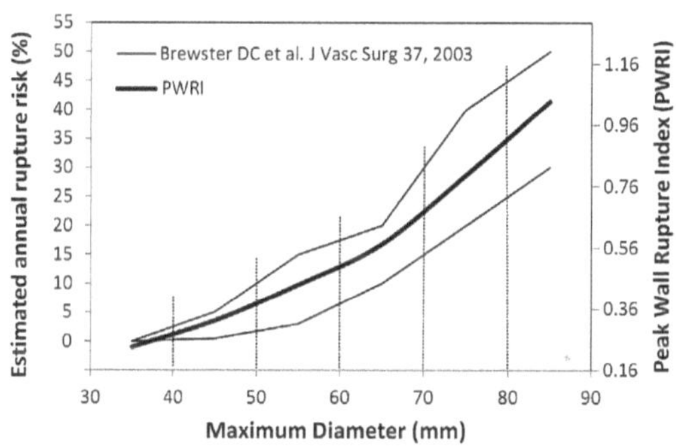

FIGURE 3.—Progressive increase of annual rupture risk of abdominal aortic aneurysm (AAA) with respect to the maximum diameter. Thin solid lines represent upper and lower estimates[2] based on reported data. The thick solid line denotes peak wall rupture index (PWRI) based on a regression analysis of our patient cohort. PWRI has been adjusted for ruptured AAAs, i.e. regression curves for ruptured and non-ruptured cases were weighted according to reported rupture prevalence.[2] Editor's Note: Please refer to original journal article for full references. (Reprinted from Gasser TC, Nchimi A, Swedenborg J, et al. A novel strategy to translate the biomechanical rupture risk of abdominal aortic aneurysms to their equivalent diameter risk: method and retrospective validation. *Eur J Vasc Endovasc Surg*. 2014;47:288-295, Copyright 2014, with permission from European Society for Vascular Surgery.)

diameter of the average AAA that has the same PWRI, i.e. is at the same biomechanical risk of rupture. Consequently, PWRI equivalent diameter facilitates a straightforward interpretation of biomechanical analysis and connects to diameter-based guidelines for AAA repair indication. PWRI equivalent diameter reflects an additional diagnostic parameter that may provide more accurate clinical data for AAA repair indication (Figs 2 and 3, Table 4).

► The indication for elective abdominal aortic aneurysm (AAA) repair is determined by the likelihood of rupture. Consequently, an accurate evaluation of

TABLE 4.—Relation Between Peak Wall Rupture Index (PWRI) and the PWRI-Equivalent Diameter D_{PWRI}. The D_{PWRI} Reflects the Maximum Diameter of the Average Abdominal Aortic Aneurysm (AAA) Patient Experiencing the Same PWRI, see also Fig. 4B for its Definition

PWRI	0.24	0.32	0.40	0.48	0.56	0.64	0.72	0.80	0.88	0.96
D_{PWRI} (mm)	32	40	48	55	62	69	75	81	87	93

rupture risk is of paramount importance in lowering aneurysm-related mortality, without substantially elevating the rate of elective AAA repair. Using a gender-specific computational method of low operator variability, these authors tested the biomechanical rupture risk assessment on the largest patient cohort to date.

Biomechanically analyzing a large patient cohort illustrated that peak wall stress (PWS) increased linearly whereas peak wall rupture index (PWRI) increased exponentially with the maximum AAA diameter (Fig 2). The average trend curves were in turn used to introduce D(PWS) and D(PWRI), which were equivalent maximal diameters of an average aneurysm that experienced the same PWS and PWRI, respectively.

The present analysis used a larger number of patients, and PWRI could significantly discriminate between male and female patients. In addition, the data predicted by their finite element models suggested that a 50-mm AAA in females has the equivalent risk of rupture as a 63-mm aneurysm in males (Table 4, Fig 3).

This article was a little difficult to understand but in the end offers the closest glimpse yet at the true rupture risk based on diameter in addition to other factors.

B. W. Starnes, MD

Comparison of outcomes following endovascular repair of abdominal aortic aneurysms based on size threshold

Keith CJ Jr, Passman MA, Gaffud MJ, et al (Univ of Alabama at Birmingham)
J Vasc Surg 58:1458-1466, 2013

Introduction.—Size threshold for operative repair of abdominal aortic aneurysms (AAAs) has been determined based on risks and outcomes of open repair vs surveillance. The influence of endovascular aneurysm repair (EVAR) on this threshold is less established. The purpose of this study is to determine whether long-term outcomes following EVAR are affected by maximum diameter at the time of treatment.

Methods.—Patients undergoing EVAR with modular stent grafts from 2000 to 2011 were identified from a prospectively maintained database and stratified by maximum aortic diameter at the time of repair: small (4.0-4.9 cm), medium (5.0-5.9 cm), and large (≥6.0 cm). Comparisons of demographics, indications for repair, perioperative complications, and long-term outcomes were made using analysis of variance, χ^2, and Kaplan-Meier plots.

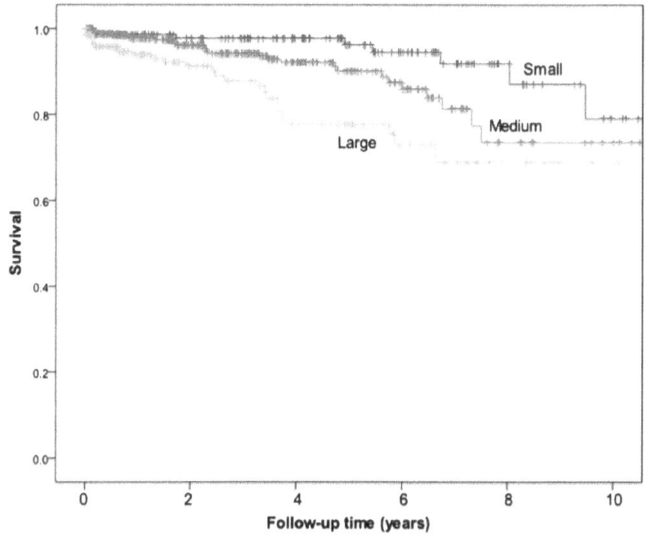

		1 y	2 y	3 y	4 y	5 y	6 y	7 y	8 y	9 y	10 y
Small	At Risk	123	109	98	78	59	47	32	19	12	6
	%	99	98	98	98	96	95	92	92	87	79
	Std error	1	1	1	1	2	3	4	4	6	9
Medium	At Risk	275	215	166	115	80	55	28	14	9	6
	%	98	96	94	92	90	86	81	74	74	74
	Std error	1	1	2	2	2	3	4	7	7	7
Large	At Risk	130	91	69	51	41	25	14	7	1	0
	%	94	91	88	78	78	73	69	69	69	69
	Std error	2	2	3	4	4	5	6	6	6	6

FIGURE 4.—Freedom from secondary intervention. (Reprinted from Keith Jr CJ, Passman MA, Gaffud MJ, et al. Comparison of outcomes following endovascular repair of abdominal aortic aneurysms based on size threshold. *J Vasc Surg.* 2013;58:1458-1466, Copyright 2013, with permission from The Society for Vascular Surgery.)

Results.—Seven hundred forty patients were identified: 157 (21.2%) small, 374 (50.5%) medium, and 209 (28.2%) large. Patients differed by mean age (69.3 ± 8.09, 71.7 ± 8.55, and 73.6 ± 8.77 years for small, medium, and large, respectively; $P < .001$), coronary artery disease (42% small, 57% medium, 51.2% large; $P = .01$), prior coronary angioplasty (14.6% small, 18.2% medium, 9.6% large; $P = .02$), congestive heart failure (5.7% small, 15.2% medium, 19.6% large; $P = .01$), prior vascular surgery (7% small, 15.8% medium, 10% large; $P = .016$), and chronic obstructive pulmonary disease (21% small, 27% medium, 33% large; $P = .038$). Small AAAs were more frequently symptomatic (19.7% small, 7.5% medium, 8.1% large; $P < .001$). There was no difference in perioperative complication rates ($P = .399$), expansion ≥5 mm (2.6% small, 5.6% medium, 7.2% large; $P = .148$), or all-type endoleak (40.8% small, 41.7% medium, 44.5% large; $P = .73$). Small AAAs developed fewer type I endoleaks (5.1% vs 6.95% medium and 14.8% large; $P = .001$). Compared with small AAAs, both medium ($P = .39$) and large

($P < .001$) required secondary intervention more frequently, with hazard ratios of 2.32 (95% confidence interval, 1.045-5.156) and 4.74 (95% confidence interval, 2.115-10.637), respectively. Ten-year survival was 72%, 63.1%, and 49.8% in the small, medium, and large groups, respectively ($P < .001$) with one rupture-related death after EVAR in the large group. All-cause mortality differed among the 75- to 84-year-old patients (30.4% small, 51.6% medium, 55.7% large; $P = .017$).

Conclusions.—EVAR for small AAAs shows improved long-term outcomes than for age-matched patients with larger aneurysms (Fig 4).

▶ Although size threshold for open repair of abdominal aortic aneurysms (AAA) has been established at 5.5 cm by evidence-based guidelines from randomized trials comparing open repair with surveillance, size threshold for endovascular aneurysm repair (EVAR) has not been established. PIVOTAL,[1] a randomized, controlled trial comparing EVAR and surveillance for small AAAs, showed no survival advantage for EVAR. However, morbidity and mortality were still very low within a relatively short follow-up interval.

This is an important study. These authors report an impressive single institution EVAR series of 740 patients with the hypothesis that long-term outcomes are improved after EVAR for small AAA (< 5 cm).

The important points of this report are:

1 The rate of type 1 endoleak is significantly higher in large aneurysms versus small ($P = .001$).

2 Secondary intervention was required for a larger percentage of medium and large aneurysms than small.

In fact, in direct comparison with small AAAs, patients with medium AAAs were 2.32 times more likely to require secondary intervention ($P = .039$; 95% confidence interval [CI], 1.045–5.156), and those with large AAAs were 4.74 times more likely ($P < .001$; 95% CI, 2.115–10.637; Fig 4).

Patients in the small AAA group were younger and had fewer medical histories of coronary artery disease, congestive heart failure, chronic obstructive pulmonary disease, and prior vascular surgery. This difference in preoperative risk profile has translated into fewer perioperative systemic complications in patients undergoing EVAR for small AAAs compared with large.

As a retrospective study, there is no control group of patients randomly assigned to EVAR versus surveillance. There is also potential for selection bias, especially for the small AAA group in that patients were selected based on favorable risk profile and more favorable AAA anatomy for EVAR, which may have influenced the results.

This study suggests that EVAR for small AAA is safe and effective. Patients with small AAAs were better surgical candidates, had lower rates of type 1 endoleak, had decreased need for secondary intervention, and had improved survival when compared with patients undergoing EVAR for medium and large AAAs.

B. W. Starnes, MD

Reference

1. Ouriel K, Clair DG, Kent KC, Zarins CK, Positive Impact of Endovascular Options for Treating Aneurysms Early (PIVOTAL) Investigators. Endovascular repair compared with surveillance for patients with small abdominal aortic aneurysms. *J Vasc Surg*. 2010;51:1081-1087.

Comparative effectiveness of endovascular versus open repair of ruptured abdominal aortic aneurysm in the Medicare population

Edwards ST, Schermerhorn ML, O'Malley AJ, et al (Beth Israel Deaconess Med Ctr, Boston, MA; Harvard Med School, Boston, MA; et al)
J Vasc Surg 59:575-582.e6, 2014

Objective.—Endovascular aortic repair (EVAR) for abdominal aortic aneurysm (AAA) is increasingly used for emergent treatment of ruptured AAA (rAAA). We sought to compare the perioperative and long-term mortality, procedure-related complications, and rates of reintervention of EVAR vs open aortic repair of rAAA in Medicare beneficiaries.

Methods.—We examined perioperative and long-term mortality and complications after EVAR or open aortic repair performed for rAAA in all traditional Medicare beneficiaries discharged from a United States hospital from 2001 to 2008. Patients were matched by propensity score on baseline demographics, coexisting conditions, admission source, and hospital volume of rAAA repair. Sensitivity analyses were performed to evaluate the effect of bias that might have resulted from unmeasured confounders.

Results.—Of 10,998 patients with repaired rAAA, 1126 underwent EVAR and 9872 underwent open repair. Propensity score matching yielded 1099 patient pairs. The average age was 78 years, and 72.4% were male. Perioperative mortality was 33.8% for EVAR and 47.7% for open repair ($P < .001$), and this difference persisted for >4 years. At 36 months, EVAR patients had higher rates of AAA-related reinterventions than open repair patients (endovascular reintervention, 10.9% vs 1.5%; $P < .001$), whereas open patients had more laparotomy-related complications (incisional hernia repair, 1.8% vs 6.2%; $P < .001$; all surgical complications, 4.4% vs 9.1%; $P < .001$). Use of EVAR for rAAA increased from 6% of cases in 2001 to 31% in 2008, whereas during the same interval, overall 30-day mortality for admission for rAAA, regardless of treatment, decreased from 55.8% to 50.9%.

Conclusions.—EVAR for rAAA is associated with lower perioperative and long-term mortality in Medicare beneficiaries. Increasing adoption of EVAR for rAAA is associated with an overall decrease in mortality of patients hospitalized for rAAA during the last decade (Figs 1 and 2, Tables 2 and 3).

▶ This is one of the best articles I have reviewed in this year's edition of the YEAR BOOK OF VASCULAR SURGERY. There have been recent early reports from

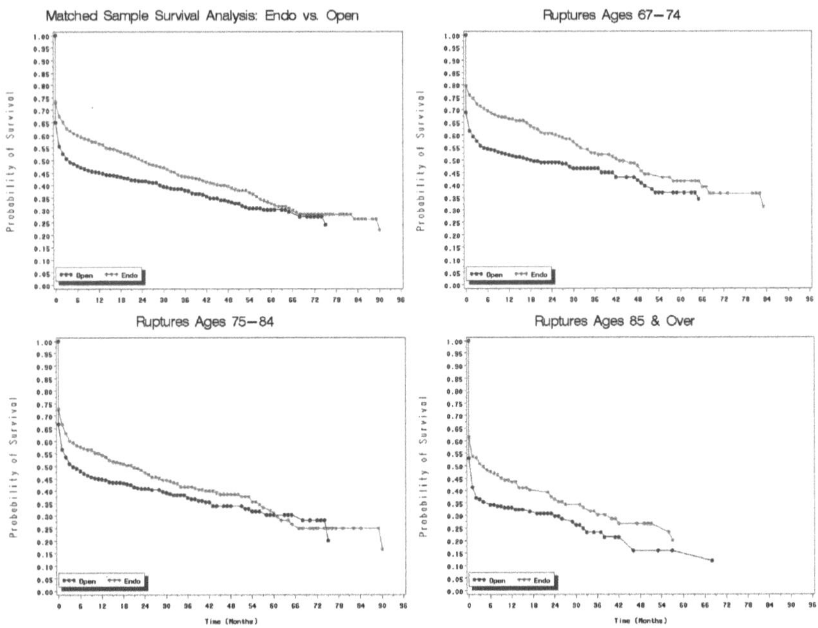

FIGURE 1.—Mortality of propensity-matched patients undergoing endovascular (*Endo*) and open repair of ruptured aortic aneurysm (rAAA) is shown overall and stratified by age. (Reprinted from Edwards ST, Schermerhorn ML, O'Malley AJ, et al. Comparative effectiveness of endovascular versus open repair of ruptured abdominal aortic aneurysm in the Medicare population. *J Vasc Surg.* 2014;59:575-582.e6, Copyright 2014, with permission from the Society for Vascular Surgery.)

small prospective, randomized trails comparing open repair with endovascular aortic repair (EVAR) for patients presenting with ruptured abdominal aortic aneurysms (AAA), suggesting that there is no difference in mortality when selection bias is eliminated from the equation. This study, although observational in nature, is extremely powerful.

These authors looked at all Medicare beneficiaries between 2001 and 2008 with a diagnosis of ruptured AAA. Of 10 998 patients undergoing repair, 1126 underwent EVAR, and 9872 underwent open repair. Propensity score analysis yielded 1099 patients in each group matched for all comorbidities. Perioperative mortality was 33.8% for EVAR and 47.7% for open repair ($P < .001$), and this difference persisted for 4 years (Table 2; Fig 1)!

During the study interval, overall mortality of patients admitted to a hospital with ruptured AAA, regardless of intervention, declined by nearly 5%, whereas the proportion of repairs performed using EVAR increased from 6% to 31%. The 1 criticism of this study would be that it remains possible that hemodynamically unstable patients would preferentially undergo open repair, which would result in higher mortality for patients treated with open repair. The authors used several unique techniques to eliminate this concern to include matched cohorts

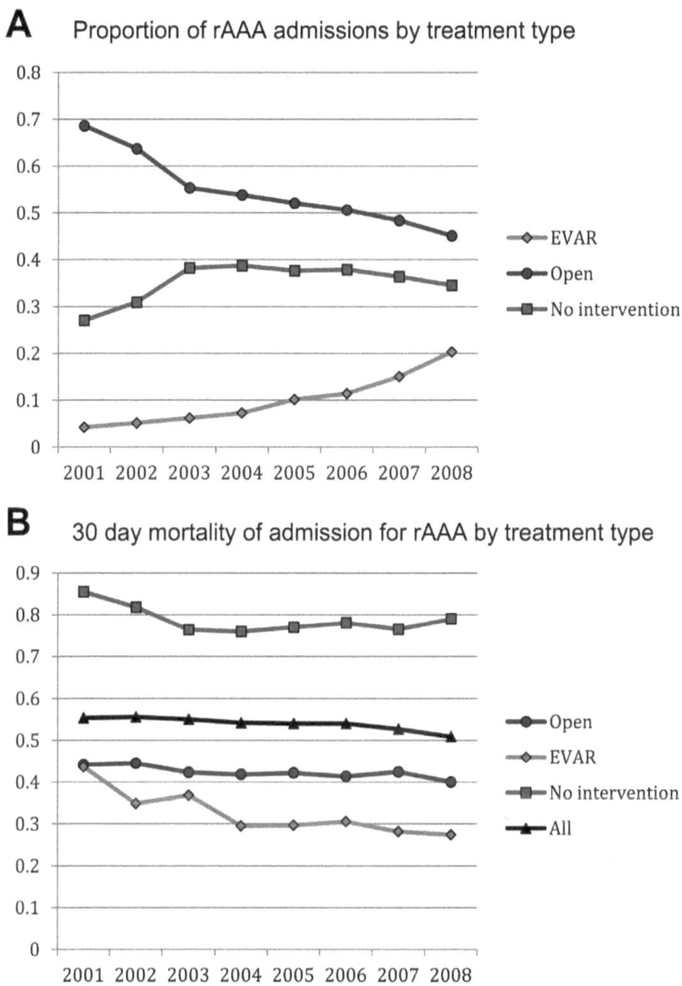

FIGURE 2.—Trends in ruptured abdominal aortic aneurysm (*rAAA*) treatment and 30-day mortality by treatment type from 2001 to 2008. **A**, Proportion of rAAA admissions by treatment type. **B**, 30-day mortality of admission for rAAA by treatment type. *EVAR*, Endovascular aortic repair. (Reprinted from Edwards ST, Schermerhorn ML, O'Malley AJ, et al. Comparative effectiveness of endovascular versus open repair of ruptured abdominal aortic aneurysm in the Medicare population. *J Vasc Surg*. 2014;59:575-582.e6, Copyright 2014, with permission from the Society for Vascular Surgery.)

and a sensitivity analysis that suggested sicker patients may be selected for EVAR, thus biasing their results in favor of open repair. Late outcomes are listed in Table 3 and trends of admissions and 30-day mortality in Fig 2. With this study, despite its observational nature, one can no longer ignore the favorable

TABLE 2.—Perioperative Outcomes

Outcome	EVAR (n = 1099)	Open (n = 1099)	*P*
Perioperative mortality, %			
All ages	33.8	47.7	<.001
67-69 years	18.8	38.7	<.001
70-74 years	27.7	41.0	<.001
75-79 years	30.1	43.0	<.001
80-84 years	39.2	53.5	<.001
≥85 years	50.0	61.5	.02
Medical complications, %			
Myocardial infarction	16.7	19.2	.13
Pneumonia	28.5	35.9	<.001
Acute renal failure	33.4	45.4	<.001
Hemodialysis	0.7	0.6	.80
Respiratory failure/tracheostomy	4.6	9.9	<.001
Venous thromboembolism	8.0	6.8	.29
Surgical complications, %			
Conversion to open repair	4.9		
Reoperation for bleeding	2.3	3.0	.24
Embolectomy	3.6	6.4	.003
Wound dehiscence	2.5	4.6	.008
Operative site hematoma	8.0	4.5	<.001
Gastrointestinal bleeding	10.3	13.8	.01
Mesenteric ischemia	7.6	14.7	<.001
Bowel obstruction or ileus	12.7	17.0	.005
Colon resection	4.4	8.5	<.001
Ostomy	2.64	5.28	.002
Discharge to home, %	62.8	40.7	<.001
LOS of survivors to hospital discharge, median (IQR) days	7 (4-24)	14 (9-23)	<.001

EVAR, endovascular aortic repair; *IQR*, interquartile range; *LOS*, length of stay.

TABLE 3.—Late Outcomes

Outcome	12 months EVAR, %	Open, %	36 months EVAR, %	Open, %	*P*[a]
Reintervention					
Open surgical[b]	1.9	0.5	3.9	0.9	.002
Endovascular[c]	4.6	0.6	10.9	1.5	<.001
Laparotomy-related complications					
Bowel obstruction					
Nonsurgical admission[d]	7.3	15.4	18.7	35.8	<.001
Surgical[e]	0.7	1.8	2.5	3.0	.157
Incisional hernia	0.3	1.2	1.8	6.2	<.001
Any surgical intervention[f]	1.0	3.0	4.4	9.1	<.001

EVAR, Endovascular aortic repair.
[a]Late outcomes were analyzed using survival analysis, and P values are those generated by the log-rank test.
[b]Conversion to open repair, open aneurysm repair, aortobifemoral bypass, axillofemoral or axillobifemoral bypass, repair of infected graft or graftenteric fistula, thrombectomy, femoral-femoral bypass.
[c]Repeat EVAR, embolization, angioplasty (aortic or iliac), extension cuff.
[d]Hospital admission with diagnosis of bowel obstruction without lysis of adhesions or bowel resection.
[e]Lysis of adhesions or bowel resection performed for diagnosis of obstruction.
[f]Surgical intervention for bowel obstruction or incisional hernia.

impact of EVAR on mortality for ruptured AAA. We don't need anymore randomized trials!

B. W. Starnes, MD

Familial abdominal aortic aneurysm is associated with more complications after endovascular aneurysm repair

van de Luijtgaarden KM, Bastos Gonçalves F, Hoeks SE, et al (Erasmus Univ Med Ctr, The Netherlands; et al)

J Vasc Surg 59:275-282, 2014

Objective.—A familial predisposition to abdominal aortic aneurysms (AAAs) is present in approximately one-fifth of patients. Nevertheless, the clinical implications of a positive family history are not known. We investigated the risk of aneurysm-related complications after endovascular aneurysm repair (EVAR) for patients with and without a positive family history of AAA.

Methods.—Patients treated with EVAR for intact AAAs in the Erasmus University Medical Center between 2000 and 2012 were included in the study. Family history was obtained by written questionnaire. Familial AAA (fAAA) was defined as patients having at least one first-degree relative affected with aortic aneurysm. The remaining patients were considered sporadic AAA. Cardiovascular risk factors, aneurysm morphology (aneurysm neck, aneurysm sac, and iliac measurements), and follow-up were obtained prospectively. The primary end point was complications after EVAR, a composite of endoleaks, need for secondary interventions, aneurysm sac growth, acute limb ischemia, and postimplantation rupture. Secondary end points were specific components of the primary end point (presence of endoleak, need for secondary intervention, and aneurysm sac growth), aneurysm neck growth, and overall survival. Kaplan-Meier estimates for the primary end point were calculated and compared using log-rank (Mantel-Cox) test of equality. A Cox-regression model was used to calculate the independent risk of complications associated with fAAA.

Results.—A total of 255 patients were included in the study (88.6% men; age 72 ± 7 years, median follow-up 3.3 years; interquartile range, 2.2-6.1). A total of 51 patients (20.0%) were classified as fAAA. Patients with fAAA were younger (69 vs 72 years; $P = .015$) and were less likely to have ever smoked (58.8% vs 73.5%; $P = .039$). Preoperative aneurysm morphology was similar in both groups. Patients with fAAA had significantly more complications after EVAR (35.3% vs 19.1%; $P = .013$), with a two fold increased risk (adjusted hazard ratio, 2.1; 95% confidence interval, 1.2-3.7). Secondary interventions (39.2% vs 20.1%; $P = .004$) and aneurysm sac growth (20.8% vs 9.5%; $P = .030$) were the most important elements accounting for the difference. Furthermore, a trend toward more type I endoleaks during follow-up was observed (15.6% vs 7.4%; $P = .063$) and no difference in overall survival.

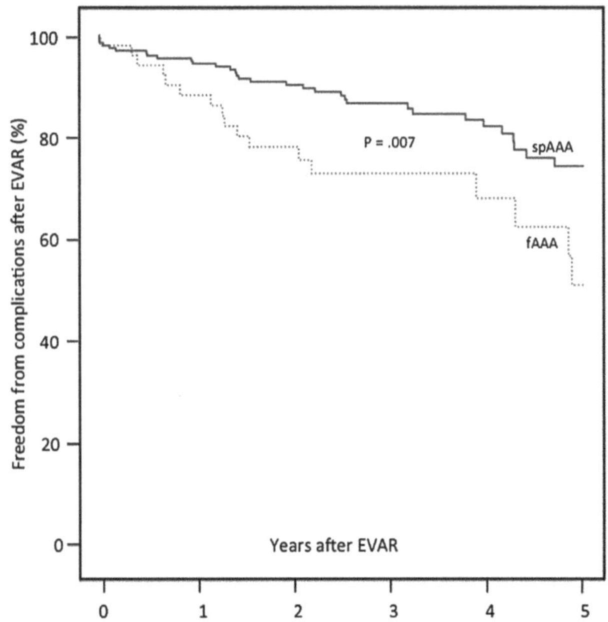

	0	1	2	3	4	5
fAAA						
Number at risk	51	44	33	23	14	9
% with events	-	88%	78%	73%	68%	51%
Standard error	(-)	.045	.058	.065	.077	.103
spAAA						
Number at risk	204	172	145	102	68	46
% with events	-	94%	90%	87%	83%	74%
Standard error	(-)	.015	.022	.026	.031	.045

FIGURE 2.—Kaplan-Meier estimates are shown for complications after endovascular aneurysm repair (*EVAR*) between familial abdominal aortic aneurysm (*AAA*) (*dashed red line*) and sporadic AAA (*solid blue line*). *fAAA*, Familial AAA; *spAAA*, sporadic AAA. For interpretation of the references to color in this figure legend, the reader is referred to web version of this article. (Reprinted from van de Luijtgaarden KM, Bastos Gonçalves F, Hoeks SE, et al. Familial abdominal aortic aneurysm is associated with more complications after endovascular aneurysm repair. *J Vasc Surg*. 2014;59:275-282, Copyright 2014, with permission from the Society for Vascular Surgery.)

Conclusions.—The current study shows that patients with a familial form of AAA develop more aneurysm-related complications after EVAR, despite similar AAA morphology at baseline. These findings suggest that patients with fAAA form a specific subpopulation and create awareness for a possible increase in the risk of complications after EVAR (Fig 2, Table 3).

▶ This is the second of 2 papers I chose on the importance of family history in the assessment and prediction of prognosis for patients harboring abdominal aortic aneurysms (AAAs). Generally, endovascular repair in patients with known genetic aortic aneurysm syndromes is not advised because these patients have a higher incidence of complications. At present, there is little known on the clinical outcomes after endovascular aneurysm repair (EVAR) for patients with an inherited risk for AAA.

TABLE 3.—Complications after Endovascular Aneurysm Repair (*EVAR*)

Variable[a]	Familial AAA (n = 51)	Sporadic AAA (n = 204)	*P* Value
Complications after EVAR, patients	18 (35.3)	39 (19.1)	.013
Endoleak during follow-up, events	8 (15.7)	18 (8.8)	.147
Type Ia	5	9	
Type Ib	3	6	
Type III	0	1	
Type undetermined	0	2	
Secondary intervention	20 (39.2)	41 (20.1)	.004
Proximal stent/cuff	4	10	
Limb extension	5	18	
Coil/glue embolization	2	2	
Open ligation of collaterals	3	4	
Conversion to AUI	1	0	
Conversion to open repair	2	5	
Relining	3	2	
Aneurysm sac growth[b]	10 (20.8)	18 (9.5)	.030
Acute limb ischemia	0	4	.313
Postimplantation aneurysm rupture	0	0	...

AAA, Abdominal aortic aneurysm; *AUI*, aorto-uni-iliac device; *CTA*, computed tomography angiography; DUS, duplex ultrasound.

[a]Categorical data are presented as number (%).

[b]Aneurysm sac measurements were available for 237 patients with ≥ two postoperative imaging examinations (ie, two CTA scans or two DUS examinations).

One may hypothesize that AAA patients with a positive family history may develop more seal and fixation problems, as well as also postprocedure sac growth because of inherited aortic wall defects. In this series of 51 patients with familial AAA compared with 204 patients with sporadic AAA, patients with familial AAA had a significantly higher secondary intervention rate after EVAR than the sporadic group (39.2% vs 20.1%; $P = .004$). Proximal stent/cuff, coil/glue embolization, open ligation of collaterals, and relining were more common in patients with familial AAA. Detailed data regarding elements of secondary intervention are presented in Table 3.

The main thrust of this study was that patients with familial AAA have a two-fold higher risk of developing aneurysm-related complications after EVAR than patients with sporadic AAA, despite similar AAA morphology (Fig 2). It may be hypothesized that an intrinsic weakness of the aortic wall results in more rapid progression of aneurysm disease and contributes to a higher need for secondary interventions in familial AAA patients. New prospective studies are needed for clarification of these findings and should help to determine which postoperative surveillance program best suits familial AAA patients.

B. W. Starnes, MD

A Pilot Study on Low-density Lipoprotein Receptor-related Protein-1 in Chinese Patients with Abdominal Aortic Aneurysm

Chan CYT, Chan YC, Cheuk BL, et al (Univ of Hong Kong Med Centre, Pokfulam)

Eur J Vasc Endovasc Surg 46:549-556, 2013

Objective.—There are no published data on the expression of low-density lipoprotein receptor-related protein 1 (LRP1) in human aortic tissues with abdominal aortic aneurysm (AAA), although some researchers have suggested that LRP1 may be a crucial regulator in the pathogenesis of AAA. The aim of this pilot study is to investigate LRP1 expression in aortic tissues from Chinese patients with AAA compared with normal control tissues.

Materials and Methods.—This study used human abdominal aortic tissues with or without AAA as a research model. Aneurysmal abdominal aortas were collected from Chinese patients with AAA ($n = 12$) during open surgical aneurysmal repair at our institution, and normal control non-aneurysmal abdominal aortas were collected from Chinese healthy organ donors ($n = 12$) during organ transplantation. Protein expression of LRP1 was analyzed by western blotting and immunohistochemistry.

Results.—LRP1 protein expression was significantly lower in AAA (mean $LRP1_{AAA}/LRP1_{Normal\ Control} = 0.51 \pm 0.28$) than in normal control aortic tissues (mean $LRP1_{Normal\ Control}/LRP1_{Normal\ Control} = 1 \pm 0.18$) in our small sample cohort ($p < .001$). No significant correlation was shown between LRP1 protein expression and the size of AAA ($p > .05$).

Conclusions.—Our pilot result suggests that a reduction in LRP1 protein expression may be associated with aneurysm progression.

▶ Abdominal aortic aneurysms (AAA) are characterized by extensive degeneration of the aortic extracellular matrix that leads to localized remodeling. Recent advances in vascular biology have led to the identification of some of the molecular pathways involved in AAA progression, with the hope of the development of a noninvasive therapeutic approach for the treatment of AAA. The use of genomics and proteomics has led to the identification of thousands of candidate genes and proteins that may be implicated in the pathogenesis of AAA formation. One such gene that has been identified as playing a potential role in the development of AAA is low-density lipoprotein receptor-related protein 1 (*LRP1*). Indeed emerging evidence has shown that mice with *LRP1* gene deletion in smooth muscle cells develop aneurysms with dilated aorta. In addition, the matrix metalloproteinase MMP-9, which degrades the extracellular matrix and is abundantly expressed in AAA tissues, is known to bind to *LRP1*. This study evaluated the expression of *LRP1* in human infrarenal aortic samples from patients with AAA compared with healthy control (organ donor) patients using Western blotting and immunohistochemistry. The results demonstrated that there was a 50% reduction in intracellular *LRP1* expression in samples from AAA patients, and this was further correlated by immunohistochemistry, where a decreased expression of LRP1 was shown in the adventitial and medial regions of the aortas from AAA patients. This may be of great importance as a potential target for the treatment of AAA; however, there are some limitations in this study that need to be addressed. In addition to the small sample number, $n = 12$, this study failed to determine colocalization of the *LRP1* gene in the immunohistochemistry experiments. *LRP1* is known to colocalize to smooth muscle cells, and because AAA progression is associated with a decrease in smooth muscle cell composition, it is possible that the reduction in expression of LRP1 observed in the current study may simply be a function of decreased smooth muscle cell content in the AAA samples.

J. Cullen, PhD

Morphologic and Biomechanical Changes of Thoracic and Abdominal Aorta in a Rat Model of Cigarette Smoke Exposure

Jaldin RG, Castardelli É, Perobelli JE, et al (São Paulo State Univ Med School, Botucatu, Brazil; Sagrado Coracao Univ, Bauru, Brazil; et al)
Ann Vasc Surg 27:791-800, 2013

Background.—Smoking is the most relevant environmental factor that affects the development of aortic aneurysm. Smokers have elevated levels of elastase activity in the arterial wall, which leads to weakening of the aorta. The aim of this study was to verify whether cigarette smoke exposure itself is capable of altering the aortic wall.

Methods.—Forty-eight Wistar rats were divided into 2-, 4-, and 6-month experimental periods and into 2 groups: smokers (submitted to smoke exposure at a rate of 40 cigarettes/day) and nonsmokers. At the end of the experimental periods, the aortas were removed and cross-sectioned to obtain histologic specimens for light microscopic and morphometric analyses. The remaining longitudinal segments were stretched to rupture and mechanical parameters were determined.

Results.—A degenerative process (i.e., a reduction in elastic fibers, the loss of lamellar arrangement, and a reduction of smooth muscle cells) was observed, and this effect was proportional in intensity to the period of tobacco exposure. We observed a progressive reduction in the yield point of the thoracic aorta over time ($P < 0.05$). There was a decrease in stiffness ($P < 0.05$) and in failure load ($P < 0.05$) at 6 months in the abdominal aorta of rats in the smoking group.

Conclusions.—Chronic exposure to tobacco smoke can affect the mechanical properties of the aorta and can also provoke substantial structural changes of the arterial wall.

▶ The causes of aortic aneurysms are multifactorial, and the end result is remodeling and weakness of the aortic wall. They are more common in men than in women, and the risk is heightened in men who smoke or used to smoke, with individuals aged 65 years and older at the greatest risk. Smoking appears to be the most common environmental factor in the development and progression of abdominal aortic aneurysm (AAA), and smokers have elevated enzyme activity in the aorta wall that may be the cause of accentuated degradation of elastic fibers and consequent weakening of the artery wall. The objective of the present study was to verify microscopic changes and the resistance of the aortic walls of rats after exposure to cigarette smoke. Their results indicate that exposure to tobacco smoke leads to deleterious effects on the aorta wall, affecting the elasticity and stiffness of the artery, and also leads to substantial structural alterations after chronic exposure; these effects were proportional in intensity to the period of tobacco exposure. Although many studies have demonstrated that tobacco smoke is associated with AAA development and progression, this is the first experimental model to show that the extent and progression of AAA development is proportional in intensity to the period of smoke exposure.

J. Cullen, PhD

Correlation of Bacterial Coinfection Versus Matrix Metalloproteinase 9 and Tissue Inhibitor of Metalloproteinase 1 Expression in Aortic Aneurysm and Atherosclerosis

Roggério A, Sambiase NV, Palomino SAP, et al (Univ of São Paulo, Brazil)
Ann Vasc Surg 27:964-971, 2013

Background.—We searched for any relationship between *Chlamydophila pneumoniae, Mycoplasma pneumoniae,* matrix metalloproteinase 9 (MMP-9), and tissue inhibitor of metalloproteinase 1 (TIMP-1) in aneurysmatic atherosclerotic lesions, and whether this relationship differed from that in atherosclerotic nonaneurysmatic lesions.

Methods.—Twenty-eight tissue samples paired by age and sex were grouped as follows: group 1 included 14 nonaneurysmal atherosclerotic fragments obtained from abdominal aortas collected from necropsies; group 2 included 14 aneurysmatic atherosclerotic aortic fragments obtained from patients during corrective surgery. Immunohistochemistry reactions were evaluated for *C pneumoniae, M pneumoniae*, MMP-9, and TIMP-1 antigens. Both groups were compared using the Mann–Whitney test, and the correlations among variables were obtained using the Spearman correlation test. $P \leq 0.05$ was considered statistically significant.

Results.—*C pneumoniae* and *M pneumoniae* antigens were detected in 100% of cases. A higher amount of *C pneumoniae* ($P = 0.005$), *M pneumoniae* ($P = 0.002$), and MMP-9 ($P = 0.021$) was found in adventitia of group 2 with aneurysm. A positive correlation was found in the aneurysm group, as follows: intima *C pneumoniae* versus adventitia thickness ($r = 0.70$; $P = 0.01$), media *C pneumoniae* versus adventitia *C pneumoniae* ($r = 0.75$; $P = 0.002$), intima *C pneumoniae* versus media *C pneumoniae* ($r = 0.8$; $P = 0.00$), and adventitia *C pneumoniae* versus intima *M pneumoniae* ($r = 0.54$; $P = 0.05$); negative correlations were as follows: adventitia thickness and adventitia *M pneumoniae* ($r = -0.65$; $P = 0.01$), media MMP-9 and media thickness ($r = -0.55$; $P = 0.04$), TIMP-1 media versus adventitia *C pneumoniae* ($r = -0.86$; $P = 0.00$), and TIMP-1 media versus *M pneumoniae* intima ($r = -0.67$; $P = 0.03$). Nonaneurysmal atherosclerotic group 1 results are as follows: adventitia *C pneumoniae* versus TIMP-1 media ($r = 0.75$; $P = 0.01$) and media *C pneumoniae* and adventitia *C pneumoniae* ($r = 0.59$; $P = 0.03$).

Conclusions.—The present work favors a role for coinfection of both *M pneumoniae* and *C pneumoniae* in the development of aortic atherosclerotic aneurysm, with increased adventitial inflammation, inhibition of TIMP-1 activity, and increased collagen degradation.

▶ Abdominal aortic aneurysms (AAA) are characterized by localized remodeling that includes the destruction of elastin and collagen combined with the inflammatory process. For many years, the development of this disease process was thought of as an "inside-out" response with the main focus on the adhesion of monocytes to the intima of the aorta. However, some studies now support a paradigm-shifting hypothesis that takes an "outside-in" approach in that the inflammatory response is initiated in the adventitia and progresses toward the intima. An association between *Chlamydophila pneumoniae* and atherosclerosis has long been described, and more recently studies have shown that viable forms of *C pneumoniae* are detectable in the AAA wall; however, antibiotic treatment has not had any effect on AAA expansion. Coinfection of *C pneumoniae* and *Mycoplasma pneumonia* has been demonstrated in ruptured atherosclerotic plaques where they are thought to cause adventitial inflammation and vessel dilation. This study examined whether coinfection by *C pneumoniae* and *M pneumonia* is present in adventitial inflammation and whether it is associated with altered matrix metalloproteinase (MMP) expression in the development of AAA compared with nonaneurysmal atherosclerosis. The authors compared nonaneurysmal aortic atherosclerotic fragments, taken at necropsies, to aortic aneurysm fusiform fragments, taken from patients undergoing surgery. Interestingly, *C pneumoniae* and *M pneumoniae* antigens were detected in 100% of the cases studied; however, significantly higher amounts were found in the adventitia of aneurysm samples in addition to the presence of profound inflammatory infiltrate and MMP-9. These findings of exacerbated inflammation and proteolytic enzymes in the adventitia, colocalized with *C pneumoniae* and *M pneumoniae* coinfection, support the "outside-in" theory of vascular inflammation and highlight the important role that coinfection may play in AAA development. This may be of significant importance in the development of novel therapeutic agents to treat AAA; not only may such agents take a novel perivascular approach to treatment, they may also target various infectious pathogens such as *C pneumoniae* and *M pneumoniae*.

J. Cullen, PhD

Exploration of the mechanisms by which 3,4-benzopyrene promotes angiotensin II-induced abdominal aortic aneurysm formation in mice

Ji K, Zhang Y, Jiang F, et al (The Second Hosp Affiliated to Wenzhou Med College, China; et al)

J Vasc Surg 59:492-499, 2014

Objective.—This study examined the influence of 3,4-benzopyrene (BaP), a compound found in cigarette smoke, on the formation of angiotensin II (Ang II)-induced abdominal aortic aneurysm (AAA) formation in mice and the underlying mechanisms.

Methods.—C57/B6n mice were divided into four groups. The control group received a weekly intraperitoneal injection of medium-chain triglycerides. The Ang II group received a daily Ang II infusion (0.72 mg/kg) and a weekly intraperitoneal injection of medium-chain triglycerides. The Ang II/BaP group received a daily Ang II infusion (0.72 mg/kg) and a weekly intraperitoneal BaP injection (10 mg/kg, dissolved in medium-chain triglycerides). The BaP group received a weekly intraperitoneal BaP injection (10 mg/kg). After 5 weeks, abdominal aortic diameter was determined. Aortic tissues underwent hematoxylin and eosin, Masson, and immunochemistry staining for evaluation of vascular wall structure, collagen, macrophage infiltration, matrix metalloproteinases (MMPs), and apoptosis.

Results.—The Ang II infusion and BaP injection induced AAAs in 41.67% of mice vs 25% in the Ang II group ($P < .05$). The average aortic diameter increased in the Ang II/BaP group compared with the Ang II group (1.40 ± 0.25 vs 1.2 ± 0.23 mm; $P < .05$). Average aortic muscular cell apoptosis was higher in the Ang II/BaP group ($31\% \pm 12\%$) than in the Ang II ($19\% \pm 5\%$; $P < .05$) or BaP groups ($23\% \pm 4\%$; $P < .05$). Aortic macrophage infiltration and expression of MMP-2, MMP-9, MMP-12, and nuclear factor-κB increased (0.56 ± 0.12, 0.47 ± 0.13, 0.49 ± 0.14, 0.49 ± 0.11, and 0.42 ± 0.12, respectively) in the Ang II/BaP group compared with the Ang II group (0.27 ± 0.08, 0.25 ± 0.06, 0.24 ± 0.09, 0.24 ± 0.09, and 0.23 ± 0.06, respectively; $P < .05$ for all).

Conclusions.—BaP promotes Ang II-induced AAA formation in mice via elevating infiltration of macrophages, activating nuclear factor-κB, upregulating the expression of MMP-2, MMP-9, and MMP-12, and increasing the apoptosis of vascular muscle cells in its synergistic effect with Ang II in aortic wall.

▶ Abdominal aortic aneurysms (AAAs) are a common but potentially fatal condition with multiple associated risk factors, including male sex, older age, smoking, family history, and atherosclerosis. The risk of developing an AAA is 8 times greater in smokers than in nonsmokers, and the risk decreases when the individual quits smoking. Indeed the US Preventive Services Task Force recommends that men aged 65 to 75 years who have ever smoked should get an ultrasound screening for abdominal aortic aneurysms, even if they have no symptoms.

3,4-benzopyrene (BaP) is one of the key components in cigarette smoke that is thought to contribute to AAA formation. This study examined the influence of BaP on the formation of angiotensin II (Ang II)-induced AAA formation in mice and the underlying mechanisms. Their results demonstrated that BaP promotes Ang II-induced AAA formation in mice via elevating infiltration of macrophages; activating nuclear factor-kB; upregulating the expression of MMP-2, MMP-9, and MMP-12; and increasing the apoptosis of vascular muscle cells in its synergistic effect with Ang II in the aortic wall. The fact that the presence of BaP increased the number of AAA-positive mice from 25% in the Ang II alone group to 42% in the Ang II + BaP group provides further evidence that tobacco smoke is a risk factor for AAA and also that it may play an important role because it increased the AAA rate by 70%. Because current therapy for AAA is limited to open surgical or endovascular repair, it is crucial that the mechanisms mediating the formation and progression of AAA are identified. The development of animal models of AAA has helped us to study the pathophysiology of the disease process and identify new therapeutic targets. Although no one model perfectly recapitulates the human disease process, this current animal model is a great starting point, and to further validate the role of BaP as a risk factor for aortic aneurysms, these experiments should be repeated in other animal models of AAA.

J. Cullen, PhD

7 Abdominal Aortic Endografting

Endovascular repair of bilateral common iliac artery aneurysms following open abdominal aortic aneurysm repair with preservation of both hypogastric arteries using commercially available stent grafts

Cuff R, Banegas S, Mansour A, et al (Spectrum Health Med Group, Grand Rapids, MI)

J Vasc Surg 59:516-519, 2014

Endovascular treatment of aneurysmal disease has become the predominant form of repair for all aneurysms. Some areas continue to pose specific challenges to stay within the general tenets of successful repair, mainly achieving adequate seal without sacrificing other arterial pathways. Following aortic aneurysm repair, the common iliac arteries can continue to have aneurysmal degeneration. We present a case of bilateral common iliac artery aneurysms that presented 9 years after open repair of

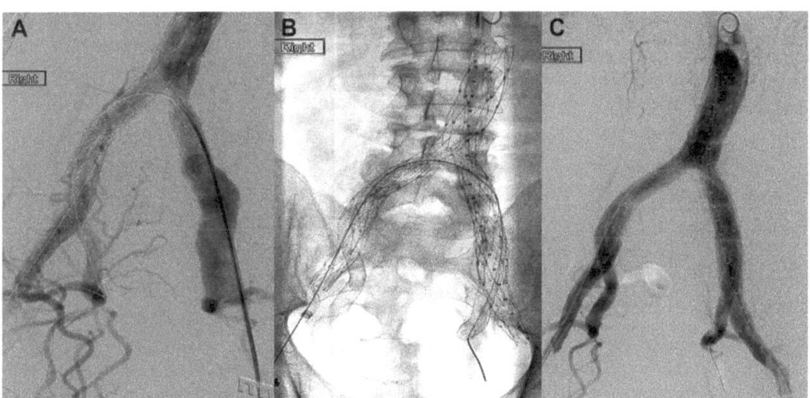

FIGURE 2.—**A**, Intraoperative angiogram following successful stent placement in the right hypogastric and external iliac arteries. **B**, Noncontrasted image following placement of bilateral internal and external iliac stent grafts. **C**, Completion angiogram demonstrating intact pelvic flow with patent stents and no endoleak. (Reprinted from Cuff R, Banegas S, Mansour A, et al. Endovascular repair of bilateral common iliac artery aneurysms following open abdominal aortic aneurysm repair with preservation of both hypogastric arteries using commercially available stent grafts. *J Vasc Surg*. 2014;59:516-519, Copyright 2014, with permission from The Society for Vascular Surgery.)

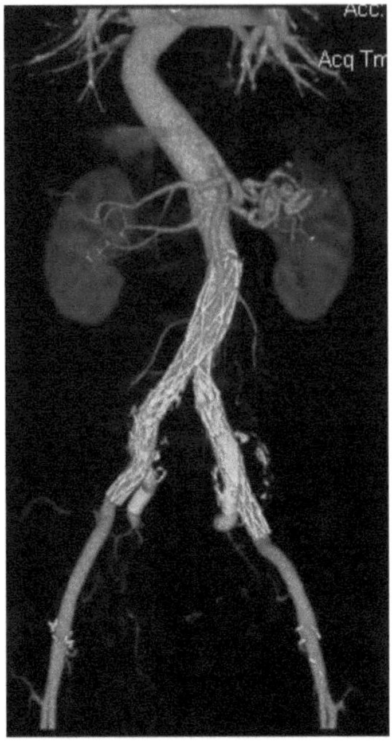

FIGURE 3.—Reconstructed image at 1-month follow-up, once again demonstrating all stents patent with no endoleak and pelvic flow. (Reprinted from Cuff R, Banegas S, Mansour A, et al. Endovascular repair of bilateral common iliac artery aneurysms following open abdominal aortic aneurysm repair with preservation of both hypogastric arteries using commercially available stent grafts. *J Vasc Surg.* 2014;59:516-519, Copyright 2014, with permission from The Society for Vascular Surgery.)

an infrarenal abdominal aortic aneurysm in conjunction with an extensive aortic dissection. These were repaired using endovascular techniques with preservation of both hypogastric arteries (Figs 2 and 3).

▶ I chose this article to comment briefly on because I feel it brings to the modestly skilled vascular surgeon a useful technique for everyday practice and emphasizes the concept of parallel endografts, including the benefits and troubles of using the Powerlink AFX device (Endologix; Irvine, CA) with Viabahn stent grafts (W.L. Gore; Flagstaff, AZ) to treat patients in need of bilateral hypogastric artery preservation (Figs 2 and 3). The unique design of the Powerlink device allows crossing of the aortic bifurcation *after* deployment of the bifurcated device, thus allowing cannulation of the hypogastric artery from the contralateral side and simultaneous deployment of a parallel graft from the ipsilateral side to successfully exclude the aneurysm.

B. W. Starnes, MD

Editor's Choice–A Shaggy Aorta is Associated with Mesenteric Embolisation in Patients Undergoing Fenestrated Endografts to Treat Paravisceral Aortic Aneurysms

Patel SD, Constantinou J, Hamilton H, et al (Royal Free Hosp NHS Foundation Trust, London, UK)

Eur J Vasc Endovasc Surg 47:374-379, 2014

Objectives.—Bowel ischaemia is a life-threatening complication of endovascular aneurysm repair. This study aims to evaluate the factors associated with mesenteric ischaemia in patients undergoing fenestrated aortic endografts to treat paravisceral aneurysms.

Methods.—Consecutive patients undergoing double or triple fenestrated stent graft insertion were retrospectively analysed. No patients were declined surgery based on anatomic complexity. Preoperative demographics, procedure-related variables, and anatomical factors were examined. Using 3D software, the aortic thrombus volume from the coeliac axis to the lowest renal, aortoiliac tortuosity, and aortic irregularity index (as graded by 3 independent assessors, graded 0–3 based on severity) were compared. Univariate analysis was performed to identify risk factors for the development of bowel ischaemia.

Results.—Ninety-nine patients underwent elective aneurysm repair (64 triple fenestrations and 35 double fenestrations), 5% of which developed bowel ischaemia, and of these 80% (4/5) died. Mesenteric ischaemia was significantly associated with increased aortic irregularity (median [range], 2 [1–3] vs. 1 [0–2], $p = .005$, ischaemia vs. no ischaemia) and increased thrombus volume (37 ± 8 vs. 21 ± 12, $p = .007$) but not aortoiliac tortuosity (1.4 [1.2–1.5] vs. 1.30 [1.2–1.7], $p = .3$), inferior mesenteric or internal iliac artery patency. Mesenteric ischaemia was also associated with a significantly higher preoperative creatinine (mean ± SD: 183 ± 74 vs. 111 ± 43, $p = .007$).

Conclusions.—The presence of aortic irregularity and increased thrombus volume in the paravisceral segment predicts the occurrence of mesenteric and renal ischaemia in patients treated with fenestrated endografts. This is likely to be related to graft manipulation and catheterisation of visceral vessels (Fig 1).

▶ The risk of mesenteric ischemia after fenestrated endovascular aneurysm repair (FEVAR) appears to be quite low on the basis of published data. This is a cautionary tale from London showing that aortic morphology may also prove to be a powerful determinant of this complication, and its incidence is higher in patients with atheromatous-laden aortic lumens.

In this series of 99 patients, those who developed mesenteric ischemia had a significantly higher thrombus volume in the paravisceral segment and higher irregularity scores. An example of the grading system that these authors came up with is depicted in Fig 1. I wish the grading scheme were more precise. The authors did have the computed tomography scans reviewed by 3 independent

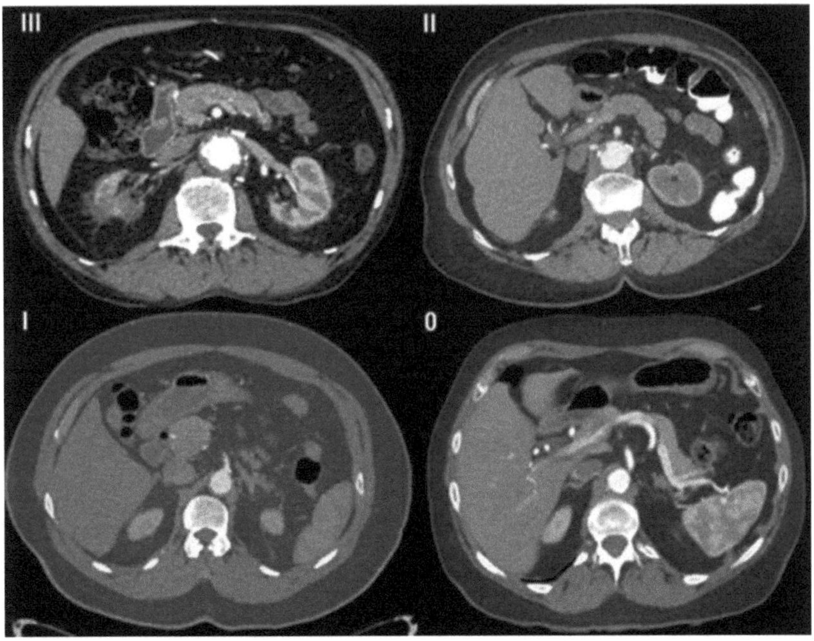

FIGURE 1.—Aortic irregularity (shaggy index). Grade III = most severe, very extensive atheromatous disease with diffuse ulcers associated with soft, loosely held debris, Grade 0 = clean non-atheromatous. (Reprinted from Patel SD, Constantinou J, Hamilton H, et al. Editor's choice – A shaggy aorta is associated with mesenteric embolisation in patients undergoing fenestrated endografts to treat paravisceral aortic aneurysms. *Eur J Vasc Endovasc Surg*. 2014;47:374-379, Copyright 2014, with permission from the European Society for Vascular Surgery.)

observers and did successfully rate interobserver error, but I don't feel this is reproducible.

That endovascular repair would lead to embolic complications seems logical given that the procedure involves the manipulation of many guidewires, sheaths, and stents inside an atherosclerotic aorta lined with thrombus. However, the rate of mesenteric ischemia after FEVAR has not been reported widely. This report of a rate of 5% should cause some concern, especially given that the overwhelming majority of patients (80%) who experience mesenteric ischemia after FEVAR die.

B. W. Starnes, MD

Inter-observer Variability in Sizing Fenestrated and/or Branched Aortic Stent-Grafts

Banno H, Kobeiter H, Brossier J, et al (Univ Paris XII, Creteil, France; et al)
Eur J Vasc Endovasc Surg 47:45-52, 2014

Background.—Several studies have examined inter-observer variability in measurements for standard EVAR, but little is known about measurements for complex aortic aneurysm.

Methods.—Two independent observers reviewed all preoperative CT scans of 268 patients in a French trial of fenestrated and/or branched aortic stent-grafts (f/b-EVAR). Those data were compared with those obtained (1) by investigators (extent of aneurysm, target vessel stenosis, and aortic diameters), and (2) from manufacturers (proximal landing zone, device diameter, and target vessel position). We assessed the reproducibility using kappa statistics for qualitative data and both Bland–Altman plot and Passing–Bablok regression analysis for quantitative data.

Results.—Reproducibility was moderate to almost perfect for all factors. However, a few critical discrepancies were found, such as target vessel clock position (≥45 minutes) and location (≥5 mm), level of proximal landing zone, and diameters of the endograft.

Conclusions.—This is the first large-scale analysis focused on inter-observer variability in sizing for f/b-EVAR. The measurement data showed

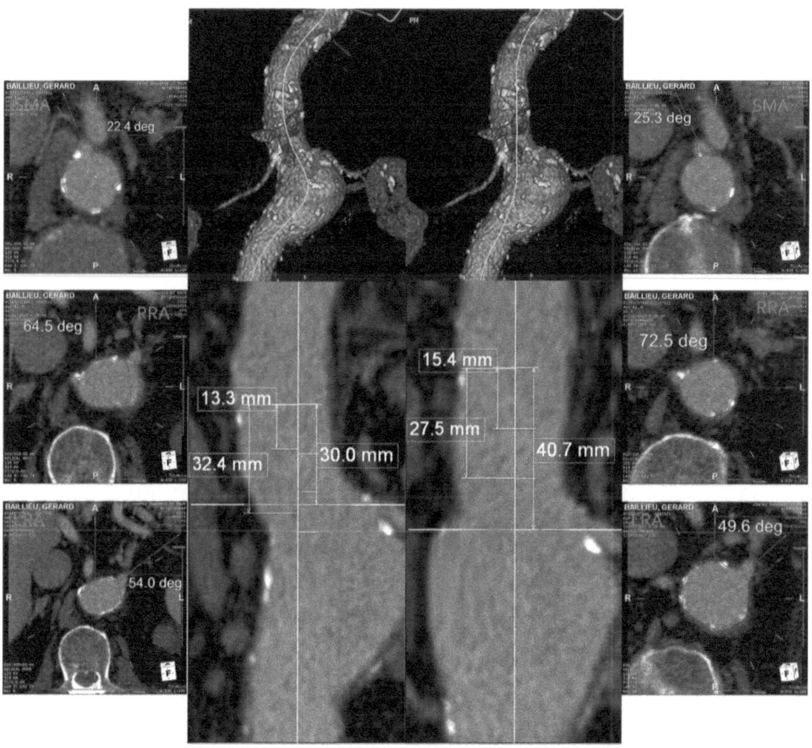

FIGURE 5.—Comparison of target vessel measurement using the centerline drawn automatically by 3D workstation (left) and the manually modified centerline (right). In this case, discrepancies of target vessel orientations were little, but there were 5 mm difference in the RRA distance and 11 mm difference in the LRA distance between the two. (Reprinted from Banno H, Kobeiter H, Brossier J, et al. Inter-observer variability in sizing fenestrated and/or branched aortic stent-grafts. *Eur J Vasc Endovasc Surg.* 2014;47:45-52, Copyright 2014, with permission from European Society for Vascular Surgery.)

good agreement, but there were some critical discrepancies between observers that may affect clinical results (Fig 5).

▶ Custom-made fenestrated devices require accurate preoperative sizing of stent grafts for technical success. The planning is critical and requires judgment and care of the operator. The possibility for significant interrater variability is not well described. This study investigated the variability between experienced endovascular surgeons' and investigator or manufacturer measuring and sizing for endovascular aneurysm repair using fenestrated and/or branched stent grafts. Both observers were well-trained and experienced vascular surgeons.

The concerning thing about this study is that there were some cases with critical discrepancies. The threshold tolerances were high at a minimum of 45 minutes on clock face and 5 mm on vessel distance from fabric edge. Some renal vessels are 5 mm in diameter, and so a whole vessel orifice distance miscalculation and the procedure will not only be difficult, it will take longer. Longer durations of intervention have been conclusively associated with higher in-hospital and 30-day mortality. Until we have better devices that are more applicable to the vast majority of patients, planning will be what separates the men from the boys.

B. W. Starnes, MD

Displacement Forces in Iliac Landing Zones and Stent Graft Interconnections in Endovascular Aortic Repair: An Experimental Study

Roos H, Ghaffari M, Falkenberg M, et al (Sahlgrenska Univ Hosp, Gothenburg, Sweden; et al)

Eur J Vasc Endovasc Surg 47:262-267, 2014

Objectives.—Stent graft migration influences the long-term durability of endovascular aortic repair. Flow-induced displacement forces acting on the attachment zones may contribute to migration. Proximal fixation of aortic stent grafts has been improved by using hooks, while distal fixation and stent graft interconnections depend on self-expansion forces only. We hypothesized that flow-induced displacement forces would be significant at the distal end, and would correlate with graft movements

Methods.—As part of an experimental study, an iliac limb stent graft was inserted in a pulsatile flow model similar to aortic in vivo conditions, and fixed—mounted at its proximal and distal ends to strain gauge load cells. Peak displacement forces at both ends and pulsatile graft movement were recorded at different graft angulations (0—90°), perfusion pressures (145/80, 170/90, or 195/100 mmHg), and stroke frequencies (60—100 b.p.m.).

Results.—Flow-induced forces were of the same magnitude at the proximal and distal end of the stent graft (peak 1.8 N). Both the forces and graft movement increased with angulation and perfusion pressure, but not with stroke rate. Graft movement reached a maximum of 0.29 ± 0.01 mm per

TABLE 2.—Sideways Movement of the Stent Graft (mm) at Different Perfusion Pressures and Stent Graft Angles. Stroke Rate 80. Mean ± Standard DEVIATION

	0°	45°	90°
145/80	0.07 ± 0.01	0.13 ± 0.003	0.22 ± 0.01
170/90	0.08 ± 0.01	0.19 ± 0.01	0.28 ± 0.01
195/100	0.10 ± 0.01	0.20 ± 0.01	0.29 ± 0.01

stroke despite fixed ends. There were strong correlations between proximal and distal displacement forces ($r = 0.97$, $p < .001$), and between displacement forces and graft movement ($r = 0.98$, $p < .001$).

Conclusions.—Pulsatile flow through a tubular untapered stent graft causes forces of similar magnitude at both ends and induces pulsatile graft movements in its unsupported mid-section. Peak forces are close to those previously reported to be required to extract a stent graft. The forces and movements increase with increasing graft angulation and perfusion pressure. Improved anchoring of the distal end of stent grafts may be considered (Table 2).

▶ The main findings of this experimental study were that flow-induced displacement forces are of the same magnitude at the proximal and distal end of a stent graft and that forces increase with graft angulation and perfusion pressure, but not with stroke rate. Pulsatile graft movements are also dependent on pressure and angulation and show a linear correlation with displacement forces. Computational studies have estimated the magnitude of migration forces on stent grafts, but none of the previous studies have directly measured flow-induced displacement forces acting on an endovascular stent graft and their relation to graft configuration and the movements of the graft (Table 2).

The ultimate conclusion of this study is that we have drastically underestimated the true extent of flow-induced forces acting on a stent graft. The forces are ultimately dependent on the perfusion pressure and the angulation between the proximal and distal landing zones. This information may aid in improvements in device design to mitigate the risk of graft migration and subsequent production of endoleak.

B. W. Starnes, MD

Endovascular management of pararenal aortic aneurysms with multiple overlapping uncovered stents

Zhang Y-X, Lu Q-S, Feng J-X, et al (Changhai Hosp, Shanghai, China)

J Vasc Surg 58:616-623, 2013

Objective.—This study aims at evaluating the safety and efficacy of a porous stent system consisting of multiple overlapping uncovered stents in the treatment of complex aortic aneurysms with vital branches.

Methods.—Data of all patients with aortic aneurysms treated in our center with multiple overlapping uncovered stents between February 2010 and December 2011 were retrospectively reviewed. Preoperative characteristics, intraoperative details, and follow-up outcomes were documented. Technical success was defined as successful deployment of the stents to target locations without procedure-related complications. Clinical success was characterized by complete shrinkage or stabilization of the aneurysm, preservation of vital branches, and absence of major complications. Patients were grouped, according to rapidity of aneurysm thrombosis, into fast-thrombosis group (complete thrombosis of aneurysmal sac was achieved in ≤6 months) and a delayed-thrombosis group (>6 months required for complete thrombosis). Possible factors affecting the speed of thrombosis were analyzed statistically with the Fisher exact test and the *t*-test.

Results.—This porous stent system was used to treat 34 patients (23 men, 11 women; mean age, 65.7 years). Technical success was achieved in all patients (100%). Regular follow-up over 6 months was achieved in 29 patients (mean length of follow-up, 11.4 months). Complete thrombosis of the aneurysm sac within 12 months was observed in 24 patients (83%). Aneurysm shrinkage was documented in seven patients (24%) and stabilization in 21 (72%). All branch arteries covered by bare stents stayed patent during follow-up. The overall clinical success rate reached 97% in the follow-up group. Risk factors for delayed thrombosis included fewer stents implanted ($P = .013$), longer sac entrance ($P = .043$), and use of antiplatelet medication ($P = .040$).

Conclusions.—An alternative method of management of complicated aortic aneurysm appears to be feasible using overlapping bare stents, which may prevent aneurysm growth while preserving vital branches. The short-term outcome of our study seems encouraging but is not sufficient to draw a robust conclusion. Further hemodynamic and clinical studies are warranted to evaluate long-term efficacy (Fig 4, Table 3).

▶ The concept of a porous stent system had been originally put forward for endovascular treatment of intracranial aneurysms. Over time, it has been gradually introduced into treatment of aneurysms at different locations and tested successfully in many patients with a satisfactory outcome for thrombosis. I still don't understand how this can be a valid or durable treatment for large--vessel aneurysmal disease, but the body of literature supporting this concept is difficult to ignore.

These authors report flow diversion and treatment of aortic disease with multiple overlapping uncovered stents. The porous system was used to treat 34 patients. However, only 8 patients had degenerative aneurysms. Most were pseudoaneurysms or dissections. More than 30% of patients had residual flow at 6-month follow-up. Risk factors for prolonged thrombosis are presented in Table 3. Fig 4 shows a patient with an unsuccessful outcome, which should cause concern to anyone reading this.

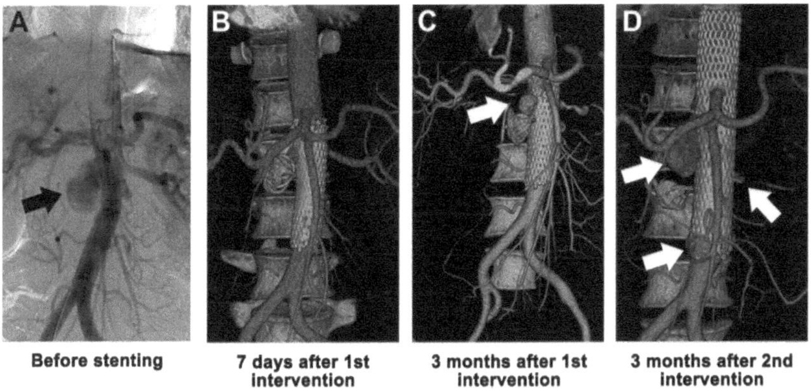

FIGURE 4.—A patient with a new aneurysm within the stented zone. **A**, Presenting angiography revealed a saccular aortic aneurysm in the renovisceral segment (*black arrow*). **B**, The aneurysm was treated with the combined use of multiple bare stents and coiling, and computed tomography angiography (CTA) before discharge revealed satisfactory exclusion. **C**, At the 3-month follow-up, a new aneurysm was detected above the original one (*white arrow*); thus, a reintervention was performed, adding two more stents to cover the new aneurysm. **D**, However, the CTA 3 months later revealed more aneurysms (*white arrows*). (Reprinted from Zhang Y-X, Lu Q-S, Feng J-X, et al. Endovascular management of pararenal aortic aneurysms with multiple overlapping uncovered stents. *J Vasc Surg*. 2013;58:616-623, with permission from The Society for Vascular Surgery.)

TABLE 3.—Risk Factors for a Prolonged Thrombosis Process

Variable[a]	Fast Thrombosis (n = 20)	Delayed Thrombosis (n = 8)	*P*
Aneurysm diameter	57.20 ± 4.81	54.85 ± 5.76	.279
Proximal aortic neck	20.65 ± 2.83	22.25 ± 2.12	.162
Sac entrance	14.95 ± 12.57	27.50 ± 17.94	.045
Stents number	3.25 ± 0.44	2.75 ± 0.46	.013
APTT	35.97 ± 2.09	36.96 ± 2.43	.286
Platelet count	208.30 ± 30.66	189.13 ± 33.93	.159
Antiplatelet therapy[b]	4 (20)	5 (62.5)	.044

APTT, Activated partial thromboplastin time.
[a]Continuous data are presented as mean 6 standard deviation and categoric data (antiplatelet therapy) as number (%).
[b]Including acetylsalicylic acid or clopidogrel, or both.

I recently had a call from my friend Marcelo Ferreira in Rio de Janeiro, Brazil who had a patient with an aortic aneurysm whom he had treated 1 year previously with a multilayer uncovered stent approach. On 1-year follow-up, the aneurysm had grown by 1.5 cm. His question was "now what?!" My question exactly!

B. W. Starnes, MD

A new staged hybrid total arch repair procedure using a branched proximal elephant trunk technique with implantation of stent grafts to the ascending aorta

Watanabe Y, Shimamura K, Shirakawa Y, et al (Osaka Univ Graduate School of Medicine, Japan)

J Vasc Surg 58:1700-1704, 2013

We report a new hybrid aortic arch repair procedure for the treatment of extensive thoracic aortic aneurysms involving the ascending aorta, arch, and descending aorta. In the first stage of this procedure, a "double-barrel tube graft" was inserted into the ascending aorta and fixed to the sinotubular junction under short-duration cardiopulmonary bypass in normothermia. In the next stage, after debranching of the left common carotid artery and left subclavian artery, stent grafts were deployed from the double-barrel tube graft to the descending aorta and the brachiocephalic artery to exclude the aneurysms. The patient's postoperative course was uneventful, with no endoleaks. The successful initial result suggests that this procedure could be an attractive treatment option for extensive aortic aneurysms (Figs 2 and 3).

► This technique is an attractive hybrid treatment option for extensive aortic aneurysms that include the ascending aorta (Fig 3). The most interesting part of the operation is reprinted in Fig 2.

Through a median sternotomy, the brachiocephalic artery and the ascending aorta were exposed. Cardiopulmonary bypass (CPB) was established with right axillary perfusion under normothermia. After the ascending aorta was cross-clamped just proximal to the brachiocephalic artery, the ascending aorta was

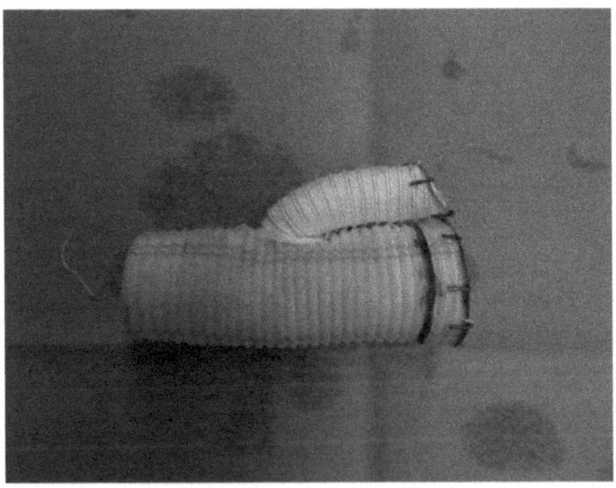

FIGURE 2.—A double-barrel tube graft was made of two graft components: a ringed Gore-Tex 12-mm graft (W. L. Gore & Associates) was used for the branch graft and a 28-mm Triplex graft (Vascutek Terumo) made of Dacron (DuPont) was used for the main graft. Radiopaque markers were placed at the distal rim of each graft and at the bifurcation. (Reprinted from Watanabe Y, Shimamura K, Shirakawa Y, et al. A new staged hybrid total arch repair procedure using a branched proximal elephant trunk technique with implantation of stent grafts to the ascending aorta. *J Vasc Surg*. 2013;58:1700-1704, Copyright 2013, with permission from The Society for Vascular Surgery.)

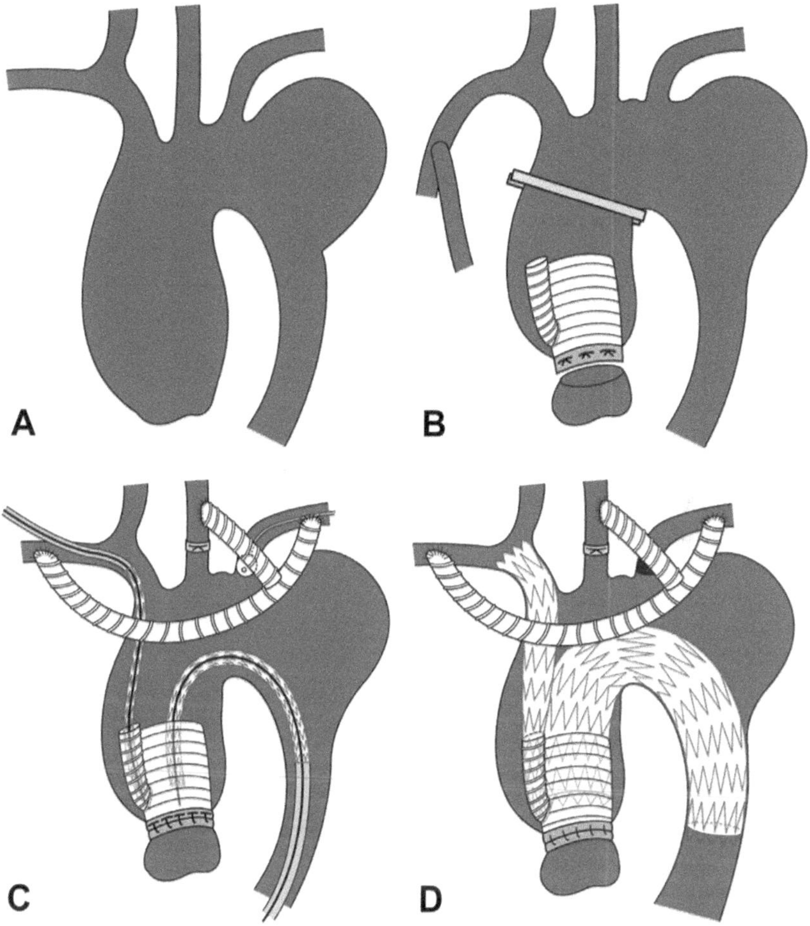

FIGURE 3.—Diagrams show the procedure. A, An aortic aneurysm extends from the ascending aorta to the descending aorta. B, The double-barreled tube graft is inserted into the ascending aorta. C, The right subclavian artery is connected to the left common carotid artery and the left subclavian artery with a ringed Gore-Tex 8-mm bifurcated graft (W. L. Gore & Associates). D, Stent grafting from the double-barreled tube graft to the descending aorta and brachiocephalic artery. (Reprinted from Watanabe Y, Shimamura K, Shirakawa Y, et al. A new staged hybrid total arch repair procedure using a branched proximal elephant trunk technique with implantation of stent grafts to the ascending aorta. *J Vasc Surg*. 2013;58:1700-1704, Copyright 2013, with permission from The Society for Vascular Surgery.)

transected just distal to the sinotubular junction. The double-barrel graft (DBG) was inserted into the ascending aorta, oriented with the branch graft directed toward the brachiocephalic artery. The proximal end of the DBG was sutured to the distal end of the transected aorta around the whole circumference, with a felt strip outer surface for reinforcement. Subsequently, this distal stump and proximal end of the transected aorta were resutured around the entire circumference. The aorta was declamped after the air and debris had been eliminated. The CPB time was 65 minutes, and cross-clamp time was

36 minutes. After hemostasis and sternal closure had been achieved, the patient was admitted to the intensive care unit.

This technique, like many others, uses the strategy of creating a landing zone for endovascular grafts. I only have one criticism of the technique. Would it not have been a simpler debranching option to perform a retropharyngeal right common carotid to left subclavian artery bypass with reimplantation of the left common carotid onto the traversing bypass graft? Food for thought!

B. W. Starnes, MD

Ambulatory percutaneous endovascular abdominal aortic aneurysm repair

Dosluoglu HH, Lall P, Blochle R, et al (Veterans Affairs Western New York Healthcare System, Buffaloa; State Univ of New York at Buffalo)
J Vasc Surg 59:58-64, 2014

Objective.—Percutaneous endovascular abdominal aortic aneurysm repair (PEVAR) has been associated with fewer groin wound complications and shorter operative times, but same-day discharge (SDD) has not been reported. The goal of our article is to assess the feasibility and safety of ambulatory PEVAR and identify patient characteristics that are eligible for this approach.

Methods.—Consecutive patients who underwent elective endovascular abdominal aortic aneurysm repair (EVAR) between March 2011 and December 2012 were reviewed. SDD was discussed during the preoperative visit with patients who were functionally independent, without significant comorbidities, and had favorable anatomy. These patients were given the option to be discharged in the evening of the PEVAR after 6 hours of bed rest if the procedure was uneventful. Causes for discharge delay and early outcomes were analyzed.

Results.—During the study period, 79 patients underwent abdominal aortic aneurysm (AAA) repair, 64 of whom (mean age, 70.2 ± 9.9; range, 59-97) had elective EVAR (3 ruptures, 5 acute presentations, 3 fenestrated EVARs, 4 elective open AAA repairs were excluded). Fifty-three patients (83%) had bilateral percutaneous access, seven had unilateral percutaneous (11%) access, and the remaining four (6%) had bilateral femoral endarterectomies. The percutaneous closure success rate was 96% in 113 attempts (three conversions for inadequate hemostasis, one for inability to deploy device). Mean length of stay was 1.3 ± 1.4 days (median, 1 day) with no 30-day mortality. Twenty-one patients (33%) were discharged the same day (SDD group), 24 (37%) on postoperative day (POD) 1, 16 (25%) on POD 2/3, and 3 (5%) stayed ≥4 days. One patient in the SDD group was readmitted on POD 3 after EVAR for severe postimplantation syndrome. Of the 23 patients who were discharged on POD 1, 10 were kept overnight due to severe chronic obstructive pulmonary disease, coronary artery disease, or advanced age, three transportation issues, two inability to void, two patient preference, two for renal protection, and four due to unplanned femoral cutdown. Patients in the SDD group were significantly younger (66.5 ± 5.4 years vs 72.0 ± 10.6 years; $P = .029$), had smaller AAAs (5.3 ± 0.5 cm vs 5.9 ± 1.0 cm; $P = .013$), less blood loss (115 ± 90 mL vs 232 ± 198 mL; $P = .012$), and shorter operating time (79 ± 24 minutes vs 121 ± 73 minutes; $P = .013$). There were fewer American Society of Anesthesiologists 4 patients in the SDD group (24% vs 48%; $P = .056$). The majority (81%) of patients in all groups had general anesthesia (86% vs 79% SDD vs others; $P = .523$).

Conclusions.—Ambulatory PEVAR was found to be feasible and safe in one-third of patients undergoing elective EVAR who did not have excessive medical risk, had good functional capacity, and underwent an uneventful procedure. The impact of SDD on cost-effectiveness needs to be further assessed and may not be feasible in hospitals reimbursed based on admission status.

▶ I have long been a champion for totally percutaneous aneurysm repair (PEVAR).[1] PEVAR is becoming increasingly popular and somewhat the standard of care in some institutions. What is not known is the safety of same-day discharge (SDD) after PEVAR. Dr Dosluoglu and colleagues provide us with an important contribution. Upon review of their EVAR series in a Veterans Affairs setting, they learned that one-third of their patients were eligible for SDD after PEVAR. The authors offered SDD to patients with the following characteristics:

1 Favorable anatomy
2 Good renal function with no plans for hydration postoperatively
3 Not medically high risk (absence of congestive heart failure, chronic obstructive pulmonary disease, age > 80)
4 Good functional capacity
5 Lived independently
6 Have someone to take care of them the night of surgery

Eighty-one percent of the procedures were performed under general anesthesia, and only one patient of 23 in the SDD group required re-admission on postoperative day 3 for postimplantation syndrome. Interestingly, in this series, nearly 20% of patients reported postoperative symptoms consistent with postimplantation syndrome, with the incidence being higher with Dacron-based implants versus polytetrafluoroethylene.

Unfortunately, this strategy—although better for patients and associated with less cost—is not applicable in the private sector and may actually be associated with a financial loss to most institutions. Until Centers for Medicare and Medicaid Services allow coding for these devices in an outpatient setting, ambulatory PEVAR will not be feasible, as hospitals won't be reimbursed for outpatient devices.

B. W. Starnes, MD

Reference

1. Starnes BW, Andersen CA, Ronsivalle JA, Stockmaster NR, Mullenix PS, Statler JD. Totally percutaneous aortic aneurysm repair: experience and prudence. *J Vasc Surg*. 2006;43:270-276.

A case-control study of intentional occlusion of accessory renal arteries during endovascular aortic aneurysm repair

Malgor RD, Oderich GS, Vrtiska TJ, et al (Mayo Clinic, Rochester, MN)

J Vasc Surg 58:1467-1475, 2013

Objective.—The purpose of this study was to evaluate outcomes of patients treated by intentional coverage of accessory renal artery (ARA) during endovascular abdominal aneurysm repair (EVAR).

Methods.—The clinical data of 119 patients (110 male and nine female; mean age, 75 years) from a cohort of 811 patients treated by EVAR from 1998 to 2009 was reviewed. Patients who had intentional coverage of at least one ARA (group A) were compared with two control groups, which included patients with no ARA (group B) and those who had ARA preserved during EVAR (group C). All three groups of patients were matched for age, gender, hypertension, and preoperative estimated glomerular filtration rate (eGFR). Paired pre- and postoperative computed tomography angiography was analyzed for the presence and volume of kidney infarction. End points were changes in eGFR, chronic kidney disease (CKD) stage, blood pressure measurements, presence and volume of kidney infarction, freedom from reintervention, and endoleak.

Results.—There were 42 patients in group A, 42 in group B, and 35 in group C. Demographics, cardiovascular risk factors, and CKD classification were similar in all three groups. Among patients in group A, 44 ARAs were intentionally covered with ARAs originating from the proximal neck in 22 patients, the aneurysm sac in 20, and the iliac arteries in two. There was one (1%) early death in the entire study. Early morbidity was similar in all three groups, including four patients (9%) in group A, four (9%) in group B, and four (11%) in group C ($P = .9$). Six (5%) patients had >25% decrease in eGFR, including two who had ARA coverage. None of the patients required dialysis. After a mean follow-up of 37 months, there were no differences in late renal function deterioration, changes in eGFR, CKD stage, or blood pressure measurements among the three groups. Three of the 18 patients (17%) with ARA >3 mm arising from the aneurysm sac developed a type II endoleak requiring coil embolization. Kidney infarction was noted in 28 patients (67%) in group A. Freedom from reintervention at 2 years was similar in groups A (64%), B (80%), and C (96%; $P = .09$).

Conclusions.—Intentional ARA occlusion during EVAR was not associated with changes in renal function or blood pressure measurements, even when performed in patients with more advanced renal dysfunction. Type II

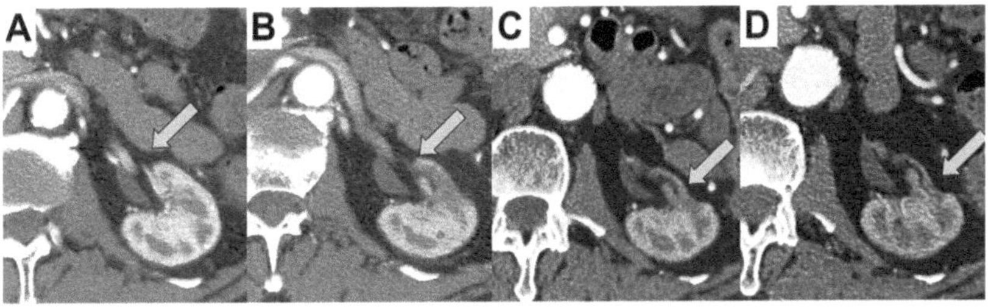

FIGURE 2.—A, Preoperative computed tomography (CT) scan shows a patent accessory renal artery (ARA) supplying the left upper pole of the kidney. B, Two months later, the same area is infarcted; no loss of parenchyma mass. C, After 4 years, the right upper pole parenchymal mass is decreased in size. D, At 7-year follow-up, a CT scan demonstrated a progressive loss of parenchymal mass despite stable estimated glomerular filtration rate (eGFR) since the procedure. (Reprinted from Malgor RD, Oderich GS, Vrtiska TJ, et al. A case-control study of intentional occlusion of accessory renal arteries during endovascular aortic aneurysm repair. *J Vasc Surg*. 2013;58:1467-1475, Copyright 2013, with permission from The Society for Vascular Surgery.)

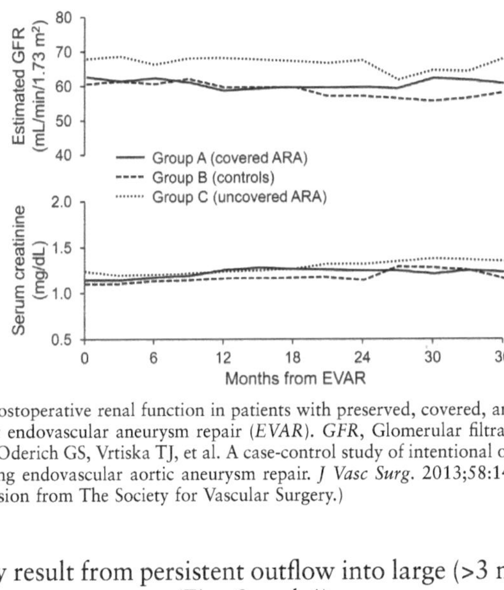

FIGURE 4.—Postoperative renal function in patients with preserved, covered, and no accessory renal artery (*ARA*) after endovascular aneurysm repair (*EVAR*). *GFR*, Glomerular filtration rate. (Reprinted from Malgor RD, Oderich GS, Vrtiska TJ, et al. A case-control study of intentional occlusion of accessory renal arteries during endovascular aortic aneurysm repair. *J Vasc Surg*. 2013;58:1467-1475, Copyright 2013, with permission from The Society for Vascular Surgery.)

endoleak may result from persistent outflow into large (>3 mm) ARAs that arise from the aneurysm sac (Figs 2 and 4).

▶ In this case-control study, endovascular abdominal aneurysm repair (EVAR) with accessory renal artery (ARA) coverage carried no negative impact on renal function or blood pressure management, even when applied to patients with more advanced stages of chronic kidney disease (CKD). Kidney infarction occurred in 67% of the patients who had an ARA covered and in none of the patients who underwent EVAR with total kidney preservation.

ARA is an anatomic variation found in 25% to 50% of the general population. The finding that one-third of the patients who had an ARA intentionally covered by a stent graft did not have any evidence of infarction indicates that other retroperitoneal or ureteral branches provide collateral flow to the kidney. The data from this well-conducted study are consistent with those of prior reports but add to the literature a more important and critical analysis of clinical, laboratory, and anatomic outcomes with a control group and longer follow-up.

These authors convincingly showed that intentional coverage of ARAs does not significantly impair renal function within the first 3 years after EVAR, even when applied to patients with advanced stages of CKD (Figs 2 and 4). Furthermore, based on their experience, they recommended that preoperative embolization should be considered in patients with ARA greater than 3 mm arising from the aneurysm sac, provided this can be performed with a low risk of embolic complications.

B. W. Starnes, MD

Visceral stent patency in fenestrated stent grafting for abdominal aortic aneurysm repair

Grimme FAB, Zeebregts CJ, Verhoeven ELG, et al (Univ of Groningen, The Netherlands; Univ Hosp Leuven, Belgium)

J Vasc Surg 59:298-306, 2014

Objective.—Fenestrated endovascular abdominal aortic aneurysm repair (F-EVAR) has been introduced for treatment of aneurysms in which visceral arteries are incorporated. Patency of target vessels has been reported to be excellent. Results of the use of stent grafts to accommodate visceral arteries in F-EVAR are presented in this study, including an overview of factors that affect outcome.

Methods.—All patients treated with fenestrated stent grafts in a single center between November 2001 and October 2011 were reviewed. Patients treated for suprarenal, juxtarenal, and infrarenal short-necked aortic aneurysms were included. Patients with thoraco-abdominal aneurysms or aneurysms treated with grafts with fixed side branches were excluded. Polytetrafluoroethylene covered stents were used routinely since June 2005. Target vessels and stents were examined using computed tomography angiography reconstructions. Primary end points were primary patency, defined as the absence of occlusion, and loss of renal function. Secondary end points were technical success, stenosis (defined as a ≥50% angiographic diameter reduction), stent fracture, and mortality.

Results.—A total of 138 patients with a median age of 73 years (range, 50-91 years) met the inclusion criteria. Median computed tomography angiography follow-up was 13 months (range, 1-97 months). In total, 392 target vessels were provided with 140 scallops and 252 fenestrations. Visceral stents (−grafts) were placed in 254 target vessels. Technical success was obtained in 249 arteries (98.0%). Overall stent patency of target vessels was 95.7% at 1 year and 88.6% at 4 years. Renal artery stent patency was 97.4% at 1 year and 91.2% at 4 years (96.8% and 89.1% for uncovered stents; 97.3% and 92.4% for covered stents, respectively). There was no significant difference in patency between covered and uncovered stents in renal arteries ($P = .71$). Renal artery stenosis occurred in 26 stented arteries (11.3%) and occlusion in seven arteries. Renal artery stent stenosis occurred significantly more in uncovered than in covered stents ($P = .04$). Stent fractures occurred more in uncovered than in covered stents ($P = .01$) and was associated with a significantly lower visceral stent patency rate ($P < .01$). During follow-up, 13 patients developed permanent renal function impairment (9.4%), of which two required permanent dialysis (1.4%). Renal dysfunction was significantly associated with renal stent occlusion or stenosis ($P < .01$).

Conclusions.—Patency rates of visceral artery stent (–grafts) in F-EVAR were 95.7% at 1 year and 88.6% at 4 years. Patency rates were affected by stent fractures, which occurred more in uncovered compared with covered stents. Renal artery stent stenosis occurred more in uncovered compared with covered stents. Renal dysfunction was significantly associated with renal stent occlusion or stenosis (Fig 5).

► Few reports describe the details on the outcome of visceral artery stenting in fenestrated endovascular abdominal aortic aneurysm repair (F-EVAR). Overall estimated 1-year patency of visceral target vessels has been reported up to 92%, with renal artery patency rates of 85%. These authors from Europe, highly experienced in F-EVAR, report their experience with branch vessel patency. FEVAR was performed in 138 patients. Thirty-day mortality was 1.4%. Two patients died within the first month, both due to bowel ischemia.

There are a couple of important lessons here worth mentioning. Stent fractures were significantly associated with reduced stent patency rates ($P < .01$; Fig 5). The overall target-vessel patency rate at 5 years was 93%.

I believe that this report represents the learning curve of these investigators and that we will actually see improved target vessel patency in the years to

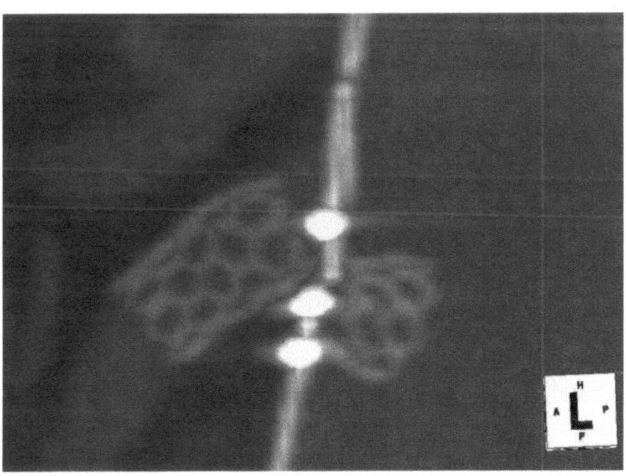

FIGURE 5.—Fractured uncovered stent in superior mesenteric artery (SMA) of 72-year-old man. Since the patient had no abdominal complaints, no intervention was performed. (Reprinted from Grimme FAB, Zeebregts CJ, Verhoeven ELG, et al. Visceral stent patency in fenestrated stent grafting for abdominal aortic aneurysm repair. *J Vasc Surg*. 2014;59:298-306, Copyright 2014, with permission from the Society for Vascular Surgery.)

come with better patient selection and stent technology. These authors state that their experience with F-EVAR began in 2001. This is interesting because the first reported F-EVAR from John Anderson was published in 2001. This probably means that these authors were practicing physician-modified grafts and just beginning to learn that a proximal seal in healthier aortic neck led to better outcomes. The majority of celiac and superior mesenteric artery vessels were managed with scallops rather than large fenestrations, and a minority of these vessels were stented.

B. W. Starnes, MD

The Morphological Applicability of a Novel Endovascular Aneurysm Sealing (EVAS) System (Nellix) in Patients with Abdominal Aortic Aneurysms

Karthikesalingam A, Cobb RJ, Khoury A, et al (St George's Vascular Inst, London, UK; et al)

Eur J Vasc Endovasc Surg 46:440-445, 2013

Objective.—Endovascular aneurysm sealing (EVAS) using the Nellix system is a promising alternative to endovascular repair (EVR) and open surgery for abdominal aortic aneurysms (AAA). The aim of this study was to investigate the proportion of patients with AAA who are morphologically suitable for treatment with Nellix.

Methods.—Patients presenting with AAA were investigated at two regionalised vascular units. Separate cohorts were identified, who had undergone infrarenal EVR, open aneurysm repair, fenestrated endovascular repair (FEVR) or non-operative management. Pre-operative morphology was quantified using three-dimensional computed tomography according to a validated protocol. Each aneurysm was assessed for compliance with the instructions for use (IFU) of Nellix.

Results.—776 patients were identified with mean age 75 ± 9 years. 730/776 (94.1%) had undergone infrarenal EVR, 6/776 (0.8%) open repair, 27/776 (3.5%) FEVR and 13/776 (1.7%) had been managed non-operatively. 544/776 (70.1%) of all AAA were morphologically suitable for Nellix. 533/730 (73.0%) of patients who had undergone infrarenal EVR were compliant with Nellix IFU, compared with 497/730 (68.1%), 379/730 (51.9%) and 214/730 (29.3%) with the IFU for Medtronic Endurant ($p = .04$) or Cook Zenith ($p < .01$) and Gore C3 Excluder ($p < .01$) endografts respectively.

Conclusions.—Nellix technology appears widely applicable to contemporary infrarenal AAA practice, and may provide an option for patients that are outside current EVR device instructions for use. However, formal outcomes study is still required, and will ultimately dictate the clinical relevance of this feasibility study. The major limitation to anatomic suitability

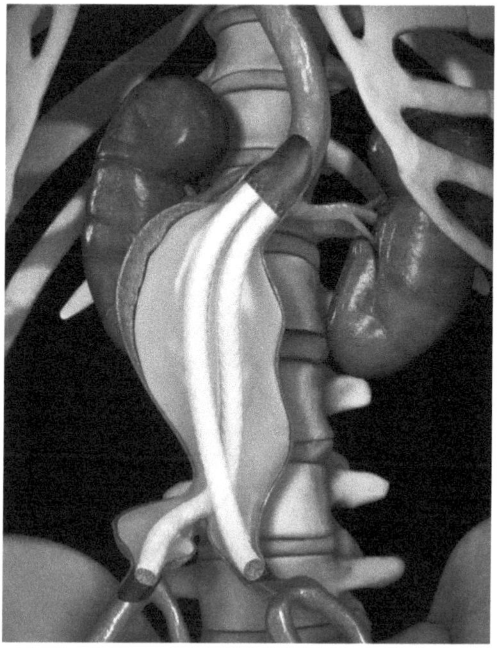

FIGURE 1.—Nellix Endovascular device from http://www.endologix.com/investigational_devices/nellix/. (Reprinted from Karthikesalingam A, Cobb RJ, Khoury A, et al. The morphological applicability of a novel endovascular aneurysm sealing (EVAS) system (Nellix) in patients with abdominal aortic aneurysms. *Eur J Vasc Endovasc Surg*. 2013;46:440-445, Copyright 2013, with permission from the European Society for Vascular Surgery.)

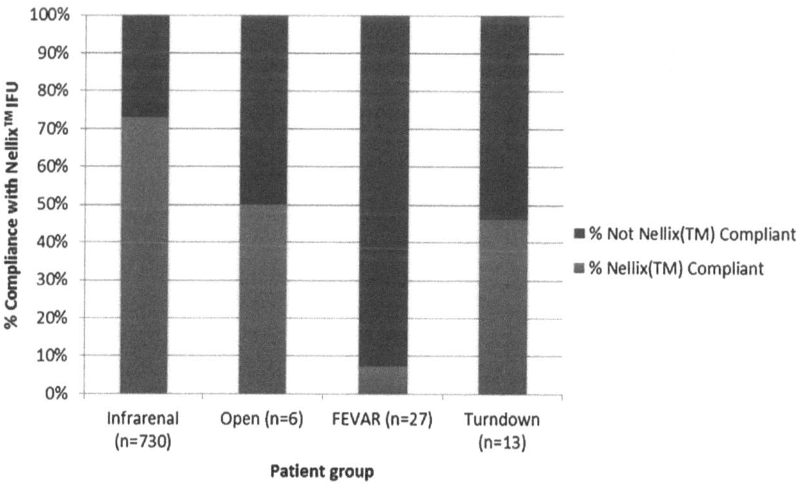

FIGURE 2.—Differing suitability for Nellix among four groups of patients. FEVR = fenestrated endovascular repair. (Reprinted from Karthikesalingam A, Cobb RJ, Khoury A, et al. The morphological applicability of a novel endovascular aneurysm sealing (EVAS) system (Nellix) in patients with abdominal aortic aneurysms. *Eur J Vasc Endovasc Surg*. 2013;46:440-445, Copyright 2013, with permission from the European Society for Vascular Surgery.)

TABLE 1.—Instructions for use for Nellix and Contemporary Endovascular Aortic Repair Devices

	Nellix	Cook Zenith	Medtronic	Gore
Non-aneurysmal AN length	≥10 mm	≥15 mm	≥10 mm	≥15 mm
Non-aneurysmal AN diameter	18–32 mm	18–32 mm	19–32 mm	19–29 mm
Maximum aortic blood flow lumen diameter	≤60 mm	–	–	–
Maximum common iliac artery diameter	8–35 mm	7.5–20 mm	8–25 mm	8–18.5 mm
Angle from neck to sac	<60	<45	If AN length 10–15 mm, then ≤45 If AN length >15 mm, then ≤60	–
Angle from suprarenal aorta to neck	–	<60	If AN length 10–15 mm, then ≤60 If AN length >15 mm, then ≤75	≤60

AN = aortic neck.

for Nellix is currently the maximum patent lumen diameter of large AAA (Figs 1 and 2, Table 1).

▶ Aneurysm morphology remains a key challenge for endovascular aneurysm repair (EVAR) and is a key determinant of eventual long-term success. This study evaluated the applicability of the Nellix device (Endologix, Irvine, CA; Fig 1) to 776 patients already treated with a variety of commercially available endovascular grafts. The primary outcome measure for each of 4 procedure groups was compliance with anatomic instructions for use supplied by the manufacturers of the Nellix device and 3 other manufacturers (Table 1).

Differing suitability for Nellix among 4 groups of patients is depicted in Fig 2. Approximately two-thirds of patients were suitable for the Nellix device within the instructions for use. Individual assessment of each morphologic criterion revealed that the most common obstacle to the use of the Nellix device was the presence of a large maximum patent lumen diameter within the aneurysm sac. The Nellix device was notably not applicable to juxtarenal aneurysms.

Clinical data are required to describe the performance of Nellix in terms of its procedural complexity, short-term morbidity, and long-term safety. It remains to be seen how Nellix technology will compare with other endografts because clinical data are currently lacking for this device.

B. W. Starnes, MD

Endovascular repair of aortoiliac aneurysmal disease with the helical iliac bifurcation device and the bifurcated-bifurcated iliac bifurcation device

Wong S, Greenberg RK, Brown CR, et al (Cleveland Clinic, OH)

J Vasc Surg 58:861-869, 2013

Background.—Iliac branch device (IBD) treatment of common and internal iliac artery (CIA and IIA) aneurysms has been controversial in the context of available embolization techniques or off-label adjunctive procedures. Two devices exist, a straight IBD (S-IBD) and a helical IBD (H-IBD). We report our midterm results with the latter and present outcomes with a third device intended to treat disease in the presence of short CIAs termed the bifurcated-bifurcated IBD (BB-IBD).

Methods.—Data were prospectively collected from IBD-treated patients with infrarenal aortoiliac or thoracoabdominal aortoiliac aneurysms. Preoperative aneurysmal characteristics were collected in accordance with the endovascular reporting standards document, including presence of IIA stenosis, CIA diameters, and the presence of an IIA aneurysm. Technical success was defined as IBD device placement, branch placement, and patency without type I or III endoleak at implantation in addition to 24 hours survival. Follow-up computed tomography scans at 1, 6 (optional), 12 months, and annually thereafter were performed and reinterventions, sac morphology changes, and endoleaks noted. Survival and patency were evaluated with life-table analyses, and differences among anatomic groups were compared with log-rank tests, whereas *t*-tests and Fisher exact tests were used to compare simple variables.

Results.—Between 2003 and 2012, 138 IBD devices were placed into 130 patients (98 H-IBD and 40 BB-IBD). Median follow-up was 20.3 months (range, 1-72 months) with 30- day, 12-month, 3- and 5-year survival rates of 99%, 90%, 79%, and 62%, respectively. Technical success was 94%, and branch patency was 94.6% at 30 days and 81.8% at 5 years. Thirty-five percent (35%) of branches were placed into patients with IIA aneurysms (in addition to their proximal disease), 20% into stenotic IIAs, and 46% into iliac systems with narrow (<16 mm) CIAs. Technical success was significantly lower in patients with IIA stenosis (81.5 vs 96.4%; Fisher exact test, $P = .015$) but not affected by the presence of an IIA aneurysm or narrow CIA. Branch patency was similar in all groups throughout follow-up. No stent fractures or component separations were noted in the IBDs or mating devices throughout the study period.

Conclusions.—The H-IBD and BB-IBD configurations have high technical success and acceptable long-term patency for the treatment of CIA and IIA aneurysms, including those with challenging anatomy difficult to treat with the straight branch design (Figs 1 and 5).

▶ In aorto-iliac aneurysm repair, the preservation of hypogastric blood flow has an important role in preventing buttock claudication and less common complications such as gluteal necrosis, ischemic colitis, spinal cord ischemia, and sexual dysfunction. Multiple endovascular techniques have been used to preserve

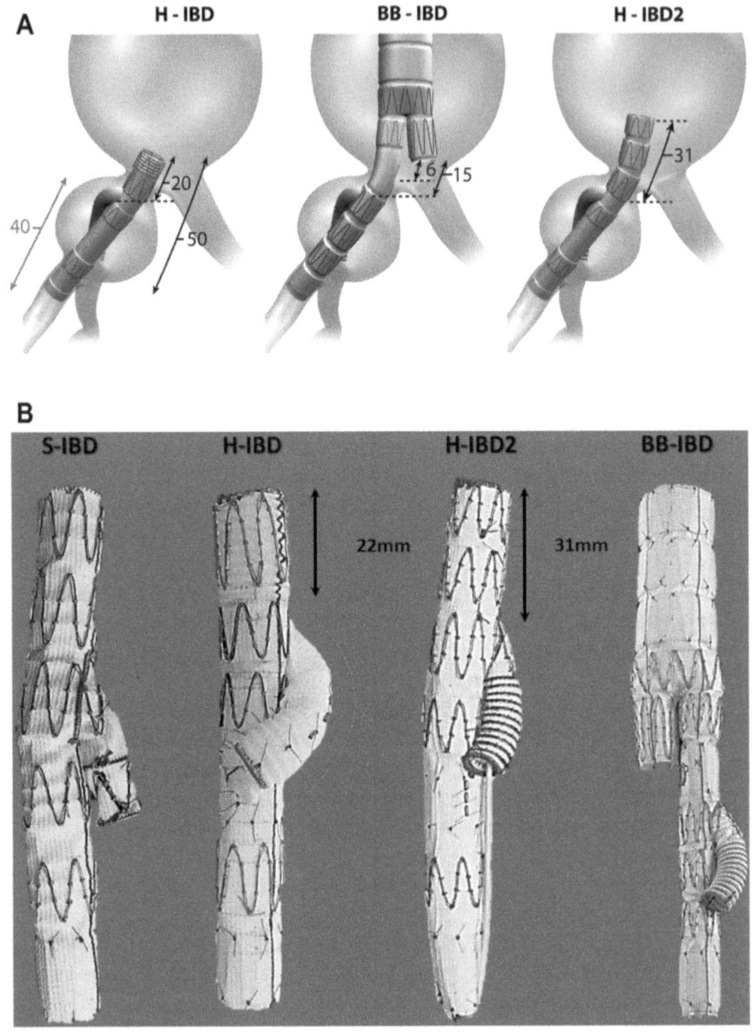

FIGURE 1.—A, This figure demonstrates the differences between the three devices. The helical iliac branch device (*H-IBD*) is about 5 cm long and, thus, extends 1 cm into the aortic portion on an abdominal aortic aneurysm if the common iliac artery (CIA) is slightly longer than 4 cm, placing two modular joints within a potentially large volume. If the CIA is shorter, then the device is even higher potentially compromising durability more and making the procedure much more challenging. The bifurcated-bifurcated IBD (*BB-IBD*) is designed for shorter CIAs, by allowing for the treatment of aneurysms involving CIAs as short as 2 to 2.5 cm without difficulty. Longer CIA aneurysms can also be treated, but the mating device to reach the internal iliac artery (IIA) landing zone must then be longer as well. Once the BB-IBD was developed, the need to treat CIAs that were shorter than 5.5 to 6 cm was obliviated, so the H-IBD2 was developed by lengthening the overlap with the aortic component to add more security to the joint. B, These images represent the actual devices. The straight IBD (*S-IBD*) is depicted first; note the minimal (10-15 mm) overlap zone in contrast to the H-IBD where the wrap of the branch around the device extends the overlap zone to 27 mm. The H-IBD2 has the extended overlap zone with the mating component increasing it from 22 mm in the H-IBD1 to 31 mm in the H-IBD2. The BBIBD is designed to mate with a 24-mm-diameter tubular graft in the distal aorta. This is identical to the distal components used in fenestrated and branched grafts, making this an ideal distal component for such cases, replacing the distal bifurcated component that would have to be combined with an IBD to achieve treatment of a CIA or IIA aneurysm. (Reprinted from Wong S, Greenberg RK, Brown CR, et al. Endovascular repair of aortoiliac aneurysmal disease with the helical iliac bifurcation device and the bifurcated-bifurcated iliac bifurcation device. *J Vasc Surg*. 2013;58:861-869, Copyright 2013, with permission from The Society for Vascular Surgery.)

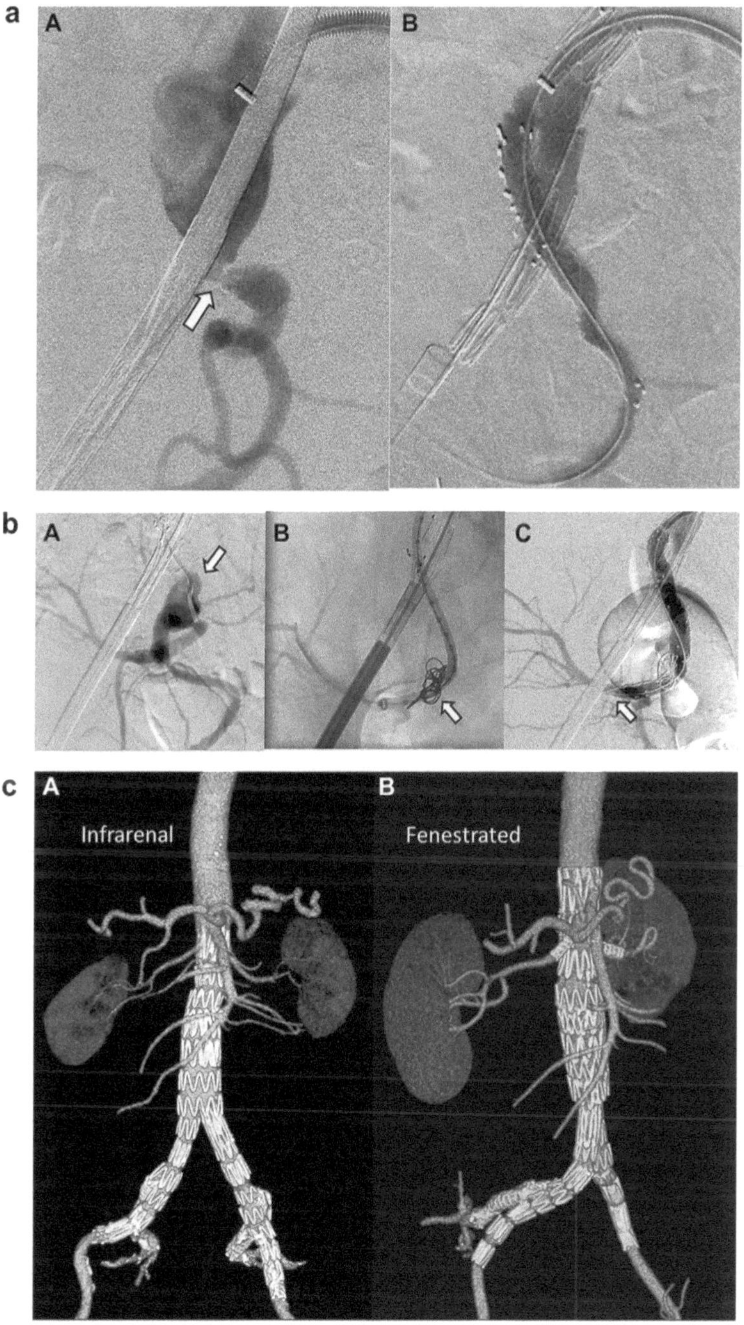

FIGURE 5.—Intraoperative pictures. **a**, Tight ostial lesion (**A**) and stent graft in situ (**B**). **b**, Internal iliac artery (IIA) aneurysm (**A**), coiling of anterior divisional branch (**B**), and placement of mating stent into the posterior divisional branch (**C**). **c**, Completed repair: infrarenal device (**A**) and fenestrated proximal device (**B**). (Reprinted from Wong S, Greenberg RK, Brown CR, et al. Endovascular repair of aortoiliac aneurysmal disease with the helical iliac bifurcation device and the bifurcated-bifurcated iliac bifurcation device. *J Vasc Surg*. 2013;58:861-869, Copyright 2013, with permission from The Society for Vascular Surgery.)

antegrade internal iliac artery (IIA) blood flow but none with the specific device design and intent to achieve the intended purpose.

Two separate physician-sponsored investigational device exemption trials at the Cleveland Clinic incorporated the use of an Iliac Branch Device (IBD) beginning in 2003 for patients with concomitant common iliac artery (CIA) or IIA aneurysms (Fig 1). Technical success was achieved in 94% of cases, and there were 9 technical failures. A total of 18 occlusions were noted in the follow-up period, of which, 11 occurred within 30 days of implantation.

The important lesson learned from this study is that an IBD is most likely the optimal means of endovascular exclusion of CIA and IIA aneurysms, helping us to extend repairs from healthy arteries proximally to healthy arteries distally (Fig 5). The helical IBD seemed to have more flexibility in terms of application to a broader number of patients. The long overlap with the helical design allows one to focus almost entirely on the accuracy of stent graft deployment at the distal IIA landing zone.

The actual proficiency of any given clinician with the implantation of IBDs can be difficult to pinpoint. The required skill set mostly revolves around endografting, but it also includes the ability to snare wires, IIA embolization techniques, and challenging ostial IIA cannulations in the setting of tight stenosis.

Lastly, this report is a tribute to the unparalleled vision of the late Roy Greenberg, a good friend and colleague of mine for more than a decade, who conceived of and began studying this device design in 2003!

B. W. Starnes, MD

The fate of untreated concomitant suprarenal aortic aneurysms after endovascular aneurysm repair of infrarenal aortic aneurysms

Herdrich BJ, Murphy EH, Wang GJ, et al (The Perelman School of Medicine the Univ of Pennsylvania, Philadelphia)
J Vasc Surg 58:1201-1207, 2013

Objective.—Many patients treated with endovascular aortic repair (EVAR) have a concomitant suprarenal abdominal aortic aneurysm (sAAA). The natural history of these sAAAs and whether they require intervention after EVAR is unknown.

Methods.—We identified 470 patients from the M2S database (M2S Inc, West Lebanon, NH) as having an infrarenal AAA (iAAA) with a concomitant sAAA (diameter, 2.9-4.7 cm). The analysis included 217 patients with preoperative computed tomography angiography and follow-up imaging of ≥12 months. Patients who did not undergo EVAR (n = 65) served as a control. Patients with EVAR were subdivided into 90 with suprarenal fixation (SR) and 62 with infrarenal fixation (IR). Standard measurements from the M2S images were extracted, and growth rates were calculated for different abdominal aortic segments.

Results.—The average follow-up was 33.0 ± 18.8 months. The average sAAA initial size and growth rate were 34.6 ± 3.0 and 0.6 ± 1.1 mm/y for SR, 34.0 ± 3.3 and 0.6 ± 1.3 mm/y for IR, and 36.6 ± 3.4 and

1.2 ± 1.5 mm/y for controls (SR vs IR, $P > .05$; SR or IR vs control, $P < .05$). After EVAR, two of 152 (1.3%) sAAAs grew to ≥50 mm, which was not statistically different from four of 65 (6.2%) in the control group ($P = .07$). At 48 months, the Kaplan-Meier freedom from sAAA growth to ≥50 mm was 99.3% for patients undergoing EVAR and 95.2% for controls ($P = .061$). Patients with starting sAAAs sized ≥40 mm had a higher growth rate (1.4 ± 2.1 mm/y) and frequency of growth to ≥50 mm (14.3%) than patients with starting sAAAs sized <40 mm (0.7 ± 1.2 mm/y and 1.5%; $P < .05$).

Conclusions.—Isolated treatment of iAAAs via EVAR with a concomitant sAAA is acceptable because endografts with or without SR do not affect sAAA growth rates. Routine EVAR follow-up is sufficient for sAAAs of <40 mm, and more intensive follow-up should be considered for sAAAs of 40 to 50 mm. For sAAAs approaching 50 mm, an endograft with IR should be considered in case sAAA repair is required in the future (Fig 2).

▶ I've always wondered if we were doing the right thing when we performed endovascular aortic repair (EVAR), particularly with transrenal fixation, in patients harboring what seemed to be an infrarenal aortic aneurysm and some

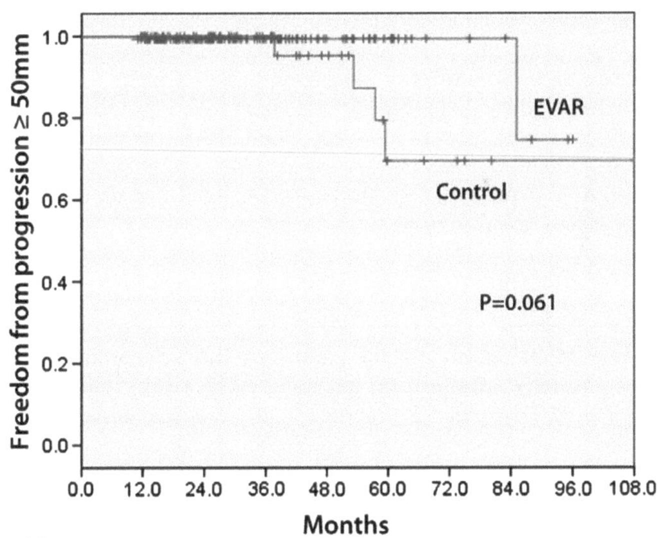

Pt at risk

EVAR	152	149	92	54	27	15	6	4	1	
Control	65	62	43	25	15	5	4	1	1	1

FIGURE 2.—Kaplan-Meier analysis of freedom from suprarenal abdominal aortic aneurysm (sAAA) growth to ≥50 mm in patients undergoing endovascular aortic repair (*EVAR*) and in controls. (Reprinted from Herdrich BJ, Murphy EH, Wang GJ, et al. The fate of untreated concomitant suprarenal aortic aneurysms after endovascular aneurysm repair of infrarenal aortic aneurysms. *J Vasc Surg.* 2013;58:1201-1207, with permission from The Society for Vascular Surgery.)

component of a suprarenal aneurysm. Should these patients be treated like those with thoraco-abdominal aortic aneurysms? What is the fate of the untreated suprarenal aortic aneurysm? This is a nice report detailing the answers to these questions.

The study included 470 patients in the M2S Inc (West Lebanon, NH) database who were identified as having and infrarenal abdominal aortic aneurysm (iAAA) with a concomitant suprarenal AAA (sAAA) 3 to 5 cm in size. A size for the sAAA of 50 mm was chosen as a cutoff because it was considered the smallest justifiable size criteria for treating sAAA in a patient with an acceptable surgical risk.

What this anatomic study found was that after EVAR, there is a low rate of growth of concomitant sAAAs to a size that may require intervention. This is an important finding because it shows that it is appropriate to treat the iAAA and observe the sAAA, and many patients will never require an intervention for their sAAA. These data further suggest that EVAR with or without transrenal fixation does not lead to faster sAAA growth. It is interesting that there is a trend toward improved freedom from sAAA growth to greater than 50 mm in the EVAR-treated patients going out to 4 years after EVAR (Fig 2).

In this study, sAAA growth to greater than 50 mm was only seen in 2.8% of patients, and the average time for this to occur was 50.4 months. Many of these patients have a limited life expectancy, and for those few patients whose sAAAs grew to greater than 50 mm, there may be a significant period after EVAR before an intervention is required for the sAAA. Because of the small number of patients with follow-up greater than 5 years, it is hard to draw conclusions about the fate of these sAAAs in patients with a prolonged life expectancy.

On the basis of these data, the authors recommend that for patients with an iAAA requiring intervention and a concomitant sAAA less than 50 mm in diameter, it is appropriate to treat the iAAA with EVAR, when anatomically suitable, and monitor the sAAA. Stent grafts with transrenal fixation do not appear to affect the growth rate of sAAAs.

B. W. Starnes, MD

In situ laser fenestration during emergent thoracic endovascular aortic repair is an effective method for left subclavian artery revascularization

Redlinger RE Jr, Ahanchi SS, Panneton JM (Eastern Virginia Med School, Norfolk, VA)

J Vasc Surg 58:1171-1177, 2013

Background.—Retrograde laser fenestration of the left subclavian artery (LSA) during emergent thoracic endovascular aortic repair (TEVAR) uses a relatively simple intraoperative method of endograft modification to revascularize aortic branches for a variety of acute thoracic aortic pathologies. This study presents our expanded experience and midterm outcomes of TEVAR with laser fenestration to revascularize the LSA as an alternative to debranching.

Methods.—Patients who underwent TEVAR with LSA revascularization by laser graft fenestration from September 2009 through August 2012 were retrospectively reviewed. TEVAR was performed with deployment of a Dacron (DuPont, Wilmington, Del) endograft over the LSA orifice. Laser catheter fenestration of the graft was performed through retrograde brachial access, followed by balloon-expandable covered stent deployment through the fenestration to traverse the endograft and LSA. Routine postoperative follow-up imaging with computed tomography angiography was performed to assess TEVAR and LSA fenestration patency, endoleak, and aneurysm/dissection exclusion.

Results.—TEVAR with laser fenestration was successfully performed in 22 patients (12 men; mean age, 57 years) in an urgent or emergent setting secondary to unremitting symptoms or rupture. Twelve patients had large symptomatic thoracic aortic aneurysms (eight secondary to chronic dissection); four patients had acute symptomatic type B aortic dissection, and six patients had an intramural hematoma or penetrating aortic ulcer, or both. An average of two endografts (range, 1-4) were deployed. LSA-covered stents were 8 to 10 mm in diameter. Mean operative time was 154 ± 65 minutes. Average hospital length of stay was 12 ± 7 days. No major fenestration-related complications occurred. One patient developed postoperative paraplegia. One patient died in the postoperative period, for an in-hospital mortality rate of 4.5%. Two patients died of non-TEVAR-related causes at a mean follow-up of 10 months (range, 1-40 months). Follow-up computed tomography angiography imaging demonstrated a 100% primary patency for the LSA stents. One patient had an asymptomatic LSA stent stenosis. Type II endoleaks from the LSA in two patients required endovascular coil embolization. No fenestration-related type I or III endoleaks were noted.

Conclusions.—In situ retrograde laser fenestration is a feasible and effective option for LSA revascularization during TEVAR involving a spectrum of acute thoracic aortic pathology. Laser fenestration provides a rapid, reproducible method of fenestrating the endograft material. The high technical success, low fenestration-related morbidity, and excellent midterm patency support this technique of intraoperative endograft modification.

▶ As stated in this article, conventional open thoracic aortic repair in an urgent or emergent setting has been demonstrated to have mortality rates close to 20% and significant morbidity, including a risk of spinal cord ischemia that can affect 18.6% of patients. Intentional coverage of the left subclavian artery (LSA), although initially thought to be benign, is now being shown to have an increased risk of subclavian steal, arm claudication, vertebral artery stroke, and spinal cord ischemia. This article from the group at Eastern Virginia Medical School retrospectively reviewed their experience using laser catheter fenestration via a retrograde brachial artery approach performed in association with thoracic endovascular aortic repair. Fenestrations took on average < 5 minutes to create in Dacron-based Cook and Medtronic thoracic endografts. All cases used a 2.0- to 2.5-mm Turbo Elite laser catheter (Spectranetics, Colorado

Springs, CO). Each fenestration was then stented open using 8- to 10-mm balloon-expandable iCast covered stents (Atrium, Hudson, NH). The authors performed concerted follow-up with computed tomographic angiography showing 100% stent primary patency at a mean of 11 months. The authors only attempted to perform in situ fenestrations if there was > 5 mm distance between the proximal endograft fabric and the LSA. The authors state that they performed in situ fenestration more commonly when using Medtronic grafts compared with Cook due to the greater distance between stents in this graft. An additional technical note they provide is that this technique is not recommended for patients with type 3 aortic arches because of the unfavorable angle the subclavian artery takes in relation to the aorta. In general, although this is a small series of patients, as the authors state, these are promising mid-term results that may be helpful in caring for our patients.

D. L. Gillespie, MD, RVT, FACS

8 Thoracic Aorta

A new staged hybrid total arch repair procedure using a branched proximal elephant trunk technique with implantation of stent grafts to the ascending aorta

Watanabe Y, Shimamura K, Shirakawa Y, et al (Osaka Univ Graduate School of Medicine, Suita, Japan)

J Vasc Surg 58:1700-1704, 2013

We report a new hybrid aortic arch repair procedure for the treatment of extensive thoracic aortic aneurysms involving the ascending aorta, arch, and descending aorta. In the first stage of this procedure, a "double-barrel tube graft" was inserted into the ascending aorta and fixed to the sinotubular junction under short-duration cardiopulmonary bypass in normothermia. In the next stage, after debranching of the left common carotid artery and left subclavian artery, stent grafts were deployed from the double-barrel tube graft to the descending aorta and the brachiocephalic artery to exclude the aneurysms. The patient's postoperative course was uneventful, with no endoleaks. The successful initial result suggests that this procedure could be an attractive treatment option for extensive aortic aneurysms.

▶ Although there have been many advances to manage complex thoracic, thoracoabdominal, and infrarenal aortic aneurysms using purely endovascular techniques, patients with diffuse aneurysmal disease starting in the ascending thoracic aorta continue to require several open reconstructions requiring total circulatory arrest to revascularize the great vessels and the descending thoracic aorta. These investigators staged a patient's repair by an initial open procedure in which they placed a staging graft that they call a double-barrel graft into the ascending aorta. Inserting this graft required a very short run on cardiopulmonary bypass (CPB). They were then able to revascularize the great vessels using extranatomic bypass and the descending aorta using a conventional thoracic stent graft docked into their staging double-barrel graft. The advantage of this hybrid treatment for extensive aortic aneurysms that include the ascending aorta is that this technique provides an adequate proximal landing zone just above the sinotubular junction with minimal open surgery. Although short-duration CPB and cardiac arrest are required, this procedure provides a reliable proximal landing zone and exclusion of the native aortic wall in the ascending aorta, which is at risk of increasing aneurysmal dilatation or dissection. These authors' operative strategy is a very important bridge until branched stent grafts for the arch become available. Although the branched devices could be an attractive treatment option for aortic arch aneurysms, an adequate proximal landing zone is needed in the ascending aorta. The technique these authors describe in which they insert a single vascular graft into the ascending aorta could provide an adequate landing zone just above the sinotubular junction, and complete exclusion of aneurysms could be accomplished by subsequent endovascular repair using branched stent grafts.

M. T. Watkins, MD

Association of race and socioeconomic status with the use of endovascular repair to treat thoracic aortic diseases

Johnston WF, Lapar DJ, Newhook TE, et al (Univ of Virginia, Charlottesville)
J Vasc Surg 58:1476-1482, 2013

Objective.—Descending thoracic aortic diseases may be treated with either open thoracic aortic repair or thoracic endovascular aortic repair (TEVAR). Previous studies have demonstrated that race and socioeconomic status (SES) affect access to care and treatment allocation in vascular surgery. We hypothesized that racial minorities and lower SES patients have decreased propensity to have their thoracic aortic disease treated with TEVAR.

Methods.—Weighted discharge records for patients who underwent either open thoracic aortic repair or TEVAR between 2005 and 2008 were evaluated using the Nationwide Inpatient Sample. Patient records were stratified by therapeutic intervention (open repair vs TEVAR). Differences in baseline comorbidities, race, and SES were compared. To account for the effects of comorbidities and other factors, hierarchical logistic regression modeling was used to determine the likelihood for TEVAR performance based on differences in patients' race and SES.

Results.—A total of 60,784 thoracic repairs were analyzed, the majority (79.4%) of which were open repairs. The most common race was white (78.2%), followed by black (9.1%), Hispanic (5.7%), Asian or Pacific Islander (2.9%), and Native American (0.7%). Patients were divided into quartiles according to SES with 20.6% of patients in the lowest SES quartile, 24.3% in the second quartile, 26.4% in the third quartile, and 28.8% in the highest SES quartile. Indications for treatment were similar for both treatment groups. After adjusting for multiple patient and hospital factors, race and SES were significantly associated with treatment modality for thoracic aortic disease. Black, Hispanic, and Native American populations had increased adjusted odds ratios of TEVAR performance compared with white patients. Similarly, lower SES correlated with increased use of TEVAR.

Conclusions.—Contrary to our initial hypothesis, racial minorities (Black, Hispanic, and Native American) and patients with lower median household incomes have a greater association with the performance for TEVAR after accounting for patient comorbid disease, indication for

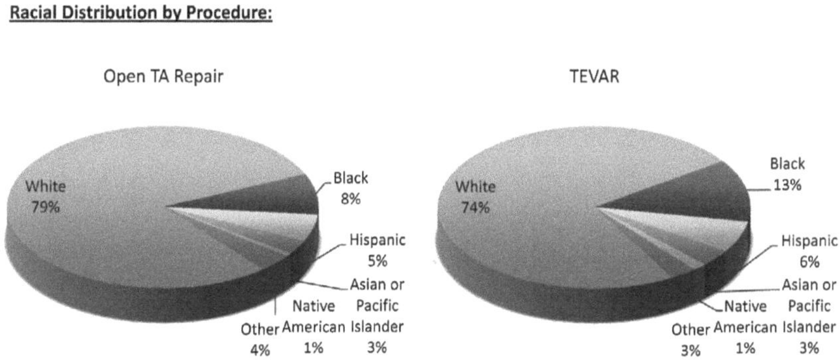

FIGURE 1.—Racial distribution of patients according to treatment for thoracic aortic disease. *TA*, Thoracic aortic; *TEVAR*, thoracic endovascular aortic repair. (Reprinted from Johnston WF, Lapar DJ, Newhook TE, et al. Association of race and socioeconomic status with the use of endovascular repair to treat thoracic aortic diseases. *J Vasc Surg*. 2013;58:1476-1482, Copyright 2013, with permission from The Society for Vascular Surgery.)

treatment, payer status, and hospital volume. These results indicate that traditional racial disparities do not persist in TEVAR allocation (Fig 1).

▶ In simply taking a look at the title of this article, one would likely think that there was significant disparity in the delivery of new technology and better quality care, with those of racial minority or low socioeconomic status (SES) receiving less quality care. Not so in this thorough review of thoracic endovascular aortic repair (TEVAR) in the Nationwide Inpatient Sample after introduction of TEVAR in America.

Throughout health care, disparities have existed between patients of different racial backgrounds, with racial minority patients often receiving substandard care, leading to worse outcomes after treatment. In organ transplantation and oncology, prior study has shown that SES independently influences treatment allocation. The difference of patient race by procedure is illustrated in Fig 1. Univariate analyses demonstrated significant differences in race and SES between patients receiving open repair and TEVAR, with 26.3% of TEVAR patients being nonwhite compared with 20.6% of open repair patients ($P < .001$). In regard to the proportion of patients receiving TEVAR according to race, 28.6% of black patients received TEVAR, whereas only 19.5% of white patients were treated with TEVAR ($P < .001$).

Racial minorities and patients with lower incomes were independently associated with an increased propensity to receive endovascular treatment for thoracic aortic disease. The increased correlation between TEVAR and racial minorities and patients from lower socioeconomic status is multifactorial and cannot be fully explained by common patient or hospital factors. Trends in TEVAR allocation indicate that treatment disparities based on race and SES are decreasing in vascular surgery.

B. W. Starnes, MD

The differences and similarities between intramural hematoma of the descending aorta and acute type B dissection

Tolenaar JL, Harris KM, Upchurch GR Jr, et al (Thoracic Aortic Res Ctr, Milan, Italy; Abbott Northwestern Hosp, Minneapolis, MN; Univ of Virginia, Charlottesville; et al)

J Vasc Surg 58:1498-1504, 2013

Introduction.—Aortic intramural hematoma type B (IMHB) is a variant of acute aortic syndrome, which presents with symptoms similar to classic type B aortic dissection (ABAD). However, the natural history of IMHB is not well understood. The purpose of this study was to better characterize IMHB, comparing its clinical characteristics, treatment, and in-hospital and long-term outcomes to those with classic ABAD.

Methods.—A total of 107 IMHB and 790 ABAD patients enrolled in the International Registry of Acute Aortic Dissection (IRAD) between January 1996 and June 2012 were analyzed. Accordingly, differences in presentation, diagnostics, therapeutic management, and outcomes were assessed.

Results.—As compared with the ABAD, IMHB presented predominantly in males (62% vs 33%; $P < .001$) at older age (69 ± 12 vs 63 ± 14; $P < .001$). IMHB patients more often had chest pain (80% vs 69%; $P = .020$) and periaortic hematoma (22% vs 13%; $P = .020$) and were more often treated medically (88% vs 62%; $P < .001$), with surgical/endovascular interventions being reserved for more complicated patients. Overall in-hospital mortality was 10% (IMHB, 7% vs ABAD, 11%; $P =$ NS). Six out of seven IMHB deaths occurred during medical treatment, two due to aortic rupture. During follow-up in IMHB, patient mortality was 7%, and no adverse events, including progression to an aortic dissection or aortic rupture, were observed. Imaging showed significantly more aortic enlargement at the level of the descending aorta in ABAD patients (39% vs 61%; $P = .034$).

Conclusions.—Most IMHB patients can be treated medically, and aortic enlargement is less common during follow-up, which may suggest that IMHB may have a slightly more benign course compared with classic ABAD in the acute setting (Fig 1).

▶ Acute intramural hematoma type B (IMHB) is a serious aortic condition characterized by a crescentic thickening of the descending thoracic aorta in the absence of an intimal flap or entry tear, resulting from hemorrhage within the aortic wall. It was initially believed that this condition was relatively rare compared with classic type B aortic dissection, although presenting with similar symptoms and morbidity and mortality rates. Recent reports suggest that IMHB has a much higher incidence of > 20% of all type B aortic dissections in some series (Fig 1).

I have become somewhat frustrated with the International Registry for Acute Aortic Dissection (IRAD) and the quality of the reports generated from these data sets. This analysis only covered 897 patients over 16 years in an international registry with 30 large referral centers. The treatment recommendations

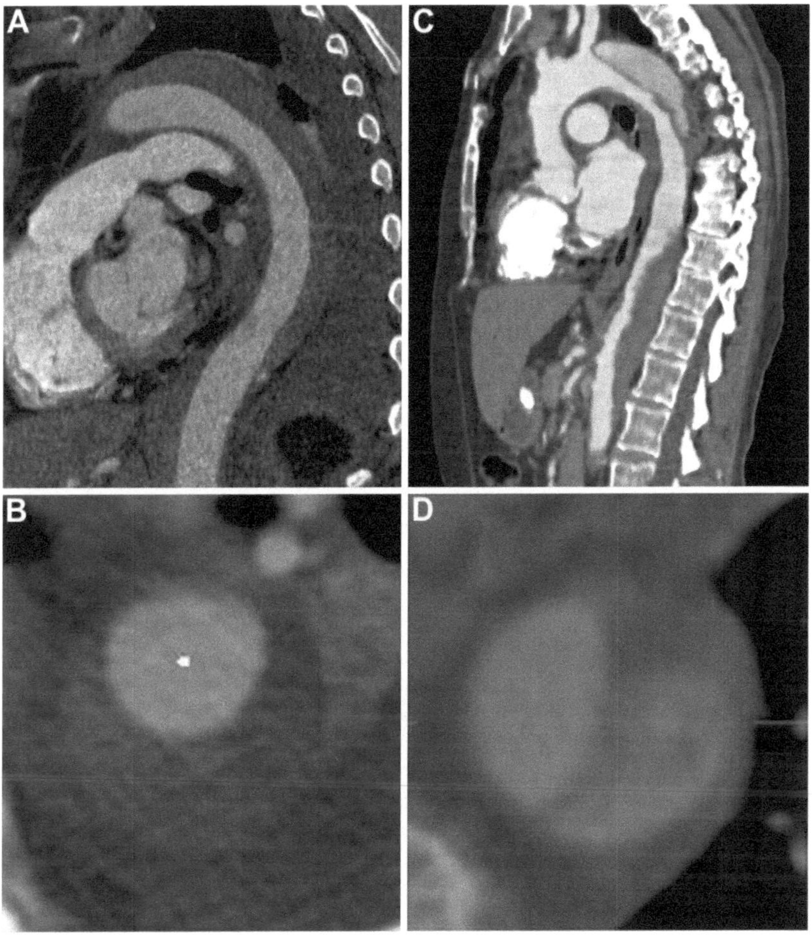

FIGURE 1.—A and B, Sagittal and transverse view of computed tomography angiogram showing an intramural hematoma of the descending aorta. C and D, Sagittal and transverse view of computed tomography angiogram showing a classic type B aortic dissection (ABAD). (Reprinted from Tolenaar JL, Harris KM, Upchurch GR Jr, et al. The differences and similarities between intramural hematoma of the descending aorta and acute type B dissection. *J Vasc Surg*. 2013;58:1498-1504, Copyright 2013, with permission from The Society for Vascular Surgery.)

put forth by these authors for the management of IMHB are primarily medical, but there remains a 10% in-hospital mortality rate! What other aortic conditions are associated with a 10% in-hospital mortality rate? Can the IRAD Investigators give us a clue as to what were the common features of those who died from IMHB? All of the patients undergoing thoracic endovascular aortic repair (TEVAR) for IMHB had a great outcome, suggesting that (1) they didn't really need treatment or (2) TEVAR is better for this aortic condition. We need a better way of tracking these conditions. IRAD was a nice try, but modern data acquisition and the Internet should allow for better datasets.

The one thing we did learn from this article was that aortic enlargement was much less common for IMHB than acute type B dissection on follow-up.

B. W. Starnes, MD

Percutaneous Closure of Large Femoral Artery Access with Prostar XL in Thoracic Endovascular Aortic Repair

Skagius E, Bosnjak M, Björck M, et al (Uppsala Univ, Sweden; et al)
Eur J Vasc Endovasc Surg 46:558-563, 2013

Objectives.—To investigate the technical success rate of Prostar XL for closure of large (≥20F) femoral vascular access sites in thoracic endovascular aortic repair (TEVAR) procedures.

Methods.—This was a single-center consecutive case series. All TEVAR procedures at Uppsala University Hospital 2006–2010 were registered prospectively. Reoperations and cases with open closure technique were excluded. Primary (early) technical failure was defined as closure failure requiring immediate (on-table) open surgical repair; late access-related complication occurred thereafter. The medical records, pre- and postoperative computed tomography images were reviewed retrospectively.

Results.—A total of 164 TEVAR procedures were identified, of which 118 (71%) had a median 22F (range 20–26F) access site sealed with tandem Prostar XL. The indications for TEVAR were dissection (47%), aneurysm (42%), trauma (8%), and miscellaneous (3%). Median follow-up time was 10 months (range 1–62). Primary technical failure occurred in 10 of 118 (8%). These cases were converted to cut-downs and surgical repair ($n = 7$), femoral fascia suturing ($n = 2$), and external compression with the Femo-Stop device ($n = 1$). Hypertension was associated with primary failure ($p = .005$), and a trend was observed for high age ($p = .078$) and increased groin subcutaneous fat layer ($p = .077$). Late access-related complications included pseudo-aneurysms ($n = 12$), small hematomas ($n = 7$), superficial groin infections ($n = 2$), and deep venous thrombosis ($n = 1$). None of the late complications required surgical treatment.

Conclusions.—The access closure technique with tandem Prostar XL for large access sites during TEVAR is safe, in experienced hands. Few technical failures and few late complications occur, and they are usually benign (Fig 1).

▶ This is yet another single-institution experience with percutaneous endovascular aneurysm repair (PEVAR; Fig 1). The unique aspects of this study are that only thoracic endovascular repairs were included with sheath sizes ranging from 20F to 26F and a mean of 22F. The other unique aspect of this article is that a "tandem" technique was used with 2 Prostar devices being used for most access sites.

Our institution and others have broad experience with the "Pre-Close" technique using both Prostar and Proglide for more than 10 years, and every large-bore access is attempted with a closure device. Even with our broad experience,

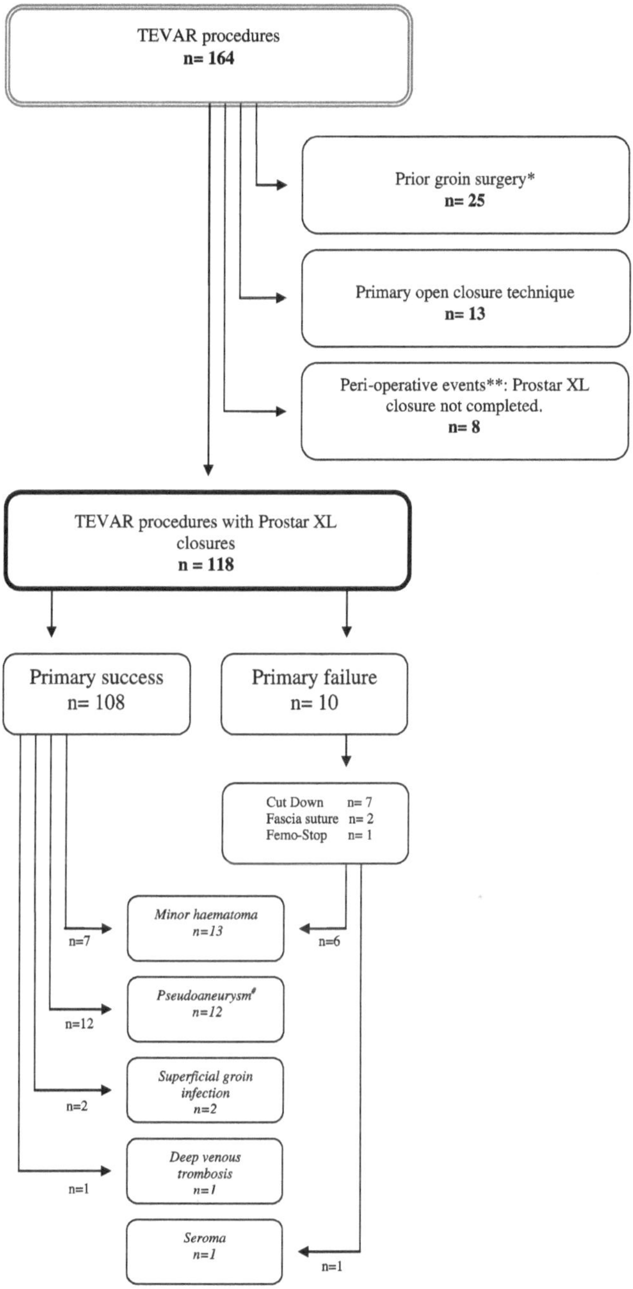

FIGURE 1.—Flowchart depicting the selection of the study population and the occurrence of early and late access-related complications. Late access-related complications are given in italics. # Eleven pseudoaneurysms were small (mean 8 mm) and treated conservatively. One patient had a 21-mm pseudoaneurysm, but due to multiple complications no treatment directed against it was initiated before she died of septicemia 3 months after the intervention. *Cut down, previous Prostar XL procedures. **Perioperative death, patient-related factors, for example iliac artery injuries. (Reprinted from Skagius E, Bosnjak M, Björck M, et al. Percutaneous closure of large femoral artery access with prostar XL in thoracic endovascular aortic repair. *Eur J Vasc Endovasc Surg*. 2013;46:558-563, with permission from European Society for Vascular Surgery.)

our failure rate still approaches 5%, slightly better than the 8% rate quoted in this paper. What that means, when only considering infrarenal endografts with bilateral large-bore sheath access, is that 1 in 20 access sites will fail, which to the patient means 1 in 10 patients will have a failure requiring surgical cutdown. Therefore, it is imperative that the capability to perform surgical cutdown and direct femoral reconstruction be available for those practitioners choosing to use this method.

We rarely have the need to use multiple Prostar devices as described in this article. Even the authors acknowledged that as their experience has matured, they tend now to use only a single device per side. I recently gave a talk at a regional meeting in which I made the bold statement that "if you are not practicing PEVAR, you are practicing in the last century *and* you are not performing standard of care!" This technique is better for patients and is associated with shorter procedure times and decreased lengths of stay.

B. W. Starnes, MD

Debate: Whether level I evidence comparing thoracic endovascular repair and medical management is necessary for uncomplicated type B aortic dissections

Brunkwall J, Lübke T, Power AH, et al (Univ of Cologne, Germany; London Health Sciences Centre and Western Univ, Ontario, Canada)

J Vasc Surg 58:836-841, 2013

Type B aortic dissections continue to be one of the most challenging clinical scenarios confronting vascular surgeons. In the era of open surgery, the therapeutic options were limited to medical management of hypertension and large open thoracoabdominal operations. In the current endovascular era, the operative strategies have become less invasive but the questions regarding therapeutic approaches have become more numerous and complex. In patients with acute uncomplicated type B aortic dissections, we are still unsure as to which patients are best treated with medical therapy alone or with the addition of early endovascular repair. Data from single centers and registries have provided some guidance; however, questions remain. Perhaps level 1 evidence from well-designed randomized controlled trials will answer all of our questions. This is the topic of the current debate.

▶ The Canadians and the Germans go at this topic in a well written and hearty debate.

German stance: Level 1 evidence comparing thoracic endovascular repair and medical management is necessary for uncomplicated type B aortic dissections.

Approximately 30% of acute type B aortic dissections are complicated by peripheral vascular ischemia or hemodynamic instability, with a subsequent high risk of death. The International Registry of Acute Aortic Dissection (IRAD) data showed that the most common cause of death was rupture (40%) followed by intestinal ischemia (17%–39%). Meanwhile, current data revealed a mortality rate of medically treated type B aortic dissections of approximately

10% within the first month. From the IRAD data, it could be concluded that calcium channel blockers were correlated with a better survival during follow-up for acute type B dissections, whereas beta-blockers improved outcomes after surgery for acute type A dissections. In the setting of acute type B dissection, 25% to 50% of patients treated medically will eventually develop late aortic-related complications that require an endovascular or open repair.

So far, there is no randomized controlled trial of thoracic endovascular aortic repair (TEVAR) for the treatment of acute complicated type B dissection. Even if underpowered for mortality, the INSTEAD trial[1] has shown that there was a remodeling of the aorta leading to an enlarged true lumen with regression of the false lumen. Aortic remodeling with thrombosis of the false lumen occurred in 91.3% of patients with TEVAR versus 19.4% of patients with best medical therapy.

Until now, there is no level 1 evidence to support the routine use of TEVAR for type B aortic dissections, and there is no level 1 evidence for the medical management either! Our strategy for managing these patients needs to be scientifically proven.

Canadian Stance: Level 1 evidence comparing thoracic endovascular repair and medical management is not necessary for uncomplicated type B aortic dissections.

There is overwhelming evidence, albeit mostly from non—level 1 data, that patients with uncomplicated acute type dissection do well with best medical therapy. We need look no further than the ADSORB trial[2] to show that clinical equipoise has not occurred, which is displayed in their slow enrollment and low recruitment.

Rather than a randomized trial that attempts to tell us whether TEVAR or best medical therapy is superior for all uncomplicated acute type B dissections, we need a study that tells us which dissections will become complicated and thus require TEVAR. As the ADSORB trial[2] has unfortunately shown, it is not possible to perform a sufficiently powered randomized controlled trial with clinically relevant end points comparing TEVAR to best medical therapy in acute type B dissection patients in a timely fashion. It took 10 years for ADSORB to complete recruitment. A randomized trial is simply not possible.

So, after extensive review of the current literature, the debaters each showed that the evidence favors medical management for uncomplicated type B dissection. However, the evidence for this strategy is weak. Considering the lack of power of the ADSORB[2] and INSTEAD[1] trials, we need large studies with long-term follow-up to provide optimal treatment guidelines.

B. W. Starnes, MD

References

1. Nienaber CA, Rousseau H, Eggebrecht H, et al. Randomized comparison of strategies for type B aortic dissection: the Investigation of Stent Grafts in Aortic Dissection (INSTEAD) trial. *Circulation.* 2009;120:2519-2528.
2. Brunkwall J, Lammer J, Verhoeven E, Taylor P. ADSORB: a study on the efficacy of endovascular grafting in uncomplicated acute dissection of the descending aorta. *Eur J Vasc Endovasc Surg.* 2012;44:31-36.

Thoracic endovascular aortic repair in management of aortoesophageal fistulas

Canaud L, Ozdemir BA, Bee WW, et al (St George's Vascular Inst, London, UK)
J Vasc Surg 59:248-254, 2014

Objective.—To provide a systematic review of the outcomes of thoracic endovascular aortic repair (TEVAR) for aortoesophageal fistula (AEF) and to identify prognostic factors associated with poor outcomes.

Methods.—Literature searches of the Embase, Medline, and Cochrane databases identified relevant articles reporting results of TEVAR for AEF. The main outcome measure was the composite of aortic mortality, recurrence of the AEF, and stent graft explantation. The secondary outcome measure was aortic-related mortality.

Results.—Fifty-five articles were integrated after a literature search identified 72 patients treated by TEVAR for AEFs. The technical success rate of TEVAR was 87.3%. The overall 30-day mortality was 19.4%. Prolonged antibiotics (>4 weeks) were administered in 80% of patients. Concomitant or staged resection or repair of the esophagus was performed in 44.4% of patients. Stent graft explantation was performed within the first month after TEVAR as a planned treatment in 11.1%. After a mean follow-up of 7.4 months (range, 1-33 months), the all-cause mortality was 40.2%, and the aortic-related mortality was 33.3. Prolonged antibiotic treatment ($P = .001$) and repair of AEFs due to a foreign body ($P = .038$) were associated with a significant lower aortic mortality. On univariate analysis, TEVAR and concomitant or staged adjunctive procedures (resection, repair of the esophagus, or a planned stent graft explantation) were associated with a significantly lower incidence of aortic-related mortality ($P = .0121$). When entered into a binary logistic regression analysis, prolonged antibiotic treatment was the only factor associated with a significant lower incidence of the endpoint ($P = .003$).

Conclusions.—Late infection or recurrence of the AEF and associated mortality rates are high when TEVAR is used as a sole therapeutic strategy. Prolonged antibiotic treatment has a strong negative association with mortality. A strategy of a temporizing endovascular procedure to stabilize the patient in extremis, and upon recovery, an open surgical esophageal repair with or without stent graft explantation is advocated.

▶ Primary and secondary aortoesophageal fistulas (AEFs) are uniformly fatal if untreated and remain a formidable surgical problem in older, high-risk patients with hemorrhagic shock or sepsis. Open repair has an extremely high operative mortality that may reach > 50%, even in centers of excellence. Thoracic endovascular aortic repair (TEVAR) has gained popularity as an emergent treatment for AEF, despite the high risk of infection. A major concern regards the durability of this strategy.

These authors looked at all published literature in the past decade regarding TEVAR for AEF. The primary outcome of interest was the composite of aortic mortality, recurrence of the AEF, and stent graft explantation. The secondary outcome measure was aortic-related mortality.

Fifty-five articles were integrated after a literature search identified 72 patients with AEF treated by TEVAR. Most patients presented with hematemesis (86.1%). Hypovolemic shock and systemic infection were present in 60.9% and 21.7%, respectively.

The overall 30-day mortality was 19.4%. Persistent postoperative sepsis was the most common early complication (23.6%). Univariate analysis demonstrated that prolonged antibiotic treatment (>4 weeks; $P=.001$) and repair of an AEF due to a foreign body ($P=.038$) were associated with a significantly lower incidence of the composite endpoint. Antibiotic treatment was the only strongly significant factor associated with a lower aortic mortality rate in the multivariate analysis.

The authors recommended that TEVAR be considered a bridge therapy followed by a delayed durable open repair when the patient has been stabilized. Clearly, any strategy in this patient population needs to be highly individualized. TEVAR for AEFs achieves the primary goal of therapy (ie, control of bleeding, prevention of fatal exsanguination). The high rate of secondary stent graft infection or recurrence of the AEF clearly prove that even combined with broad-spectrum antibiotics, TEVAR cannot replace surgical debridement and/or drainage of the infected mediastinum.

B. W. Starnes, MD

Natural history of grade I-II blunt traumatic aortic injury

Osgood MJ, Heck JM, Rellinger EJ, et al (Vanderbilt Univ Med Ctr, Nashville, TN; et al)

J Vasc Surg 59:334-342, 2014

Background.—Endovascular aortic repair has revolutionized the management of traumatic blunt aortic injury (BAI). However, debate continues about the extent of injury requiring endovascular repair, particularly with regard to minimal aortic injury. Therefore, we conducted a retrospective observational analysis of our experience with these patients.

Methods.—We retrospectively reviewed all BAI presenting to an academic level I trauma center over a 10-year period (2000-2010). Images were reviewed by a radiologist and graded according to Society for Vascular Surgery guidelines (grade I-IV). Demographics, injury severity, and outcomes were recorded.

Results.—We identified 204 patients with BAI of the thoracic or abdominal aorta. Of these, 155 were deemed operative injuries at presentation, had grade III-IV injuries or aortic dissection, and were excluded from this analysis. The remaining 49 patients had 50 grade I-II injuries. We managed 46 grade I injuries (intimal tear or flap, 95%), and four grade II injuries (intramural hematoma, 5%) nonoperatively. Of these, 41 patients had follow-up imaging at a mean of 86 days postinjury and constitute our study cohort. Mean age was 41 years, and mean length of stay was 14 days. The majority (48 of 50, 96%) were thoracic aortic injuries and the remaining two (4%) were abdominal. On follow-up imaging, 23 of 43 (55%) had complete resolution of injury, 17 (40%) had no change in aortic injury, and two (5%) had progression of injury. Of the two patients with progression, one progressed from grade I to grade II and the other progressed from grade I to grade III (pseudoaneurysm). Mean time to progression was 16 days. Neither of the patients with injury progression required operative intervention or died during follow-up.

Conclusions.—Injury progression in grade I-II BAI is rare (~5%) and did not cause death in our study cohort. Given that progression to grade III injury is possible, follow-up with repeat aortic imaging is reasonable (Figs 1 and 2).

▶ I just returned from Charing Cross in London where I debated with Dr Ali Azizzadeh on the classification of blunt aortic injury (BAI). We both have long-held different opinions regarding the classification of this injury, and this article (selfishly) supports my bias. I believe that, to serve a purpose, grading systems must help dictate therapy. The current classification was proposed in 2009 and has been adopted by the Society for Vascular Surgery. In this grading system, injuries are assigned to 1 of 4 categories: grade I (intimal tear), grade II (intramural hematoma), grade III (pseudoaneurysm), and grade IV (rupture). The current recommendations are to treat grade I injuries with observation and repeat imaging and treat grade II through IV injuries with thoracic endovascular aortic repair.

A recent trend in the management of BAI has been evolution toward nonoperative therapy of "minimal aortic injury." Grade II injuries (intramural hematoma), although still "minimal," are often managed more aggressively, reflected by current practice guidelines that recommend repair of these injuries despite lack of

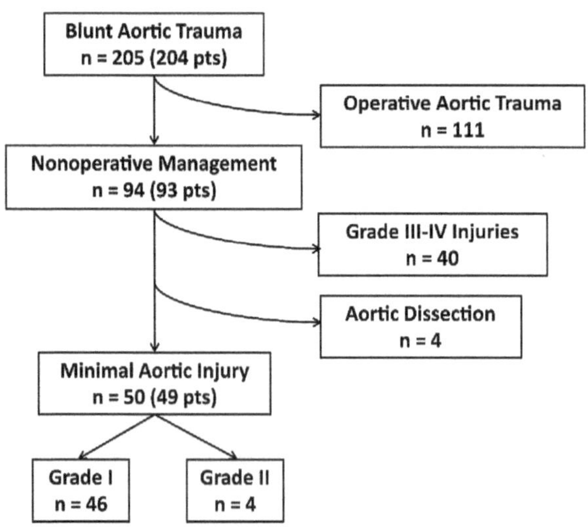

FIGURE 1.—Diagram summarizing selection of patients for inclusion in this analysis. *pts*, Patients. (Reprinted from Osgood MJ, Heck JM, Rellinger EJ, et al. Natural history of grade I-II blunt traumatic aortic injury. *J Vasc Surg*. 2014;59:334-342, Copyright 2014, with permission from the Society for Vascular Surgery.)

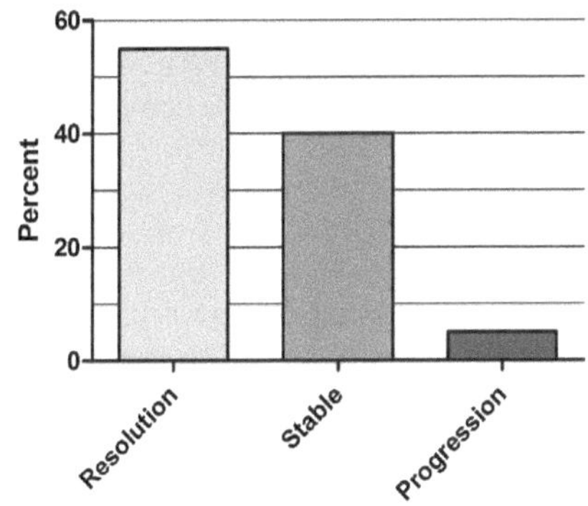

FIGURE 2.—Evolution of injury following grade I-II blunt aortic injury (BAI). Between the time of injury and last follow-up imaging, 55% of patients demonstrated complete injury resolution, 40% had stable injuries, and 5% of patients developed injury progression to higher injury grade. (Reprinted from Osgood MJ, Heck JM, Rellinger EJ, et al. Natural history of grade I-II blunt traumatic aortic injury. *J Vasc Surg*. 2014;59:334-342, Copyright 2014, with permission from the Society for Vascular Surgery.)

supportive data.[1] Our own experience with more than 140 patients with BAI is that we have *never* seen a grade II injury.[2] Therefore, I don't believe they exist. At the University of Washington, we divide these injuries into 2 categories, those with and without an external contour abnormality of the aorta. We only treat those patients who have disrupted the smooth outer lining of the aorta.

In this series of 205 patients, 50 had grade I or II injuries and were managed nonoperatively. There were only 4 grade II injuries, all (100%) of which healed on follow-up imaging. Only 2 grade I injuries progressed: 1 to a grade II injury that then healed and 1 to a grade 3 injury that was treated. Importantly, none of the 50 patients died of their BAI (Figs 1 and 2). You be the judge . . . do grade II injuries matter?

B. W. Starnes, MD

References

1. Lee WA, Matsumura JS, Mitchell RS, et al. Endovascular repair of traumatic thoracic aortic injury: clinical practice guidelines of the Society for Vascular Surgery. *J Vasc Surg*. 2011;53:187-192.
2. Starnes BW, Lundgren RS, Gunn M, et al. A new classification scheme for treating blunt aortic injury. *J Vasc Surg*. 2012;55:47-54.

Fate of patients with spinal cord ischemia complicating thoracic endovascular aortic repair

Desart K, Scali ST, Feezor RJ, et al (Univ of Florida College of Medicine, Gainesville)
J Vasc Surg 58:635-642.e2, 2013

Objective.—Spinal cord ischemia (SCI) is a potentially devastating complication of thoracic endovascular aortic repair (TEVAR) that can result in varying degrees of short-term and permanent disability. This study was undertaken to describe the clinical outcomes, long-term functional impact, and influence on survival of SCI after TEVAR.

Methods.—A retrospective review of all TEVAR patients at the University of Florida from 2000 to 2011 was performed to identify individuals experiencing SCI, defined by *any* new lower extremity neurologic deficit not attributable to another cause. SCI was dichotomized into immediate or delayed onset, with immediate onset defined as SCI noted upon awakening from anesthesia, and delayed characterized as a period of normal function, followed by development of neurologic injury. Ambulatory status was determined using database query, record review, and phone interviews with patients and/or family. Mortality was estimated using life-table analysis.

Results.—A total of 607 TEVARs were performed for various indications, with 57 patients (9.4%) noted to have postoperative SCI (4.3% permanent). SCI patients were more likely to be older (63.9 ± 15.6 vs 70.5 ± 11.2 years; $P = .002$) and have a number of comorbidities, including chronic obstructive pulmonary disease, hypertension, dyslipidemia, and cerebrovascular disease ($P < .0001$). At some point in their care, a cerebrospinal fluid drain was placed in 54 patients (95%), with 54% placed postoperatively. In-hospital mortality was 8.8% for the entire cohort (SCI vs no SCI; $P = .45$). SCI developed immediately in 12 patients, delayed onset in 40, and indeterminate in five patients due to indiscriminate timing from postoperative sedation. Three patients (25%) with immediate SCI had measurable functional improvement (FI), whereas 28 (70%) of the delayed-onset patients experienced some degree of neurologic recovery ($P = .04$). Of the 34 patients with complete data available, 26 (76%) reported quantifiable FI, but only 13 (38%) experienced return to their preoperative baseline. Estimated mean (± standard error) survival for patients with and without SCI was 37.2 ± 4.5 and 71.6 ± 3.9 months ($P < .0006$), respectively. Patients with FI had a mean survival of 53.9 ± 5.9 months compared with 9.6 ± 3.6 months for those without improvement ($P < .0001$). Survival and return of neurologic function were not significantly different when patients with preoperative and postoperative cerebrospinal fluid drains were compared.

Conclusions.—The minority of patients experience complete return to baseline function after SCI with TEVAR, and outcomes in patients without early functional recovery are particularly dismal. Patients experiencing delayed SCI are more likely to have FI and may anticipate similar life-expectancy with neurologic recovery compared with patients without SCI. Timing of drain placement does not appear to have an impact on postdischarge FI or long-term mortality (Fig 4).

▶ This is 1 of 2 important articles in this edition of Year Book of Vascular Surgery addressing the topic of spinal cord ischemia complicating thoracic endovascular aortic repair (TEVAR). This study analyzed a large cohort of TEVAR patients with and without spinal cord ischemia (SCI) and further stratified according to timing of onset of the injury and degree of functional

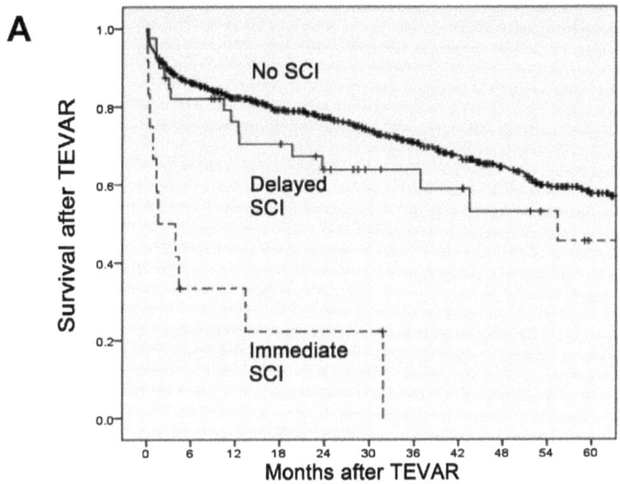

		0	6	12	18	24	30	36	42	48	54	60
No SCI	At Risk	550	451	389	341	304	269	232	197	157	126	96
	SE	.01	.02	.02	.02	.02	.02	.02	.02	.03	.03	.03
Delayed	At Risk	40	31	26	24	18	14	13	12	9	7	4
	SE	.06	.07	.07	.08	.08	.08	.09	.10	.10	.11	.11
Immed.	At Risk	12	3	3	2	2	2					
	SE	.14	.14	.12	.12	.12	.09					

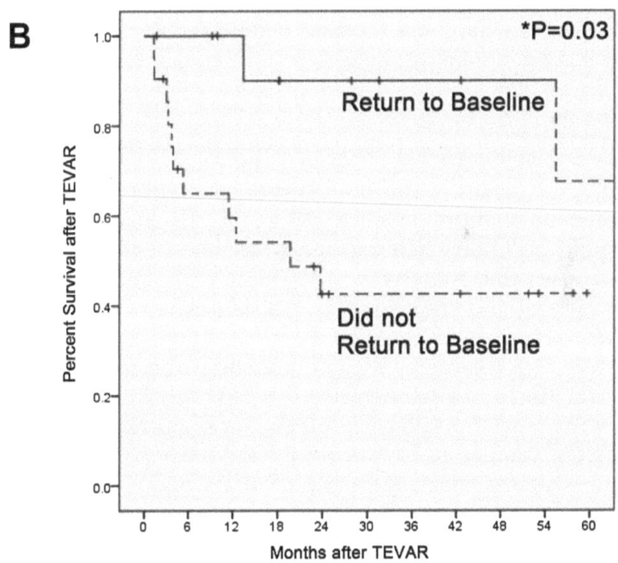

		0	6	12	18	24	30	36	42	48	54	60
RTB	At Risk	13	12	10	9	7	6	5	5	4	4	3
	SE	.00	.00	.09	.09	.09	.09	.09	.09	.09	.21	.21
No RTB	At Risk	21	12	11	10	6	5	5	5	4	2	
	SE	.11	.11	.11	.12	.12	.12	.12	.12	.12	.12	

FIGURE 4.—A, Differential survival is noted between patients with return to preoperative neurologic baseline status vs those without return to baseline if spinal cord ischemia (*SCI*) developed ($P = .03$) after thoracic endovascular aortic repair (*TEVAR*). B, Differential survival is shown between those patients without SCI vs those with immediate or delayed SCI. Delayed SCI patients can anticipate similar long-term life expectancy compared with patients without SCI. *RTB*, Return to baseline; *SE*, standard error. (Reprinted from Desart K, Scali ST, Feezor RJ, et al. Fate of patients with spinal cord ischemia complicating thoracic endovascular aortic repair. *J Vasc Surg*. 2013;58:635-642.e2, with permission from The Society for Vascular Surgery.)

impairment after this complication. Consistent with previous reports on SCI after endovascular aortic repair, these patients have a poor long-term survival. Interestingly, the timing of SCI and trajectory of functional impairment were important indicators of overall prognosis.

The incidence of SCI in this report is high at 9.4% compared with that of other contemporary series. The permanent SCI rate was 4.3%. Spinal drains were only selectively used, and there was no formal protocol. Overall functional outcome was measured by ambulatory status as follows: (1) ambulating independently, (2) ambulating with assistance (eg, cane, walker), (3) nonambulatory but mobile (stand/pivot and transfer, wheelchair use), and (4) bedridden. Perhaps the most interesting finding from this study included the prognostic significance of timing and rate of recovery after TEVAR. Most of the patients who have SCI after TEVAR present in a delayed fashion (>70%). Of these delayed presentations, most (62.5%) experienced at least some neurologic recovery and were independently ambulating or ambulating with minimal assistance at the time of discharge. Those patients with immediate-onset SCI after TEVAR and no improvement in functional status before discharge have a dismal prognosis (Fig 4).

B. W. Starnes, MD

Aortic arch debranching and thoracic endovascular repair

De Rango P, Cao P, Ferrer C, et al (Univ of Perugia, Italy; Hosp S. Camillo - Forlanini, Rome, Italy)

J Vasc Surg 59:107-114, 2014

Objective.—Currently, the best approach to the aortic arch remains unsupported by robust evidence. Most of the available data rely on small sample numbers, heterogeneous settings, and limited follow-up. The objective of this study was to evaluate early and midterm results of arch debranching and endovascular procedures.

Methods.—From 2005 through 2013, 104 consecutive patients underwent elective arch treatment with debranching and thoracic endovascular aortic repair. Rates of perioperative (30-day) mortality and neurological complications, and mortality, endoleak, supra-aortic vessel patency, and arch diameter changes at 5 years were analyzed.

Results.—Patients' mean age was 69.8 years, and 90 were males. Twenty arches were repaired for dissection. Nineteen patients required total debranching for diseases extended to zone 0. In 59, debranching and thoracic endovascular aortic repair procedures were staged. At 30 days, death, stroke, and spinal cord ischemia occurred in six, four, and three patients, respectively. Extension to ascending aorta (zone 0 landing) was the only multivariate independent predictor for perioperative mortality (odds ratio, 9.6; 95% confidence interval, 1.54-59.90; $P = .015$), but not for stroke. Four retrograde dissections, two fatal, occurred during the perioperative period. At 1, 3, and 5 years, Kaplan-Meier survival rates were 89.0%, 82.8%, and 70.9%, and freedom from persistent endoleak rates were 96.1%, 92.5%, and 88.3%, respectively. Over 5-year follow-up, 34 aneurysms shrank

≥5 mm, and four grew. Five reinterventions were required. Two supra-aortic vessel occlusions and no late aorta-related mortalities were recorded.

Conclusions.—Despite the perioperative mortality risk, the late outcome of endovascular arch repair presents a low rate of aorta-related deaths and reinterventions and acceptable midterm survival. Furthermore, more than one-third of the aneurysms' diameters decrease over 5 years as a measure of the long-term efficacy of treatment. Retrograde type A dissection remains a major concern in the perioperative period and careful arch approach is required (Fig 4, Tables 2 and 3).

▶ This study is one of the largest and most comprehensive to date describing aortic arch debranching and thoracic endovascular repair for the management of a variety of aortic pathologies. The authors report on 104 consecutive patients with follow-up out to 5 years. Patients were divided into groups based on Arch Zone.[1]

In Zone 0, all 4 supra-aortic vessels were revascularized using either total debranching through median sternotomy or partial debranching associated with branched stent graft or chimney techniques.

In Zone 1, a carotid-carotid bypass using retropharyngeal or antetrachea tunnel was performed in association with left subclavian artery revascularization by transposition or bypass.

In Zone 2, carotid subclavian bypass or transposition was performed.

Technical details are listed in Table 2. Perioperative outcomes are listed in Table 3, and cumulative survival in Fig 4.

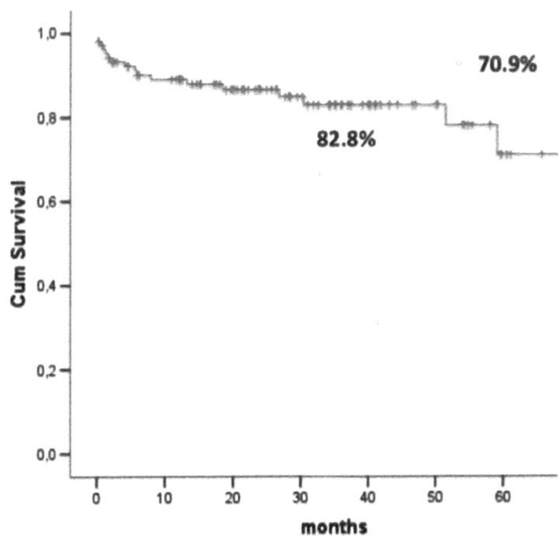

months	0	12	24	36	48	60
N at risk	104	81	55	34	19	9
Survival %	100	89	86.5	82.8	82.8	70.9
St. Error %	-	3.1	3.5	4.2	4.2	8.8

FIGURE 4.—Survival in 104 patients with aortic arch debranching. (Reprinted from De Rango P, Cao P, Ferrer C, et al. Aortic arch debranching and thoracic endovascular repair. *J Vasc Surg*. 2014; 59:107-114, with permission from The Society for Vascular Surgery.)

TABLE 2.—Technical Details in 104 Arch Debranching Procedures

Technical Details	No. (%)	Procedure Description
Staged procedure	59 (56.7)	
Zone 0	19 (18.3)	16 total surgical debranching 1 single (innominate) chimney stent graft + Car-Car-Subcl 1 single (innominate) branched stent graft + Car-Car-Subcl 1 triple chimney stent graft
Zone 1	51 (49.0)	Surgical bypass/transposition: 37 Car-Car-Subcl (20 retropharyngeal; 17 ante-trachea) 2 Car-Car (ante-trachea) 6 Car-Subcl (bovine arch) 6 bilateral Car-Subcl: 4 aberrant Subcl 2 aberrant Subcl + bovine arch
Zone 2	34 (32.7)	31 Car-Subcl 3 single (left Subcl) chimney stent graft
Number of aortic stent grafts/repairs[a]	150/103	(1 patient died after 1° stage) 59 Single stent graft 39: Two aortic stent grafts 4: Three aortic stent grafts 1: Four aortic stent grafts

Car, Carotid; *Car-Car*, right common carotid-left common carotid surgical bypass; *Car-Car-Subcl*, right common carotid-left common carotid-left subclavian surgical bypass/transposition; *Car-Subcl*, common carotid-subclavian surgical bypass/transposition; *Subcl*, subclavian; *TEVAR*, thoracic endovascular aortic repair.

In two patients, left subclavian arteries not revascularized because of urgency or direct vertebral revascularization.

[a]Device models employed in the 103 TEVARs included: 46 Cook Zenith, 22 Gore TAG-C-TAG, 26 Medtronic Talent/Valiant, 9 Bolton Relay.

TABLE 3.—Perioperative (30-day) Major Outcomes in 104 Arch Debranching Procedures

Outcome Measure	No.	%
Mortality	6	5.8
Stroke	4	3.8
Spinal cord ischemia	3	2.9
Technical success	100	97.1
Retrograde de novo type A dissection	4	3.8
• 1 intraoperative for zone 0 repair[a]		
• 3 perioperative		
○ 2 lethal for zone 0 repairs[b]		
○ 1 for zone 1 repair @10 days (successfully treated)		

[a]One intraoperative dissection occurred at the time of debranching and was successfully treated with ascending aorta replacement followed by thoracic endovascular repair (TEVAR).

[b]One lethal dissection occurred in a staged procedure after the first and TEVAR stage was not performed; the second lethal dissection occurred after a single stage procedure.

The highlight of this study is that total debranching (Zone 0 landing) accounted for a 30-day mortality risk significantly higher compared with the partial debranching group (odds ratio, 11.1; 95% confidence interval, 1.86–65.90; $P = .010$). However, the 30-day risk of stroke and of spinal cord ischemia was not significantly different among groups. Zone 0 landing was confirmed as the single independent predictor of death. Wide confidence intervals limit the predictive value of these results, but they are compelling nonetheless.

B. W. Starnes, MD

Reference

1. Mitchell RS, Ishimaru S, Ehrlich MP, et al. First international summit on thoracic aortic endografting: roundtable on thoracic aortic dissection as an indication for endografting. *J Endovasc Ther*. 2002;9:I98-II105.

Fenestrated and branched endovascular aortic repair for chronic type B aortic dissection with thoracoabdominal aneurysms

Kitagawa A, Greenberg RK, Eagleton MJ, et al (Cleveland Clinic Foundation, OH)
J Vasc Surg 58:625-634, 2013

Objective.—The treatment of patients with arch and thoracoabdominal aortic aneurysms (TAAAs) and chronic dissections is challenging. We report the results of fenestrated and branched endovascular aortic repair (FEVAR) of such aneurysms.

Methods.—A single-center prospective FEVAR trial enrolled 356 patients (2006 to 2011), of whom 30 had chronic dissections with arch aneurysm or TAAAs, or both. Patients were divided into group A, 15 patients (mean age, 58 years) with extensive dissections extending from the arch through the visceral segment, and group B, 15 patients (mean age, 74 years old) with focal dissections and no extension into the thoracic aorta. Inclusion criterion was aneurysm size > 5.5 cm in diameter. Customized grafts were implanted into the true lumen, and branches were

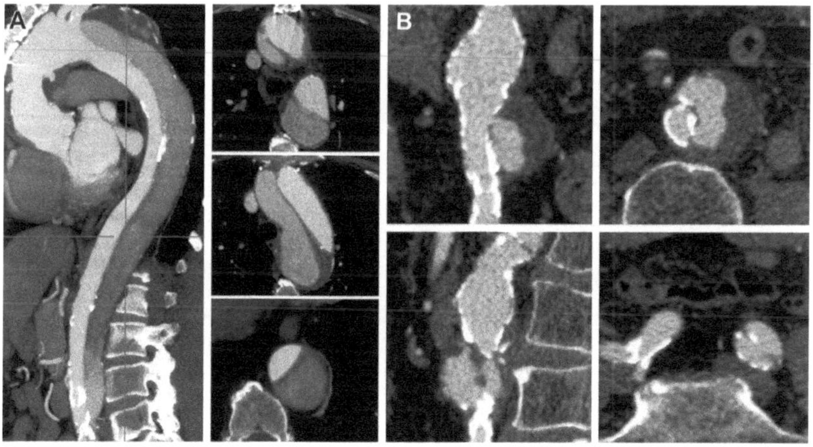

FIGURE 1.—The classification of chronic type B aortic dissection. **A**, *left panel*, Extensive dissection is defined as an aortic dissection extending from the arch (*right upper panel*) through the visceral segments (*right middle and lower panels*) with type II or type III thoracoabdominal aortic aneurysm (TAAA). If the arch was also involved in aneurysmal change with the TAAA, the extent of the aortic disease is classified as "extensive aorta." **B**, Focal dissection is defined as an aortic dissection limited to an intimal tear that abutted the visceral segment (*upper left and upper right panels*) that may extend into the iliac vessels (*lower right panel*) but not into the thoracic aorta (*lower left panel*). (Reprinted from Kitagawa A, Greenberg RK, Eagleton MJ, et al. Fenestrated and branched endovascular aortic repair for chronic type B aortic dissection with thoracoabdominal aneurysms. *J Vasc Surg*. 2013;58:625-634, Copyright 2013, with permission from The Society for Vascular Surgery.)

extended into the true lumen of the supra-aortic trunk (arch branch devices) and visceral vessels. Patients were monitored annually with clinical, imaging, and laboratory studies. Outcome analyses included survival, rupture, spinal cord ischemia, endoleak, morbidity (cardiac, renal or pulmonary), reinterventions, dissection, and aneurysm growth.

Results.—The mean time from the onset of dissection to the FEVAR performed in group A was 10.4 years. The mean maximum aneurysm diameter was 60 mm. Follow-up averaged 1.7 years. There were no perioperative

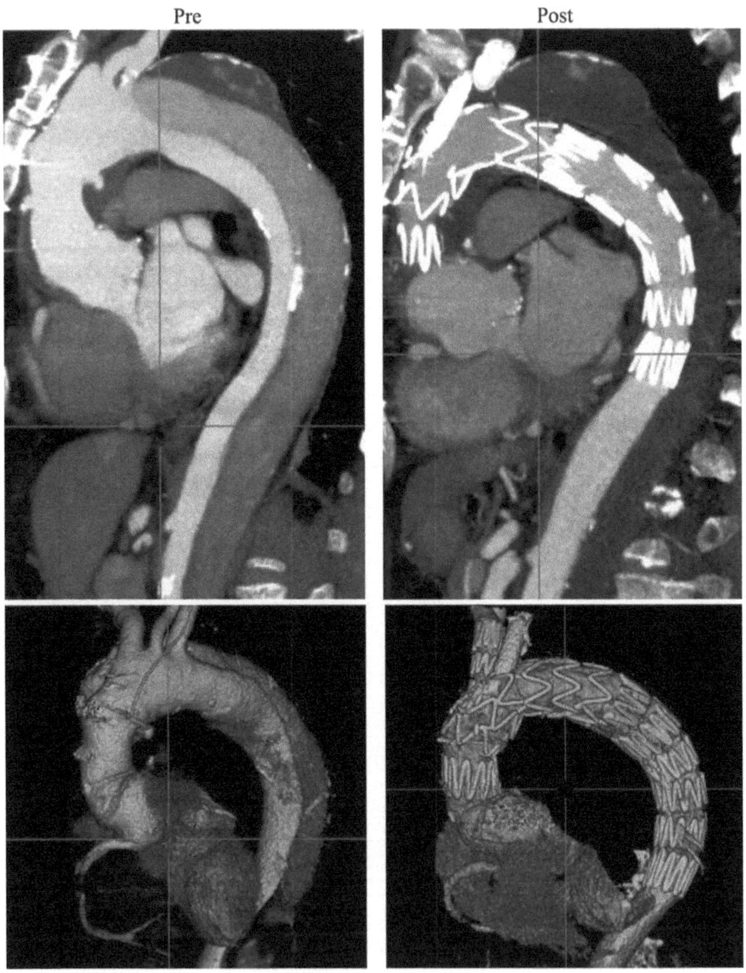

FIGURE 2.—Fenestrated and branched endovascular aortic repair (FEVAR) for chronic type B dissection extending from arch to descending thoracic and thoracoabdominal aorta (extensive dissection) with branched arch graft are shown in preoperative and postoperative (**top**) computed tomography (CT) and (**bottom**) volume-rendered images. (Reprinted from Kitagawa A, Greenberg RK, Eagleton MJ, et al. Fenestrated and branched endovascular aortic repair for chronic type B aortic dissection with thoracoabdominal aneurysms. *J Vasc Surg*. 2013;58:625-634, Copyright 2013, with permission from The Society for Vascular Surgery.)

deaths. One aortic-related death occurred at 87 days due to progression of a pre-existing untreated arch dissection. No ruptures, cardiac, renal, pulmonary, or spinal cord ischemia complications occurred. Despite the initially narrow true lumen dimensions, stent grafts expanded to their nominal diameters after implantation without any blood flow disturbance of branched visceral vessels and distal aorta. No graft compression occurred. Post-FEVAR growth was noted in two patients, related to type II endoleaks. Sac regression was similar (−6.8 vs −11.4 mm; $P = .43$), but early endovascular reinterventions were more common in group A (8 patients). Patients with extensive dissection were younger, and the dissection more likely to be associated with a defined connective tissue disease (Marfan syndrome or Loeys-Dietz mutations, 40% vs 0%; $P = .006$).

Conclusions.—FEVAR is feasible for patients with chronic dissections and TAAA. Concerns regarding visceral vessel access and graft compression resulting from narrow true lumen diameters were not relevant in our experience. Favorable sac and lumen morphologic changes, coupled with a low mortality and complication risk, makes this an attractive means of handling this clinical problem (Figs 1-3, Table 2 and 3).

▶ Our current knowledge regarding the optimal therapeutic approach in aortic dissection comes from studies involving the thoracic aorta. This is a single-center report on isolated acute abdominal aortic dissection (IAAAD)—considered a relatively rare entity. I chose this report to review because it hones in on certain features of this disease process that deserve mention and because it is the largest series, albeit small, of endovascular repair for IAAAD.

The natural history of IAAAD is unknown. IAAAD has generally been considered a rare event, accounting for only 1% to 4% of all aortic dissections.

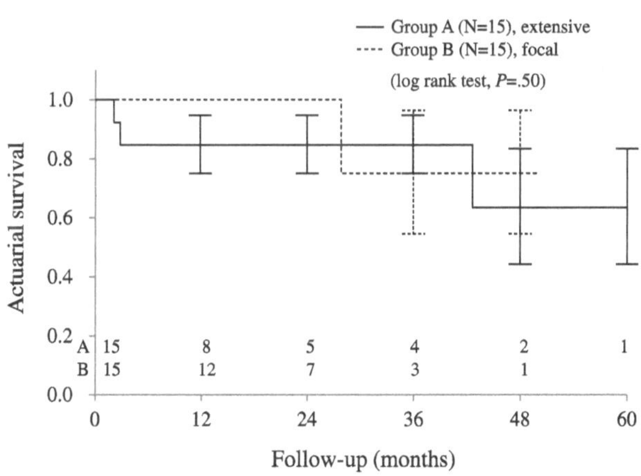

FIGURE 3.—Actuarial survival curves of fenestrated and branched endovascular aortic repair (FEVAR) in the Kaplan-Meier analysis are shown for group A (n = 15; *black line*) and group B (n = 15; *dotted line*), with the *error bars* showing the standard error. (Reprinted from Kitagawa A, Greenberg RK, Eagleton MJ, et al. Fenestrated and branched endovascular aortic repair for chronic type B aortic dissection with thoracoabdominal aneurysms. *J Vasc Surg*. 2013;58:625-634, Copyright 2013, with permission from The Society for Vascular Surgery.)

TABLE 2.—Endoleaks after Fenestrated and Branched Endovascular Aortic Repair (FEVAR) for Chronic type B Aortic Dissection in Group A (no Endoleaks in Group B)

Endoleak	Group A (Extensive) (n = 15) No. (%)	
Primary	10 (66.7)[a]	
Type I	5 (33.3)	
Type IA	1 (6.7)	Proximal landing zone
Type IB	4 (26.6)	Iliac landing zone
		Hypogastric branch distal
Type II	5 (33.3)	Renal branch
		Celiac branch
		SMA branch
Secondary	1 (6.7)	Renal branch

SMA, Superior mesenteric artery.
[a]Staged endoleaks (two endoleaks were found separately) (n = 3).

TABLE 3.—Reinterventions after Fenestrated and Branched Endovascular Aortic Repair (FEVAR) for Chronic Type B Aortic Dissection in Group A (no Reinterventions in Group B)

Reintervention	Group A (Extensive) (n = 15) No.	Repair
First reintervention	8	Iliac leg extension
Type I	5	Hypogastric interruption
		Re-TEVAR
Type III	3	Celiac artery stent
		Renal artery re-PTA
		SMA stent
Second reintervention	4	
Type III	4	Renal artery stent with IMA CE[a]
		Renal artery stent
		Renal artery re-PTA
		Translumbar CE with plug
Third reintervention	2	
Type II	2	Translumbar CE

CE, Coil embolization; *IMA*, inferior mesenteric artery; *PTA*, percutaneous transluminal angioplasty; *TEVAR*, thoracic endovascular aortic repair.
[a]Coil or glue embolization.

In this study, a whopping 37% of all patients presented with aortic dissection. Despite this aberrancy, the authors adopted an aggressive treatment protocol consisting of the following factors:

(1) unrelenting pain, defined as pain not amenable to analgesic treatment, even opioids, for more than 48 hours and

(2) size greater than 3 cm.

This is in keeping with recommendations from other notable authors. The authors used several endografts to manage IAAAD and suggest the routine use of bifurcated endografts with active fixation (Fig 3). I must admit that I have not used a size threshold of only 3 cm as an indication for elective repair in these patients but after reading the discussion of this report, I plan to do so.

B. W. Starnes, MD

9 Aortoiliac Disease and Leg Ischemia

The use of cryopreserved aortoiliac allograft for aortic reconstruction in the United States

Harlander-Locke MP, Harmon LK, Lawrence PF, et al (Univ of California Los Angeles; et al)

J Vasc Surg 59:669-674.e1, 2014

Background.—Aortic infections, even with treatment, have a high mortality and risk of recurrent infection and limb loss. Cryopreserved aortoiliac allograft (CAA) has been proposed for aortic reconstruction to improve outcomes in this high-risk population.

Methods.—A multicenter study using a standardized database was performed at 14 of the 20 highest volume institutions that used CAA for aortic reconstruction in the setting of infection or those at high risk for prosthetic graft infection.

Results.—Two hundred twenty patients (mean age, 65; male:female, 1.6/1) were treated since 2002 for culture positive aortic graft infection (60%), culture negative aortic graft infection (16%), enteric fistula/erosion (15%), infected pseudoaneurysm adjacent to the aortic graft (4%), and other (4%). Intraop cultures indicated infection in 66%. Distal anastomosis was to the femoral artery and iliac. Mean hospital length of stay was 24 days, and 30-day mortality was 9%. Complications occurred in 24% and included persistent sepsis (n = 17), CAA thrombosis (n = 9), CAA rupture (n = 8), recurrent CAA/aortic infection (n = 8), CAA pseudoaneurysm (n = 6), recurrence of aortoenteric fistula (n = 4), and compartment syndrome (n = 1). Patients with full graft excision had significantly better outcomes. Ten (5%) patients required allograft explant. Mean follow-up was 30 ± 3 months. Freedom from graft-related complications, graft explant, and limb loss was 80%, 88%, and 97%, respectively, at 5 years. Primary graft patency was 97% at 5 years, and patient survival was 75% at 1 year and 51% at 5 years.

Conclusions.—This largest study of CAA indicates that CAA allows aortic reconstruction in the setting of infection or those at high risk for infection with lower early and long-term morbidity and mortality than other previously reported treatment options. Repair with CAA is associated with low rates of aneurysm formation, recurrent infection, aortic blowout,

TABLE 1.—Initial Aortic Procedure Indications

Indication	No.	% of Total Patients
Abdominal aortic aneurysm	165	75
Suprarenal	6	
Infrarenal	159	
Occlusive disease	51	23
Aortic	9	
Aortic + iliac(s)	42	
Trauma- aorta	2	1
Atheroembolism from aorta	1	.5
Iatrogenic aortic injury	1	.5
Type of procedure		
Open reconstruction	209	95
Endovascular	11	5

TABLE 3.—Organisms Identified from Intraoperative Cultures of Resected Prior Aortic Graft

Organism	No.	% of Total Patients
Culture negative	75	34
Methicillin-sensitive *staphylococcus aureus*	21	10
Polymicrobial	21	10
Methicillin-resistant *staphylococcus aureus*	14	6
Escherichia coli	13	6
Pseudomonas	10	5
Staphylococcus sp	9	4
Enterococcus sp	8	4
Propionibacterium acnes	6	3
Vancomycin resistant enterococcus	6	3
Streptococcus sp	6	3
Salmonella	4	2
Clostridium	4	2
Klebsiella	4	2
Corynebacterium sp	4	2
Bacteroides sp	4	2
Enterobacterium sp	4	2
Other	7	3

and limb loss. We believe that CAA should be considered a first line treatment of aortic infections (Tables 1 and 3).

▶ The purposes of this study were (1) to evaluate the safety and efficacy of cryopreserved aortoiliac allograft (CAA) for inline aortic reconstruction in patients with aortic graft infection and (2) to evaluate the US experience with CAA using a standardized, multi-institutional database. I am a big fan of CAA, and like these authors, I believe it should be considered as first-line therapy for patients with aortic graft infections.

Indications and techniques for initial aortic surgery are listed in Table 1. The mean time between the initial prosthetic aortic graft procedure and CAA implant was 7 months (range, 1–22 months). I found it interesting to look at the organisms responsible for the infections (Table 3).

This is the largest series of cryopreserved aortoiliac arterial allografts and represents approximately 25% of all CAAs implanted in the United States since commercial availability. The application of current cryopreservation techniques has been shown to preserve the integrity of the collagen matrix. CAA allows for inline reconstruction in the presence of infection, with lower patient morbidity and mortality than the results of other published treatment options. Furthermore, CAA is associated with low rates of aneurysm formation, allograft rupture, recurrent infection, and limb loss.

B. W. Starnes, MD

Endovascular treatment for isolated acute abdominal aortic dissection

Kouvelos GN, Vourliotakis G, Arnaoutoglou E, et al (Univ of Ioannina, Greece; 401 General Military Hosp of Athens, Greece)

J Vasc Surg 58:1505-1511, 2013

Background.—Isolated acute abdominal aortic dissection (IAAAD) is considered an unusual clinical entity and is traditionally treated by open surgical repair. We report our single-center experience during the last 9 years, evaluating the outcomes after endovascular repair in this patient population.

Methods.—All patients with a diagnosis of IAAAD treated in our institute were included in this retrospective review. Between January 2004 and December 2012, 38 patients suffering from an acute aortic dissection were referred regionally for intervention to our department: 24 (63.2%) with a thoracic aortic dissection type B and 14 patients (36.8%, all male; median age, 65 years) with an IAAAD. Demographics, perioperative, procedure-specific, and follow-up data were prospectively aggregated in an electronic database.

Results.—Patients suffering from IAAAD presented with acute abdominal pain (n = 13) and acute lumbar pain (n = 1). Insufferable pain and enlargement of the aorta were the main indications for treatment. Mean (± standard deviation) maximal abdominal aortic diameter at presentation was 3.5 ± 0.94 cm (range, 2.6-5.1 cm). None of these patients had a concomitant thoracic aortic dissection. All patients were treated by endovascular means, with a primary technical success rate of 100%. Two patients (14%) died perioperatively from cardiac causes. Median hospital stay was 4.5 days (range, 3-16 days). During a mean follow-up period of 37.41 ± 23.56 months (range, 8-82 months; median, 32.5 months), two patients experienced primary treatment failure needing reintervention that led to a successful outcome. The cumulative free-from-reintervention rate was estimated 90.9% at 58 months (standard error, 8.7%). A full aortic remodeling without any events was noted in all other patients during the follow-up period.

Conclusions.—Based on our series, IAAAD may represent a not so rare clinical entity as generally thought, suggesting that it may be underdiagnosed. Endovascular treatment of IAAAD appears to be a feasible and

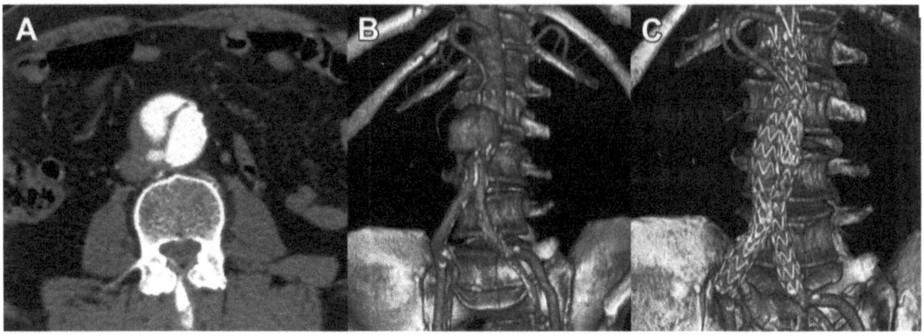

FIGURE 3.—A and B, Axial images and three-dimensional reconstruction of computed tomography angiography (CTA) showing a dissection of the infrarenal aorta. C, Postoperative result 12 months after the deployment of a stent graft with suprarenal fixation. (Reprinted from Kouvelos GN, Vourliotakis G, Arnaoutoglou E, et al. Endovascular treatment for isolated acute abdominal aortic dissection. *J Vasc Surg*. 2013;58:1505-1511, with permission from The Society for Vascular Surgery.)

efficient therapeutic approach and might be considered as the first-line treatment in all patients with suitable anatomy (Fig 3).

► Our current knowledge regarding the optimal therapeutic approach in aortic dissection comes from studies involving the thoracic aorta. This is a single-center report on isolated acute abdominal aortic dissection (IAAAD), which is considered a relatively rare entity. I chose this article to review because it hones in on certain features of this disease process that deserve mention and because it is the largest series, albeit small, of endovascular repair for IAAAD.

The natural history of IAAAD is unknown. It has generally been considered a rare event, accounting for only 1% to 4% of all aortic dissections.[1] In this study, a whopping 37% of all patients presented with aortic dissection. Despite this aberrancy, the authors adopted an aggressive treatment protocol consisting of the following factors:

(1) unrelenting pain, defined as pain not amenable to analgesic treatment, even opioids, for >48 hours and

(2) size >3 cm.

This is in keeping with recommendations from other notable authors.[2] The authors used a variety of endografts to manage IAAAD and suggest the routine use of bifurcated endografts with active fixation (Fig 3). I must admit that I have not used a size threshold of only 3 cm as an indication for elective repair in these patients, but after reading the discussion of this article, I plan to do so.

B. W. Starnes, MD

References

1. Trimarchi S, Tsai T, Eagle KA, et al. International Registry of Acute Aortic Dissection (IRAD) Investigators. Acute abdominal aortic dissection: insight from the International Registry of Acute Aortic Dissection (IRAD). *J Vasc Surg*. 2007;46:913-919.
2. Farber A, Wagner WH, Cossman DV, et al. Isolated dissection of the abdominal aorta: clinical presentation and therapeutic options. *J Vasc Surg*. 2002;36:205-210.

A new technique for reconstruction of the aortic bifurcation with saphenous vein panel graft

Mallios A, Boura B, Alomran F, et al (Institut Mutualiste Montsouris, Paris, France)

J Vasc Surg 59:511-515, 2014

A 60-year-old male patient presented with a false aneurysm of the common iliac artery and methicillin-resistant *Staphylococcus aureus* septicemia complicating previously placed kissing covered stents of the aortic bifurcation. We removed the prosthetic material and repaired the aortic bifurcation with a composite saphenous vein panel graft. To our knowledge, this technique is presented for the first time in the literature (Figs 2, 4 and 5).

▶ This is a useful technique for aortoiliac reconstruction using only saphenous vein. The neoaortoiliac system procedure using femoropopliteal vein has been used for these types of reconstructions but associated with long operative times and postoperative morbidity that is not insignificant.[1,2] The authors provide a useful formula for calculating the required length of saphenous vein needed for reconstruction (Fig 2). Sometimes pictures tell the whole story. Refer to Figs 4 and 5. Note the unique folded central patch.

B. W. Starnes, MD

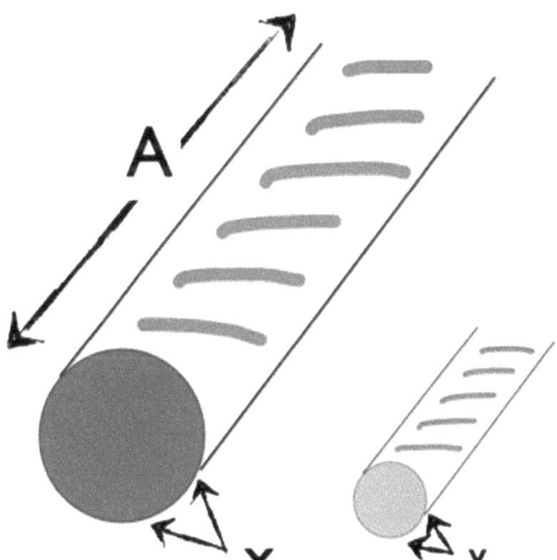

FIGURE 2.—Illustration of the parameters A, X, and Y that define the necessary length of venous graft. The length (L) of the GSV required can be estimated using the equation: L = (A)(X/Y).; where *A* is the length of the vessel or graft that needs to be replaced, *X* is the perimeter of the vessel or graft that needs to be replaced, and *Y* is the perimeter of the saphenous vein. (Reprinted from Mallios A, Boura B, Alomran F, et al. A new technique for reconstruction of the aortic bifurcation with saphenous vein panel graft. *J Vasc Surg*. 2014;59:511-515, with permission from The Society for Vascular Surgery.)

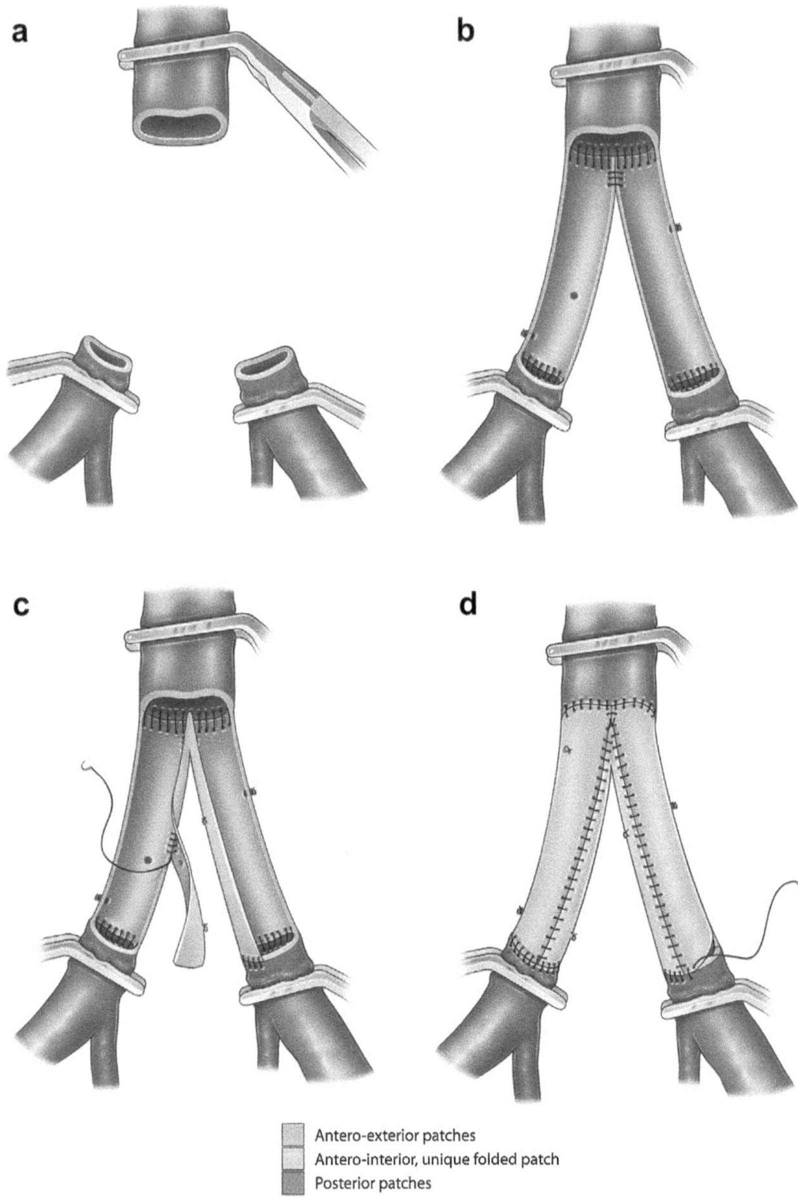

FIGURE 4.—Illustration of the reconstruction. **a**, Before suturing; **b**, after suturing the posterior patches; **c**, after suturing the unique antero-interior patch; and **d**, final view after suturing the antero-exterior patches. (Reprinted from Mallios A, Boura B, Alomran F, et al. A new technique for reconstruction of the aortic bifurcation with saphenous vein panel graft. *J Vasc Surg*. 2014;59:511-515, with permission from The Society for Vascular Surgery.)

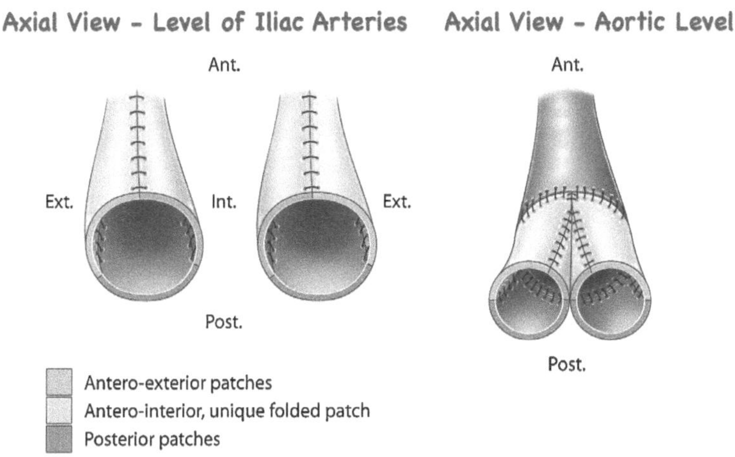

FIGURE 5.—Illustration of the reconstruction, axial view at the iliac (*left*) and aortic (*right*) level. *Ant*, Anterior; *Ext*, exterior; *Int*, interior; *Post*, posterior. (Reprinted from Mallios A, Boura B, Alomran F, et al. A new technique for reconstruction of the aortic bifurcation with saphenous vein panel graft. *J Vasc Surg*. 2014;59:511-515, with permission from The Society for Vascular Surgery.)

References

1. Beck AW, Murphy EH, Hocking JA, Timaran CH, Arko FR, Clagett GP. Aortic reconstruction with femoral-popliteal vein: graft stenosis, incidence, risk and reintervention. *J Vasc Surg*. 2008;47:36-43.
2. Ali AT, Mondrall JG, Hocking J, et al. Long term results of the treatment of aortic graft infection by in situ replacement with femoral popliteal vein grafts. *J Vasc Surg*. 2009;50:30-39.

Results of iliac stenting and aortofemoral grafting for iliac artery occlusions

Sachwani GR, Hans SS, Khoury MD, et al (St. John Providence Health System, Detroit, MI; et al)

J Vasc Surg 57:1030-1037, 2013

Objective.—To compare long-term results of percutaneous iliac artery stenting (PCIS) with aortobifemoral (ABF) grafting for patients with symptomatic iliac artery occlusions.

Methods.—A retrospective review of 229 patients (January 2000 to December 2011) with symptomatic iliac artery occlusions was performed. In 100 patients, 103 PCIS procedures were performed, and 101 patients underwent ABF grafting. Outcome data including periprocedural complications, improvement in ankle-brachial index, morbidity, and mortality were collected in a vascular registry. Kaplan-Meier estimates for patency and survival were analyzed. Univariate (Fisher exact test) and multivariate analyses of variables associated with the loss of primary patency were performed.

Results.—Patients in the ABF grafting group were younger (60 ± 0.9 years old vs 65 ± 1.2 years old; $P=.002$) and more commonly had a history of nicotine abuse (97% vs 86%; $P=.002$), chronic obstructive pulmonary disease (85% vs 70%; $P=.02$), and a greater incidence of superficial femoral artery disease (45% vs 24%; $P=.001$). The most common presenting symptoms in both groups consisted of intermittent claudication (66% ABF vs 71% PCIS), rest pain (20% ABF vs 17% PCIS), and ulceration or gangrene of toes (14% ABF vs 15% PCIS). At 72 months, the primary patency for ABF bypass was greater than for PCIS (91% vs 73%; $P=.010$). Secondary patency rates were equivalent in both groups (98% ABF vs 85% PCIS). Survival in the ABF bypass group was significantly greater than in the PCIS group (76% vs 68%; $P=.013$). Hyperlipidemia (hazard ratio, 2.55; $P=.049$) and concurrent superficial femoral artery lesion (hazard ratio, 2.61; $P=.026$) were factors associated with the loss of primary patency for the entire cohort. The average hospital stay was 7 ± 2 days in the ABF group and 1 ± 0.3 days in the PCIS group ($P=.0001$). There were no periprocedural deaths in the PCIS group; there were four deaths in the ABF group ($P=.058$). In the PCIS group, ankle-brachial index increased from 0.66 to 0.89, and in the ABF group, ankle-brachial index increased from 0.54 to 0.98 (both groups, $P<.001$).

Conclusions.—This study demonstrates that PCIS remains a suitable, less invasive first-line therapy for iliac artery occlusions. PCIS has lower morbidity, shorter hospital length of stay, and equivalent secondary patency but inferior primary patency compared with ABF.

▶ The standard considerations of percutaneous iliac intervention (PSCIS) versus open aortobifemoral surgery (ABF), vis-à-vis patient recovery versus durability, echo many of the prescient comparisons of open abdominal aortic aneurysm repair and endovascular aneurysm repair. Consequently, what does the work of Sachwani and colleagues contribute to the well-worn debate? First, a modern comparison of contemporary aortic surgery and perioperative management to endovascular techniques is needed, and herein they deliver just that. Next, on multivariate analysis, for the ABF group, there were no predictors of loss of primary patency; this would suggest a durable intervention. Next, the lack of superficial femoral artery runoff hurt primary patency only in the PCIS group, which suggests that ABF may better handle concomitant femoral disease. Secondary patency is achieved equally by ABF and PCIS. The study has some time biases given that 70% of the ABFs were performed in the first 6 years of the study interval, but refinements in open surgery are likely minimal in the decade. Ultimately, the choice to proceed from ABF to PCIS is often driven by the patient, and this article lends credence to the value of both propositions.

J. Black, MD, FACS

Antegrade Eversion Endarterectomy of the External Iliac Artery

Nagy GC, Wunsch M, Jordan A, et al (St. Bernward Hosp, Hildesheim, Germany; Queen Elisabeth Hosp, Berlin, Germany; DRK Kliniken Berlin Köpenick, Germany; et al)

Eur J Vasc Endovasc Surg 46:103-109, 2013

Objective.—We describe and present the results of our novel technique for eversion endarterectomy of the external iliac artery (EIA).

Methods.—For our prospective follow-up study, antegrade eversion endarterectomy (AEEA) of the EIA was mostly performed as a bail-out procedure, if (endovascular-assisted) remote endarterectomy from the groin had failed. Postoperative clinical and hemodynamic changes were reported according to the recommendations of the Society for Vascular Surgery. To evaluate the data, we used the Kaplan-Meier product limit method.

Results.—Thirty patients (mean age 65.5 years) underwent AEEA on 33 EIAs for atherosclerotic occlusive disease over a 10-year period. The mean follow-up was 50 months. The primary technical success rate was 100%. The 30-day mortality was 0. There were no early occlusions. Two patients required redo surgery for retroperitoneal haematomas. Postoperative improvement was marked in 30%, moderate in 64% and minimal in 6%, explained by 21 (64%) concomitant occlusions of the superficial femoral arteries. The 1-, 3- and 5-year primary patency rates were 100%, 96% and 90%, and primary assisted patency rates were 100%, 96% and 96% respectively. Fourteen patients (47%) died during the long follow-up period from unrelated causes.

Conclusion.—AEEA is a safe autologous surgical technique with promising results.

▶ The technique of iliac endarterectomy has evolved over the decades, and the increasing use of aortoiliac endovascular therapy has further limited the role of direct surgical reconstruction. Yet there are many situations in which the authors' technique of performing antegrade iliac eversion endarterectomy may have merit over extra-anatomic bypass. First, in the older patient with diffuse iliac disease, using a contralateral iliac for inflow for femoral-femoral bypass may yield onset of symptoms in the other leg. Second, eversion techniques use the external iliac artery, and in reoperative groin surgery in which there is a risk of infection and lymphatic fistula, the autogenous reconstruction is advantageous. As with any eversion technique, control of the endpoint is the key, and this technique is easily married to common femoral endarterectomy and patching. I do suspect caution is to be considered in proximal control, and the diffuse nature of iliac occlusive disease can limit safe clamping of a severely calcified distal common iliac artery to start the eversion technique.

J. Black, MD

Cutting-Balloon Angioplasty Versus Balloon Angioplasty as Treatment for Short Atherosclerotic Lesions in the Superficial Femoral Artery: Randomized Controlled Trial

Poncyljusz W, Falkowski A, Safranow K, et al (Pomeranian Med Univ, Szczecin, Poland; et al)

Cardiovasc Intervent Radiol 36:1500-1507, 2013

Purpose.—To evaluate the treatments of a short-segment atherosclerotic stenosis in the superficial femoral arteries with the cutting balloon angioplasty (CBA) versus conventional balloon angioplasty [percutaneous transluminal angioplasty (PTA)] in a randomized controlled trial.

Material and Methods.—The study group comprised 60 patients (33 men, 27 women; average age 64 years) with a short (≤5 cm) focal SFA *de novo* atherosclerotic stenosis associated with a history of intermittent claudication or rest pain. The primary end point of this study was the rate of binary restenosis in the treated segment 12 months after the intervention. All patients were evenly randomized to either the PTA or CBA treatment arms. Follow-up angiograms and ankle–brachial index (ABI) measurements were performed after 12 months. The evaluation of the restenosis rates and factors influencing its occurrence were calculated by logistic regression analysis.

Results.—In the intention-to-treat analysis, restenosis rates after 2-month follow-up were 9 of 30 (30 %) in the PTA group and 4 of 30 (13 %) in the CBA group ($p = 0.117$). In the actual treatment analysis, after exclusion of patients who required nitinol stent placement for a suboptimal result after angioplasty alone (5 patients in the PTA group and none in the CBA group), restenosis rates were 9 of 25 (36 %) and 4 of 30 (13 %), respectively ($p = 0.049$). In the intention-to-treat analysis there were also significant differences in ABI values between the PTA and CBA groups at 0.77 ± 0.11 versus 0.82 ± 0.12, respectively ($p = 0.039$), at 12 months.

Conclusion.—Based on the presented results of the trial, CBA seems to be a safer and more effective than PTA for treatment of short atherosclerotic lesions in the superior femoral artery.

▶ Percutaneous balloon angioplasty (PTA) with selective stenting has long been the initial treatment of choice for short segment lesions (< 5 cm) in the superficial femoral artery (SFA). In fact, Trans-Atlantic Inter-Society Consensus II recommendations are largely based on PTA with selective stenting. In this study, the authors compare PTA with cutting balloon angioplasty (CBA) to treat de novo, short segment lesions of the SFA in patients with claudication or rest pain. Patients underwent ABIs at 1 month and repeat angiography at 12 months to assess patency.

In the PTA group ($n = 30$), 5 patients (13%) required stents at the initial procedure for suboptimal results. In the CBA group ($n = 30$), no patients required stents at the initial procedure. Comparing the PTA alone and the CBA group at 1 year, angiography demonstrated a restenosis rate of 36% in the PTA alone group and 13% in the CBA group ($P = .049$). Additionally, ABI values were

0.77 and 0.82 for the PTA and CBA groups, respectively ($P = .039$). The authors suggest that a more controlled laceration of the plaque in the CBA group leads to a decreased inflammatory response and neointimal formation than the PTA alone group.

These results are promising and suggest that CBA should be considered as first-line therapy when treating short-segment lesions of the SFA. CBA has largely been ignored compared with the more glamorous drug-eluting balloon technology, but as suggested in this study, perhaps CBA should be included in larger studies focusing on the treatment of isolated, short lesions of the SFA.

B. Peterson, MD

A Quantitative Method for Evaluating Local Perfusion Using Indocyanine Green Fluorescence Imaging

Terasaki H, Inoue Y, Sugano N, et al (Tokyo Med and Dental Univ, Japan)
Ann Vasc Surg 27:1154-1161, 2013

Background.—The purpose of this study is to introduce a new method, indocyanine green fluorescence imaging (ICG-FI), as an adjunct to distal pressure measurements in patients with peripheral arterial disease and symptomatic lower limb ischemia.

Methods.—A total of 34 patients with peripheral arterial disease, including 11 with claudication (Fontaine II), 7 with rest pain (FIII), and 16 with an ulcer or gangrene (FIV), were enrolled. After an intravenous injection of ICG (0.1 mg/kg), foot perfusion was recorded by an infrared light camera. Fluorescence intensity was plotted on a time–intensity curve using recorded images, allowing the calculation of new parameters. Severity of ischemia was assessed as the duration between the rising point and half value of maximum brightness ($T_{½}$). The difference in the fluorescence intensity between 10 seconds after the rising point and baseline (PDE_{10}) was compared with the transcutaneous oxygen pressure ($tcPO_2$) at the same site ($n = 51$).

Results.—Median $T_{½}$ was 23 seconds in FII, 41 seconds in FIII ($P < 0.05$), and 17 seconds in FIV patients. PDE_{10} correlated moderately with $tcpO_2$ ($r^2 = 0.5$). A cut-off value ($PDE_{10} = 28$) predicted a critically ischemic limb (FIII and FIV), defined as $tcpO_2$ <30 mm Hg with a sensitivity of 100% and specificity of 86.6%.

Conclusions.—Local tissue perfusion can be quantitatively evaluated by using ICG fluorescence imaging. It is a safe, fast, noncontact method of imaging, which may be useful even at the ulcer itself and in the circumferential area.

▶ The purpose of this study was to determine whether indocyanine green (ICG) fluorescence imaging, would be a useful adjunct to distal pressure measurements in patients with peripheral arterial disease and symptomatic lower limb ischemia. The rationale for this analysis is based on the fact that toe pressure and tissue oxygen levels rely on contact with skin that may be jeopardized.

This technique requires intravenous injection of ICG, the intensity of which can be imaged noninvasively. These investigators show that there are statistically different characteristics in imaging intensity and washout in different levels of ischemia (claudication vs rest pain). Among the advantages of this new method is that it provides a dynamic image of the perfusion of the foot and shows ischemic patches in the foot area. It also provides a perfusion estimate for 1 specific site, as does transcutaneous oxygen tension, but does it without actually making contact with the skin. It may be most important to determine whether there is anatomic correlation between perfusion in the feet with the patency of the tibial vessels as detected with noninvasive imaging. Although these results are promising, the low numbers of patients studied limits my confidence that these data will be applicable to a larger patient population.

M. T. Watkins, MD

Agreement among observers in the assignment of TransAtlantic Inter-Society Consensus classification and runoff score

Wu TY, Giesler G, Herscu G, et al (Univ of Southern California, Pasadena, CA)
J Vasc Surg 58:1254-1258, 2013

Objective.—Productive communication among clinical practitioners is essential if recommendations regarding practice are to exist. The durability of vascular procedures is often influenced by factors such as lesion classification and runoff quality. It is the purpose of this article to determine how reproducible these measures are in the hands of various specialists who deal extensively with peripheral arterial disease.

Methods.—The peripheral arteriograms of 100 patients undergoing percutaneous intervention were distributed to six specialists (three vascular surgeons, two interventional radiologists, and one interventional cardiologist). Each was provided with the reference document describing TASC II classification, Society for Vascular Surgery (SVS) runoff score, and simplified runoff score. With no further instruction, each individual was asked to assign each angiogram a TASC II class, SVS runoff score, and a simplified runoff score. Comparisons between the scores assigned were made using kappa statistic.

Results.—When using the simplified runoff score for grading peripheral arterial disease, there was excellent correlation among readers ($k = 0.81$; $P = .001$), even across different specialties. When using TASC II class to grade lesions, there was a greater degree of variation when compared with the simplified runoff score ($k = 0.44$; $P < .05$). Finally, there was poor correlation between readers when using the SVS runoff score ($k = 0.10$; $P < .05$) and the modified SVS runoff score ($k = 0.26$; $P = .001$).

Conclusions.—Descriptors of clinical disease severity are not universally reproducible. The simplified runoff score is reproducible when interpreted by multiple readers across different specialties and can be used without further modification. The TASC II classification may need minor alterations in description to obtain good correlation among readers. Before the SVS runoff score can be universally adapted, it will need to be described in much better detail or significantly modified.

▶ It has been shown that lesion characteristics and distal runoff largely determine the outcome and long-term durability of peripheral open and endovascular interventions. Various lesion classification systems and distal runoffs scores exist, and this study attempts to evaluate the precision and accuracy of these classification systems. Specifically, this study evaluates the following: the simplified runoff score, the Trans-Atlantic Inter-Society Consensus (TASC) II classification, and the Society for Vascular Surgery (SVS) runoff score.

Eighty-eight angiograms from a single operator were reviewed by 6 physicians. Three of these physicians were vascular surgeons, 2 were interventional radiologists, and 1 was an interventional cardiologist. The kappa statistic measures precision and quantitatively reports the amount of agreement between observers. Using this methodology, the following results were reported. The overall agreement between observers using the simplified runoff score was 90.5%. The overall agreement between observers using the TASC II classification was 58.3%. Finally, the overall agreement between observers using the SVS scoring system was 17.4%.

This study clearly points out that considering the TASC II classification and SVS runoff scoring systems the gold standards for describing lower extremity lesion characteristics needs to be reevaluated. A significant amount of interobserver variation calls into question the validity of these classification systems and perhaps argues for the use of the simplified runoff score as the new gold standard.

B. Peterson, MD

Agreement among observers in the assignment of TransAtlantic Inter-Society Consensus classification and runoff score

Wu TY, Giesler G, Herscu G, et al (Univ of Southern California, Pasadena, CA)
J Vasc Surg 58:1254-1258, 2013

Objective.—Productive communication among clinical practitioners is essential if recommendations regarding practice are to exist. The durability of vascular procedures is often influenced by factors such as lesion classification and runoff quality. It is the purpose of this article to determine how reproducible these measures are in the hands of various specialists who deal extensively with peripheral arterial disease.

Methods.—The peripheral arteriograms of 100 patients undergoing percutaneous intervention were distributed to six specialists (three vascular surgeons, two interventional radiologists, and one interventional cardiologist). Each was provided with the reference document describing TASC II classification, Society for Vascular Surgery (SVS) runoff score, and simplified runoff score. With no further instruction, each individual was asked to assign each angiogram a TASC II class, SVS runoff score, and a simplified runoff score. Comparisons between the scores assigned were made using kappa statistic.

Results.—When using the simplified runoff score for grading peripheral arterial disease, there was excellent correlation among readers (k = 0.81; $P = .001$), even across different specialties. When using TASC II class to grade lesions, there was a greater degree of variation when compared with the simplified runoff score (k = 0.44; $P < .05$). Finally, there was poor correlation between readers when using the SVS runoff score (k = 0.10; $P < .05$) and the modified SVS runoff score (k = 0.26; $P = .001$).

Conclusions.—Descriptors of clinical disease severity are not universally reproducible. The simplified runoff score is reproducible when interpreted by multiple readers across different specialties and can be used without further modification. The TASC II classification may need minor alterations in description to obtain good correlation among readers. Before the SVS runoff score can be universally adapted, it will need to be described in much better detail or significantly modified (Table 2).

▶ Anatomic classification of peripheral arterial disease (PAD) is a topic that frequently generates lively discussion between providers, particularly when different systems are being used by individuals from different specialty backgrounds. The level of anatomic complexity for any given classification system is a key determinant of both reproducibility and clinical applicability. Simple approaches may have high levels of interobserver agreement but more limited ability to stratify likelihood of a treatment's success or durability. On the other hand, more detailed classification systems may provide greater precision at the expense of greater complexity and a corresponding increase in the number of opportunities for disagreement. Although the authors' assertion that simplicity should be favored unless a clear benefit is gained through greater complexity certainly makes sense, it is important to bear in mind that interobserver agreement does not necessarily reflect clinical utility or predictive value and that the scores being evaluated represent disease classification systems rather than simple diagnostic tests.

The results of this study underscore the significant limitations of existing approaches to anatomic PAD classification, which warrant consideration when these scores are used to stratify risk or guide treatment selection. Interobserver agreement was substantial for the simplified runoff score described by Ahn et al[1] but underwhelming for both the TransAtlantic Inter-Society Consensus (TASC) classification and Society for Vascular Surgery (SVS) runoff score

TABLE 2.—Agreement among the Different Specialties in the Assignment of TASC II Classification and Runoff Scores

	Simple	TASC II	Modified SVS
Vascular surgeons' kappa	0.891	0.473	0.202
Nonsurgeons' kappa	0.742	0.380	0.330
P value	.032	.289	.208

SVS, Society for Vascular Surgery; *TASC*, TransAtlantic Inter-Society Consensus.

(Table 2). The authors correctly note that agreement between unmodified SVS scores was only slightly better than would be expected from random number assignment, but it is important to remember that the kappa statistic does not account for the level of disagreement between observers; accordingly, SVS scores that were close but not identical might not represent the same level of disagreement as different scores within other systems with fewer ordinal categories. The apparent learning effect observed for the standard and modified SVS runoff scores (with greater percent agreement within the second half of angiograms interpreted) was not identified for the TASC II classification, possibly reflecting greater baseline provider familiarity with this approach.

Although many providers who treat PAD likely would not be surprised by the mediocre interobserver agreement observed in this study, the best approach to achieving greater consistency and reproducibility remains unclear. As suggested in the discussion, modification of the source documents for each scoring system to minimize ambiguity would potentially lead to decreased variability through improved user comprehension, but the systems were presumably developed with this consideration in mind, and no specific changes are suggested within the article. In addition to the systems themselves, some discrepancies are likely also the result of observer-specific factors such as specialty, experience, and relative enthusiasm toward various treatment alternatives. Although the authors attempt to address this question by comparing scores between observers from surgical versus nonsurgical training backgrounds, specialty representation among the small number of observers was 2:1 (3 surgeons, 2 interventional radiologists, and 1 cardiologist), limiting conclusions that can be made related to observer-specific factors and potentially biasing the results in favor of a vascular surgeon perspective.

M. Corriere, MD, MS

Reference

1. Ahn SS, Rutherford RB, Becker GJ, et al. Reporting standards for lower extremity arterial endovascular procedures. Society for Vascular Surgery/International Society for Cardiovascular Surgery. *J Vasc Surg*. 1993;17:1103-1107.

A Randomized Trial of Exercise Training in Abdominal Aortic Aneurysm Disease

Myers J, Mcelrath M, Jaffe A, et al (Veterans Affairs Palo Alto Health Care System, CA; et al)
Med Sci Sports Exerc 46:2-9, 2014

Purpose.—Screening programs and greater public awareness have increased the recognition of early abdominal aortic aneurysm (AAA) disease. No medical therapy has proven effective in limiting AAA progression, and little is known regarding the safety and efficacy of exercise training in these patients. We evaluated the safety and efficacy of up to 3 yr of training in patients with early (≤5.5 cm) AAA disease.

Methods.—One hundred and forty patients with small AAAs (72 ± 8 yr) were randomized to exercise training ($n = 72$) or usual care ($n = 68$). Exercise subjects participated in a combination of in-house and home training for up to 3 yr. Cardiopulmonary exercise testing (CPX) was performed at baseline and 3, 12, 24, and 36 months. Comparisons were made for AAA expansion, safety, CPX responses, and weekly energy expenditure.

Results.—The average duration of participation was 23.4 ± 9.6 months; 81% of subjects completed ≥1 year. No adverse clinical events or excessive AAA growth rates related to training occurred. Exercise subjects expended a mean 1999 ± 1030 $kcal \cdot wk^{-1}$. Increases in peak exercise time and estimated METs occurred at the 3-month and 1-, 2-, and 3-yr evaluations ($P < 0.01$ between groups). A significant between-group interaction occurred for $\dot{V}O2$ at the ventilatory threshold ($P = 0.02$), and submaximal heart rate was significantly reduced among exercise subjects. Neither exercise status nor level of fitness significantly influenced rate of AAA enlargement.

Conclusions.—These results support the safety and efficacy of training in patients with small AAA, a population for which few previous data are available. Despite advanced age and comorbidities, training up to 3 yr was well tolerated and sustainable in AAA patients. Training did not influence rate of AAA enlargement.

▶ Consensus guidelines recommend supervised exercise programs for patients with intermittent claudication. This study was designed to investigate the impact of treadmill-based supervised exercise training alone or in combination with lower limb resistance training on the primary outcome of pain-free walking distance and secondary outcomes of 6-minute walking distance, skeletal muscle mass, and calpain activity (measured by muscle biopsy). Calpain activity is known to be correlated with damage to muscle morphology and cell death. This study showed that supervised exercise training actually resulted in increased calpain activity and a reduction in skeletal muscle mass, which has potential detrimental long-term health outcomes. The addition of resistance training did not improve the walking distance but did ameliorate the reduction in skeletal muscle mass that was observed during supervised exercise training without resistance training. Calpain activity was not increased when resistance training was added to the regimen. Although this is a small study, these results suggest that supervised treadmill-based exercise as a treatment for intermittent claudication may be detrimental owing to the induction of catabolic muscle wasting. Resistance training, when added to the supervised exercise regimen, may decrease the muscle wasting. This study also showed that walking distance did not increase with or without resistance training. Thus, there appears to be a need for more extensive analysis of the effect of supervised walking regimens and consideration of local and systemic consequences of therapeutic ischemia reperfusion injury.

M. T. Watkins, MD

Comparison of two treadmill training programs on walking ability and endothelial function in intermittent claudication

Mika P, Konik A, Januszek R, et al (Univ School of Physical Education, Cracow, Poland; Jagiellonian Univ School of Medicine, Cracow, Poland; et al)

Int J Cardiol 168:838-842, 2013

Background.—In this randomized trial we compared two treadmill trainings, based on exercises performed to moderate claudication pain vs pain-free training, with respect to their effects on walking ability and endothelial function.

Methods.—A total of sixty patients with stable intermittent claudication were randomized to the pain-free treadmill training (repetitive intervals to onset of claudication pain) or moderate treadmill training (repetitive intervals to moderate claudication pain). In both groups exercises were performed 3 times a week for 3 months. Changes in flow mediated dilatation (FMD) and treadmill walking performance as well as plasma levels of C-reactive protein (hs-CRP) and fibrinogen were assessed before and after the program.

Results.—Fifty-two patients completed the training program. Post-training maximal walking time was prolonged by 100% ($p < 0.001$) vs 98% ($p < 0.001$), and pain-free walking time by 120% ($p < 0.001$) vs 93% ($p < 0.001$) in the moderate training group as compared to the pain-free training group, respectively. FMD increased by 56% ($p < 0.001$) in the moderate training group and by 36% ($p < 0.01$) in the pain-free training group. No significant changes in the levels of hs-CRP and fibrinogen were seen after treadmill program in either group.

Conclusions.—Both pain-free treadmill training and the moderate treadmill training have similar efficacy on walking ability in patients with claudication. The improvement of post-training FMD indicates systemic effect of both treadmill programs on endothelial function. Both programs appear to be safe therapeutic modes, since none of them escalates the inflammation. Pain-free treadmill training seems useful and effective therapeutic option for patients with claudication.

▶ This randomized controlled trial of the 2 types of exercise programs (pain-free walking [PFT] versus maximal time [MT]) shows similar improvement of endothelial function and walking ability regardless of the training method. The rationale for the study was prompted by the suggestion that repeated episodes of leg muscle pain followed by rest may lead to cumulative inflammatory response and disease progression in patients with claudication. The acute inflammatory response to strenuous exercise may also exacerbate endothelial dysfunction in patients with claudication, which paralleled with an increase of inflammation markers. In light of these, the pain-free treadmill training with exercises interrupted at the onset of claudication pain has been proposed as an effective and safe option for the treatment of patients with claudication. However, it has also been noticed that less optimal training response occurs when the patients stop at the onset of claudication before any pain develops. This study addressed the fact that no direct comparison between treadmill programs had been reported. This study showed significant improvement of 120% pain-free walking time (PFWT) and 100% maximal walking time (MWT) in the MT group as well as 93% PFWT and 98% MWT in the PFT group. This improvement of walking abilities did not statistically differ between groups. Similar findings were detected with respect to flow-mediated dilation between the 2 exercise regimens. The authors acknowledge that a major limitation of this study is the lack of a no-training control group and potential confounding effects of patients' medications on endothelial reactivity and walking ability. Nevertheless, this is an important report and needs to be repeated with appropriate controls.

M. T. Watkins, MD

Evaluation of Superficial Femoral Artery Remote Endarterectomy for Treatment of Critical Limb Ischemia in Patients with Limited Autogenous Conduit

Sheng N, Chiriano J, Teruya TH, et al (Loma Linda Univ Med Ctr, CA)
Ann Vasc Surg 28:262.e1-262.e7, 2014

Background.—Many patients with critical limb ischemia require infrageniculate bypass with a prosthetic graft due to the limited availability of autogenous vein. Prosthetic grafts have been shown to have inferior patency and subject the patient to increased infection rates when compared to bypass with autogenous conduit for lower extremity revascularization. In an effort to avoid the use of prosthetic material, we evaluated the use of remote superficial femoral artery endarterectomy (RSFAE) with distal autogenous revascularization in patients with critical limb ischemia and limited conduit.

Methods.—This study is a retrospective review of a prospectively maintained database from January 2009 to September 2011. All patients undergoing RSFAE for critical limb ischemia were identified. Patients undergoing RSFAE with simultaneous distal revascularization constituted the study group. Outcome variables, including patency, time to healing, limb salvage, ambulatory status, and survival, were analyzed.

Results.—Twenty-one patients underwent RSFAE at our institution. The study group was comprised of 5 patients undergoing RSFAE and adjunct distal revascularization for critical limb ischemia during the study period. Four patients (80%) presented with tissue loss, and 1 (20%) presented with ischemic rest pain. Three (60%) required simultaneous outflow sequential vein bypass and 2 (40%) required distal endovascular revascularization. The distal target vessels for bypass included the infrageniculate popliteal artery, posterior tibial artery, and peroneal artery. The mean operative time was 5.3 hours. The mean length of hospital stay was 8 days. Technical success was 100%, and there were no early reconstruction failures. There was 1 popliteal wound complication, and no groin wound complications during the study follow-up. At 6 months postoperatively, 4 of 5 reconstructions were patent. Two of 5 patients (40%) required percutaneous reintervention for restenosis at 10 and 11 months, respectively. Primary assisted patency was 80% with a mean follow-up of 12.6 months (range 8–22 months). The 4 patients with tissue loss achieved initial wound healing at a mean time of 4.8 months. The limb salvage rate was 80% and there have been no deaths.

Conclusions.—Remote superficial femoral artery endarterectomy with distal revascularization allows for autogenous reconstruction in patients with critical limb ischemia and compromised conduit by shortening bypass length. This procedure constitutes an appealing alternative to the use of synthetic material for lower extremity revascularization. Further study is needed to determine whether the long-term results are superior to distal composite bypass or polytetrafluoroethylene bypass alone.

▶ In this study, the authors present interesting data from a small group of patients in whom they used remote superficial femoral artery endarterectomy (RSFAE) with a distal revascularization procedure (either endovascular or short bypass) in patients with critical limb ischemia and limited autogenous conduit. Previous RSFAE studies did not focus on patient with critical limb ischemia, nor did they routinely include a distal revascularization procedure.

Here, the authors present a series of 5 patients with critical limb ischemia but without suitable saphenous vein conduit treated with RSFAE and distal revascularization. Characteristics of the lesions treated included flush SFA occlusions with reconstitution of the distal SFA or popliteal artery or mid-SFA and popliteal artery occlusions with tibial artery reconstitution. The results demonstrate primary patency at 6 months of 80% with the 1 occlusion leading to above-knee amputation. Two of the 5 patients developed restenosis requiring percutaneous reintervention at 10 and 11 months, leading to a primary assisted patency at 1 year of 80% and limb salvage rate of 80%.

Although this series is quite small, this article does present an interesting alternative for treating patients with critical limb ischemia and limited autogenous conduit. The authors present some helpful tips to improve initial technical success rates with remote endarterectomy. Specifically, they avoid RSFAE in patients with heavily calcified SFAs; they routinely address the distal endarterectomy site with angioplasty or stenting. Furthermore, if plaque retrieval is difficult despite using the endohelix instrument, they do not hesitate to perform a popliteal cutdown and complete the endarterectomy via a retrograde approach.

The limited number of patients in this series does not allow for significant conclusions to be made regarding this treatment approach, but this article does present an interesting alternative for this often difficult-to-treat patient population. Clearly, larger studies with comparison to endovascular treatment only, prosthetic or composite bypass, and upper extremity venous conduit are needed before more definitive treatment algorithms can be established.

B. Peterson, MD

Lower extremity arterial reconstruction for critical limb ischemia in diabetes

Ballotta E, Toniato A, Piatto G, et al (Univ of Padua, Padova, Italy)

J Vasc Surg 59:708-719, 2014

Background.—The impact of diabetes mellitus on the technical and clinical outcomes of infrainguinal arterial reconstruction (IAR) for critical limb ischemia (CLI) remains controversial. This study analyzed the outcome of IAR in diabetic patients with CLI over a 17-year period.

Methods.—Details on all consecutive patients undergoing primary IAR at our institution were stored prospectively in a vascular registry from 1995 to 2011. Demographics, risk factors, indications for surgery, inflow sources and outflow target vessels, types of conduit, and adverse outcomes were analyzed. Postoperative surveillance included clinical examination, duplex scans, and ankle-brachial index measurements in all patients at discharge, 1 and 6 months after surgery, and every 6 months thereafter. End points were patency, limb salvage, survival, and amputation-free survival rates, and were assessed using Kaplan-Meier life-table analysis. The χ^2 or Fisher exact, Student *t*, and log-rank tests were used to establish statistical significance.

Results.—Overall, 1407 IARs were performed in 1310 patients with CLI by the same surgeon, 705 (50.2%) in 643 diabetic patients and 702 in 667 nondiabetic patients. Autogenous vein conduits were used in 87% of the IARs. There were no perioperative deaths. Diabetic patients had significantly more major (16.7% vs 11.8%; $P = .02$) and minor complications (9.7% vs 6.5%; $P = .02$) than nondiabetic patients. At 5 and 10 years, there were no significant differences between diabetic and nondiabetic patients in the rates of primary patency (65% and 46% vs 69.5% and 57%; log-rank test, $P = .09$), secondary patency (76% and 60% vs 80% and 68%; log-rank test, $P = .20$), limb salvage (88% and 76% vs 91% and 83%; log-rank test, $P = .12$) survival (51% and 34% vs 57% and 38%; log-rank test, $P = .41$), or amputation-free survival (45.5% and 27% vs 51% and 29%; log-rank test, $P = .19$). The type of conduit did not affect patency or limb salvage rates in either group.

Conclusions.—Diabetic patients receiving IAR for CLI can have the same survival and amputation-free survival rates as nondiabetic patients. Their comparable technical and clinical outcomes strongly demonstrate that diabetics with CLI can expect the same quantity and quality of life as nondiabetics with CLI, and aggressive attempts at limb salvage in patients with diabetes mellitus, including distal and foot level bypass grafting, should not be discouraged.

▶ This report is of interest in that it prompts more questions than it answers. In an extensive study of outcomes after open infrainguinal reconstruction in more than 1400 patients for at least 7 years, these authors have an admirable outcome with respect to amputation-free survival, limb loss, complications, and mortality. These authors found no significant difference between diabetic and nondiabetic patients with respect to these important variables. Even with respect to perioperative cardiac events, there was no difference in the incidence between the diabetic and nondiabetic patients. This is likely because cardiac enzymes were only evaluated if there were obvious changes in the electrocardiogram. This is an insensitive measure of perioperative cardiac morbidity. It is possible that some of the reasons their outcomes were so good were that only 10% of the patients had reconstruction with prosthetic grafts. Their analysis was limited because some of the data were collected retrospectively from one institution and reflect a single surgeon's experience. I found it very curious that consideration of the kind of anesthesia used for these patients was not discussed until the very last paragraph of the report. All of these operations were done under regional anesthesia. The authors mention that this might have led to fewer cardiovascular events and quicker procedures. I cannot understand how the kind of anesthesia contributed to quicker operations.

M. T. Watkins, MD

Sustained Safety and Effectiveness of Paclitaxel-Eluting Stents for Femoropopliteal Lesions: 2-Year Follow-Up From the Zilver PTX Randomized and Single-Arm Clinical Studies

Dake MD, Ansel GM, Jaff MR, et al (Stanford Univ Med Ctr, CA; Riverside Methodist Hosp, Columbus, OH; Massachusetts General Hosp, Boston; et al)
J Am Coll Cardiol 61:2417-2427, 2013

Objectives.—A prospective, multinational randomized controlled trial (RCT) and a complementary single-arm study evaluated the 2-year safety and effectiveness of a paclitaxel-coated drug-eluting stent (DES) in patients with superficial femoral artery lesions. The RCT compared the DES with percutaneous transluminal angioplasty (PTA) and provisional bare-metal stent (BMS) placement.

Background.—Local drug delivery for superficial femoral artery lesions has been investigated with the intent of limiting restenosis similarly to DES for the coronary arteries. One-year outcomes of DES in the superficial femoral artery are promising, but longer-term benefits have not been established.

Methods.—In the RCT, patients were randomly assigned to primary DES implantation (n = 236) or PTA (n = 238). Acute PTA failure occurred in 120 patients, who underwent secondary randomization to DES (n = 61) or BMS (n = 59) placement. The single-arm study enrolled 787 patients with DES treatment.

Results.—Compared with the control group, the primary DES group demonstrated significantly superior 2-year event-free survival (86.6% vs. 77.9%, $p = 0.02$) and primary patency (74.8% vs. 26.5%, $p < 0.01$). In addition, the provisional DES group exhibited superior 2-year primary patency compared with the provisional BMS group (83.4% vs. 64.1%, $p < 0.01$) and achieved higher sustained clinical benefit (83.9% vs.

68.4%, $p = 0.05$). Two-year freedom from target lesion revascularization with primary DES placement was 80.5% in the single-arm study and 86.6% in the RCT.

Conclusions.—Two-year outcomes with the paclitaxel-eluting stent support its sustained safety and effectiveness in patients with femoropopliteal artery disease, including the long-term superiority of the DES to PTA and to provisional BMS placement. (Evaluation of the Zilver PTX Drug-Eluting Stent in the Above-the-Knee Femoropopliteal Artery; NCT00120406; Zilver® PTX™ Global Registry; NCT01094678).

▶ The 2-year results of the Zilver PTX randomized trial were among the most awaited trial results of 2013. The Zilver PTX outperformed PTA with primary patency of 83% at 2 years versus only 26% for PTA. Provisional bare metal stenting fell short of provisional Zilver stenting for primary patency at 2 years (90% vs 72%). Importantly, adherence to dual antiplatelet therapy at 1 month significantly promoted Zilver patency, which was not found at a 3-month comparison. Thus, the convention of duration of dual antiplatelet therapy remains a significant question. In addition, lesion length was cautious in the trial at mean length of 66 mm, so applicability of Zilver PTX to longer lesions is not known. Some element of reassurance is provided by the accompanying results of the single-arm study of Zilver PTX wherein the lesion length was 99 mm with similar result. In this era of cost containment, readmission for target lesion revascularization can potentially be lessened with this drug-eluting device. Consequently, cost data regarding such health care system expense reductions will importantly motivate its adoption but only for those who are wise in such matters.

J. Black, MD

Preliminary results of the initial United States experience with the Supera woven nitinol stent in the popliteal artery

León LR Jr, Dieter RS, Gadd CL, et al (Tucson Med Ctr, AZ; Loyola Univ Med Ctr, Maywood, IL; Univ of Arizona Health Science Ctr, Tucson)

J Vasc Surg 57:1014-1022, 2013

Background.—Popliteal artery stenting is not routinely performed due to concerns related to the high mobility of the knee joint and the potential for external stent compression, fractures, and occlusion. Open bypass is traditionally considered the gold standard for popliteal artery atherosclerotic lesions. The Supera stent (IDEV Technologies Inc, Webster, Tex) was developed to provide superior radial strength, fracture resistance, and flexibility compared with laser-cut nitinol stents. This study represents the initial United States experience in the management of popliteal artery atherosclerotic disease with the Supera interwoven wire stent.

Methods.—Patients undergoing stent implantation in the 20-month period after the 2008 Food and Drug Administration clearance were included. Medical records, radiographic imaging, and procedural data were examined. Procedural angiograms were classified according to Trans-Atlantic Inter-Society Consensus criteria. Patency and limb loss rates were calculated using Kaplan-Meier analysis.

Results.—A total of 39 stents were placed in 34 patients due to isolated popliteal artery occlusive disease. Clinical follow-up was a mean of 12.7 months (range, 0.2-33.7 months), and radiologic follow-up was a mean of 8.4 months (range, 0-26.8 months). Most patients had critical limb ischemia (CLI), with tissue loss (38.2%) or rest pain (35.3%) as the indication for intervention. In 20 patients (58.8%), the most distal end of the stent(s) landed in the below-the-knee popliteal segment, 12 (35.3%) landed in the above-the-knee segment, and two (5.9%) landed precisely at the knee. Other than angioplasty and stenting, 47% of patients did not receive any adjuvant concomitant therapy in the treated leg. Two patients underwent concomitant atherectomy of the popliteal segment. Primary, primary assisted, and secondary patency rates by duplex ultrasound imaging were 79.2%, 88.1% and 93%, respectively, by Kaplan-Meier estimates, with a mean stented length of 12 cm. Six instances of stent occlusion were noted, and six patients were identified with hemodynamically significant in-stent stenosis. Three patients sustained limb loss (8.8%), two related to uncontrolled infections, and one due to perioperative ischemic complications (both with patent stents at the time of limb loss). The overall mortality was 8.8% during the study period. Knee roentgenography was performed in all but one patient, and no stent fractures were identified.

Conclusions.—Stenting of the popliteal artery using the Supera stent system appears to be safe and effective. The interwoven stent design may better serve areas under extreme mechanical stress. Our results with this highly diseased patient population justify a prospective trial in this subject.

▶ This report represents the initial US experience with the Supera stent used in the popliteal artery. The mean stent length is 12 cm, which would generally imply the 12-month primary patency should be at least 70%, which is achieved admirably in 79%, considering close to 60% of stents extended to the below-knee popliteal segment. The details on stent occlusion are provided on Table 5 in the original article, but noticeably absent is the detail on operator for 2 of the 6 instances; does this imply difficulty in visualization or delivery to target lesions? In the popliteal artery, avoidance of stent fracture is key, and the lack of occurrence of stent fracture is identified at follow-up. The Supera stent is part of the arsenal for popliteal intervention and may have durable benefit after failed percutaneous transluminal angioplasty or atherectomy.

J. Black, MD

Ten-year technical and clinical outcomes in TransAtlantic Inter-Society Consensus II infrainguinal C/D lesions using duplex ultrasound arterial mapping as the sole imaging modality for critical lower limb ischemia

Sultan S, Tawfick W, Hynes N (Galway Univ Hosp, Ireland; Galway Clinic, Ireland)

J Vasc Surg 57:1038-1045, 2013

Objective.—The aim of this study was to evaluate duplex ultrasound arterial mapping (DUAM) as the sole imaging modality when planning for bypass surgery (BS) and endovascular revascularization (EvR) in patients with critical limb ischemia for TransAtlantic Inter-Society Consensus (TASC) II C/D infrainguinal lesions.

Methods.—This was a retrospective review evaluating the accuracy of DUAM as the sole imaging tool in determining patient suitability for BS vs EvR. Primary outcomes were the sensitivity and specificity of DUAM compared with intraoperative digital subtraction angiography. Secondary outcomes were procedural, hemodynamic, and clinical outcomes, amputation-free survival, and freedom from major adverse clinical events.

Results.—From 2002 to 2012, a total of 4783 patients with peripheral arterial disease were referred, of whom 622 critical limb ischemia patients underwent revascularization for TASC C and D lesions (EvR: n = 423; BS: n = 199). Seventy-four percent of EvR and 82% of BS were performed for TASC D ($P = .218$). The DUAM showed sensitivity of 97% and specificity of 98% in identifying lesions requiring intervention. Of the 520 procedures performed with DUAM alone, there was no difference regarding the number of procedures performed for occlusive or de novo lesions (EvR: 65% and 71%; BS: 87% and 78%; $P = .056$). Immediate clinical improvement to the Rutherford category ≤3 was 96% for EvR and 97% for BS ($P = .78$). Hemodynamic success was 79% for EvR and 77% for BS ($P = .72$). Six-year freedom from binary restenosis was 71.6% for EvR and 67.4% for BS ($P = .724$). Six-year freedom from target lesion revascularization was 81.1% for EvR and 70.3% for BS ($P = .3571$). Six-year sustained clinical improvement was 79.5% for EvR and 66.7% for BS ($P = .294$). Six-year amputation-free survival was 77.2% for EvR and 74.6% for BS ($P = .837$). There was a significant difference in risk of major adverse clinical events between EvR and BS (51% vs 70%; $P = .034$). Only 16.4% of patients required magnetic resonance angiography, which tended to overestimate lesions with 84% agreement with intraoperative findings. Six-year binary restenosis was 71% for DUAM procedures compared with 55% for magnetic resonance angiography procedures ($P = .001$), which was solely based on the prospective modality.

Conclusions.—The DUAM epitomizes a minimally invasive, economically proficient modality for road mapping procedural outcome in BS and EvR. It allows for high patient turnover with procedural and clinical success without compromising hemodynamic outcome. The DUAM is superior to other available modalities as the sole preoperative imaging tool in a successful limb salvage program.

▶ Duplex ultrasound of peripheral vascular disease is a well-established modality for follow-up of vascular intervention, and in some centers, it is used to determine targets for peripheral bypass surgery. A comprehensive duplex ultrasound mapping of the lower extremity must balance the requisite operator skill and the accuracy of the information. In this regard, Dr Sultan et al demonstrate in an experienced center that duplex ultrasound mapping can provide diagnostic accuracy rivaling axial imaging and angiography. The results are admirable, and the question of generalizability would have been answered if the early and later groups were cohorted and compared.

J. Black, MD

Twenty-Year Analysis of Trends in the Incidence and In-Hospital Mortality for Lower-Extremity Arterial Thromboembolism

Korabathina R, Weintraub AR, Price LL, et al (Tufts Med Ctr, Boston, MA; et al)
Circulation 128:115-121, 2013

Background.—Epidemiology data for lower-extremity arterial thromboembolism (LET) are limited and may result from either acute limb ischemia or an acute exacerbation of critical limb ischemia. Given marked changes in both diagnosis and therapy over the last 2 decades, we hypothesized that this time period would have witnessed reductions in both the incidence and in-hospital mortality of LET.

Methods and Results.—Data from 1988 through 2007 from the National Hospital Discharge Survey were analyzed. All admissions for patients with LET were extracted, and the respective *International Classification of Diseases, Ninth Revision, Clinical Modification* codes were internally validated for both LET and acute limb ischemia. Descriptive statistics were used. The validity of the codes was good for identifying LET cases but poor for identifying acute limb ischemia cases because many of these acute presentations were attributable to critical limb ischemia. Over the 20-year span, there were 1.76 million cases of LET. The incidence of LET decreased significantly from 42.4 per 100 000 persons between 1988 and 1997 to 23.3 per 100 000 persons between 1998 and 2007. The in-hospital mortality for LET decreased significantly from 8.28% between 1988 and 1997 to 6.34% between 1998 and 2007, and male patients achieved greater mortality reduction compared with female patients. Treatments for acute limb ischemia showed decreasing use of surgical bypass and amputation and increasing rates of catheter-based thrombolysis.

Conclusions.—Over the 20-year study period, there have been significant reductions in both LET incidence and in-hospital mortality. Unfortunately, LET admissions extracted from an administrative database comprise a diverse group of individuals, including those with acute and chronic forms of limb ischemia and iatrogenic arterial injury, limiting the true assessment of ALI incidence.

▶ Acute limb ischemia can manifest secondary to acute emboli or acute chronic vascular disease. This study demonstrates a significant reduction in the incidence of the condition and lower mortality related to it. The overall incidence of arterial thromboembolism in the study is overestimated in the data extracted from an administrative database because the current coding cannot separate acute ischemia from thromboembolism versus acute exacerbation of chronic underlying disease. Regardless, the exact causes for the reduced incidence of arterial thromboembolism are likely related to validated risk models to demonstrate safety of oral anticoagulation that have reduced cardiac emboli formation. Prevention is thus better than the cure, given that the severity of the condition is belied by the realization of the study that 25% of patients do not undergo revascularization, likely secondary to comorbidities or nonviable limbs.

J. Black, MD

Comparative effectiveness study of self-directed walking exercise, lower extremity revascularization, and functional decline in peripheral artery disease

McDermott MM, Kibbe M, Guralnik JM, et al (Northwestern Univ Feinberg School of Medicine, Chicago, IL; Univ of Maryland School of Medicine, Baltimore; et al)

J Vasc Surg 57:990-996.e1, 2013

Objective.—Among individuals with peripheral artery disease (PAD), we compared annual change in 6-minute walk performance between participants who neither underwent lower extremity revascularization nor walked for exercise (group 1, reference), those who walked regularly for exercise (group 2), and those who underwent lower extremity revascularization (group 3).

Methods.—Participants were recruited from Chicago-area vascular laboratories and followed annually. Change in 6-minute walk was calculated beginning at the study visit preceding lower extremity revascularization or exercise behavior and continuing for 1 additional year after the therapy was reported. Results are adjusted for age, sex, race, comorbidities, and other confounders.

Results.—Of 348 PAD participants, 43 underwent revascularization during median follow-up of 84 months. Adjusted annual declines in 6-minute walk were -96.6 feet/year for group 1, −49.9 feet/year for group 2, and −32.6 feet/year for group 3 ($P < .001$). Forty-one percent of revascularizations were not associated with ankle-brachial index (ABI) improvement. When group 3 was limited to participants with ABI improvement ≥0.15 after revascularization, annual adjusted changes in 6-minute walk were −97.7 feet/year for group 1, −46.5 feet/year for group 2, and +68.1

feet/year for group 3 ($P < .001$). When group 3 was limited to participants without ABI improvement ≥0.15 after revascularization, annual adjusted changes in 6-minute walk were −99.2 feet/year for group 1, −48.0 feet/year for group 2, and −61.7 feet/year for group 3 ($P < .001$).

Conclusions.—A large proportion of PAD participants did not have ABI improvement of at least 0.15 at follow-up study visit after revascularization. The benefits of lower extremity revascularization in patients with PAD appear closely tied to improvements in the ABI after revascularization.

▶ Patients with peripheral arterial disease comprise a heterogeneous population, and treatments include widely disparate treatment strategies and high costs. In a health care delivery environment that is under examination to prove benefit, this study is enlightening and should motivate careful clinical decision making. The results include patient self-report, so detail on the revascularization procedures is lacking, but the finding that 72% of patients did not experience an increase in ankle-brachial index >0.15 (the Society for Vascular Surgery standard for hemodynamic success) after self-reported revascularization impugns our ability to decipher procedural benefit. Indeed, if a vascular surgeon was under pay-for-performance restrictions, the fact that only 30% of our patients benefitted from a revascularization to stem their functional decline would effectively end the specialty. As such, the study suggests that research is needed to determine which procedures are most likely to produce hemodynamic success. In effect, the paradigm that less is more is not operant, and a true comprehensive revascularization may be best for functional results.

J. Black, MD

Distal anastomotic vein adjunct usage in infrainguinal prosthetic bypasses

McPhee JT, Goodney PP, Schanzer A, et al (Brigham and Women's Hosp, Boston, MA; Dartmouth Hitchcock Med Ctr, Lebanon, NH; UMass Memorial Med Ctr, Worcester, MA; et al)

J Vasc Surg 57:982-989, 2013

Objective.—Single-segment saphenous vein remains the optimal conduit for infrainguinal revascularization. In its absence, prosthetic conduit may be used. Existing data regarding the significance of anastomotic distal vein adjunct (DVA) usage with prosthetic grafts are based on small series.

Methods.—This is a retrospective cohort analysis derived from the regional Vascular Study Group of New England as well as the Brigham and Women's hospital database. A total of 1018 infrainguinal prosthetic bypass grafts were captured in the dataset from 73 surgeons at 15 participating institutions. Propensity scoring and 3:1 matching was performed to create similar exposure groups for analysis. Outcome measures of interest included: primary patency, freedom from major adverse limb events (MALEs), and amputation free survival at 1 year as a function of vein patch utilization. Time to event data were compared with the log-rank test; multivariable Cox proportional hazard models were used to evaluate the adjusted association between vein cuff usage and the primary end points. DVA was defined as a vein patch, cuff, or boot in any configuration.

Results.—Of the 1018 bypass operations, 94 (9.2%) had a DVA whereas 924 (90.8%) did not (no DVA). After propensity score matching, 88 DVAs (25%) and 264 no DVAs (75%) were analyzed. On univariate analysis of the matched cohort, the DVA and no DVA groups were similar in terms of mean age (70.0 vs 69.0; $P = .55$), male sex (58.0% vs 58.3%; $P > .99$), and preoperative characteristics such as living at home (93.2% vs 94.3%; $P = .79$) and independent ambulatory status (72.7% vs 75.7%; $P = .64$). The DVA and no DVA groups had similar rates of major comorbidities such as hypertension chronic obstructive pulmonary disease, diabetes mellitus, coronary artery disease, and dialysis dependence ($P > .05$ for all). Likewise, they had similar rates of distal origin grafts (13.6% vs 12.5%; $P = .85$), critical limb ischemia indications ($P = .53$), and prior arterial bypass (58% vs 47%; $P = .08$). The DVA group had a higher rate of completion angiogram performed (55.7% vs 37.5%; $P = .002$) and were more likely to be discharged on coumadin (53.4% vs 37.1%; $P = .01$). By multivariable analysis, use of a distal DVA was protective against MALEs (hazard ratio, 0.36; 95% confidence interval, 0.14-0.90; $P = .03$).

Conclusions.—This contemporary multi-institutional propensity-matched study demonstrates that patients that receive distal anastomotic vein adjuncts as part of infrainguinal prosthetic bypass operations in general have more extreme comorbidities and more technically challenging operations based on level of target vessel and prior bypass attempts. After propensity-matched analysis, the use of a DVA may protect against MALEs in prosthetic bypass surgery and should be considered when feasible.

▶ Distal anastomotic adjuncts in infrainguinal prosthetic bypasses can take many forms and incur extra operative time. Their usage is highly variable and often reported in single-center series. This report from the Vascular Study Group of New England (VSGNE) draws a large study population and propensity matching for further analysis. The main finding of the report is with 1-year follow-up infrainguinal bypass grafts performed with distal anastomotic adjuncts, which were associated with lower rates of major adverse limb events. The study invites some selection biases in that those with adjuncts were more likely to be discharged on Coumadin, which is known to reduce the acuity of failures. Nonetheless, it is worth considering distal anastomotic adjuncts when feasible and in those thought at high risk for failure.

J. Black, MD, FACS

Predictive value of angiographic scores for the integrated management of the ischemic diabetic foot

Bargellini I, Piaggesi A, Cicorelli A, et al (Univ of Pisa, Italy)

J Vasc Surg 57:1204-1212, 2013

Objective.—To retrospectively evaluate the agreement between the angiographic scores and the clinical outcomes after endoluminal revascularization in diabetic patients with Fontaine stage IV critical limb ischemia (CLI).

Methods.—Clinical and procedural data were retrospectively collected of consecutive diabetic patients with Fontaine stage IV CLI who underwent percutaneous lower limb endoluminal revascularization from January 2009 to June 2011. Pre- and postprocedural angiographic images were retrospectively reviewed to classify lower limb arterial involvement according to four systems: (1) TransAtlantic Inter-Society Consensus [TASC] I; (2) TASC II; (3) Graziani's morphologic classification; and (4) Joint Vascular Society Council calf and foot scores. Foot lesions were graded according to the University of Texas wound classification system. Clinical results (healing, nonhealing, or major amputation) were compared with baseline clinical data and angiographic results.

Results.—In the study period, 202 percutaneous procedures were performed, with an immediate technical success rate of 94%. Preprocedurally, the mean ± standard deviation calf and foot scores were 7.8 ± 1.6 and 7.3 ± 2.3, respectively; 132 patients (65%) were in Graziani's morphologic classes from 4 to 7; in 112 (55%) cases, TASC II was considered inapplicable, for the absence of femoropopliteal lesions; and finally, 93% of limbs were classified as TASC I type D lesions. After the procedure, mean calf and foot scores were 4.8 ± 2.3 and 5.9 ± 2.6, respectively, and 87% of cases were in Graziani's classes 1 and 2; TASC II was inapplicable in all cases, whereas 80% of cases remained TASC I type D lesions. Healing rate was 67% and major amputation rate was 4%. Among all the clinical and angiographic variables included in the analysis, only pre- and postprocedural foot scores were significantly associated to the clinical outcome ($P < .05$).

Conclusions.—Endoluminal revascularization represents a valuable treatment option in diabetic patients with CLI. TASC classifications are inadequate to describe peripheral arterial involvement in the vast majority of diabetic patients with CLI. Pre- and postprocedural foot scores represent the most significant angiographic parameters to evaluate treatment success.

▶ Dedicated vascular care to manage the diabetic foot is critical for long-term salvage. The association of macrovascular diabetic tibial disease is currently equally considered with the microvascular damage from long-term cellular changes. This study highlights the critical importance of not seeking an "optimal cosmetic" angiographic result at the calf level as the goal of revascularization; the primary effort should be focused on improving blood flow to the wound area. Thus, the paper reinforces the angiosome model, and the foot score modeling of this article is worth consideration, however tedious. Equally critical is the long time to wound healing, with a mean healing time of 6 months, and the authors' major amputation rate of only 4% for a diabetic critical limb ischemia population is testimony to the value of multidisciplinary and dedicated diabetic foot care programs.

J. Black, MD

Predictors and outcomes of restenosis following tibial artery endovascular interventions for critical limb ischemia

Saqib NU, Domenick N, Cho JS, et al (Univ of Pittsburgh School of Medicine, PA)

J Vasc Surg 57:692-699, 2013

Objective.—Restenosis following tibial artery endovascular interventions (TAEIs) is thought to be benign but is not well characterized. This study examines the consequences and predictors of recurrent stenosis of TAEIs for critical limb ischemia.

Methods.—All TAEIs for critical limb ischemia performed between 2004 and 2010 were retrospectively reviewed. Restenosis was detected by noninvasive imaging and angiography when indicated. Restenoses were identified and the limb outcomes recorded. Tibial reinterventions were performed only for persistent, worsening, or recurrent tissue loss or rest pain with evidence of recurrence on duplex ultrasound or hemodynamic imaging. The χ^2 test and logistic regression were applied as indicated. One-year patency rates were calculated using the Kaplan-Meier method.

Results.—A total of 235 limbs in 210 patients were treated for critical limb ischemia (70% tissue loss, 30% rest pain). Tissue loss included gangrene (49%) and ulcers (51%), and involved the forefoot (80%), the heel (14%), or both (6%). Seventy-eight percent of limbs had Trans-Atlantic InterSociety Consensus C/D lesions, with mean preoperative runoff score of 12. Interventions were isolated tibial (45%) or multilevel (55%) (including tibial). Mean postoperative runoff score improved to 6.6, but restenosis occurred in 96 limbs (41%) at a mean of 4 months. The 1-year primary patency was 59% with a mean follow-up of 9 months. Restenosis presented with a persistent wound (32%), worsened wound (42%), rest pain (16%), or no symptoms (10%). A repeat TAEI was performed in 42 (44%), major amputation in 26 (27%), open bypass in 20 (21%), and observation in eight (8%). The overall amputation rate was 13%, but limb loss was significantly higher in patients with restenosis (n = 26 [27%]) than in patients with no restenosis (n = 5 [4%]; $P < .001$). Patients with restenosis and tissue loss were more likely to have presented with gangrene (63% vs 38%; $P = .0003$) but had comparable wound distribution ($P =$ NS). There was a trend toward a higher restenosis rate in patients with renal insufficiency (odds ratio, 5.57; $P = .08$), but this was unaffected by diabetes, statin therapy, or smoking (P = NS). The rate of repeat intervention after the first reintervention was 36%, with an 87% overall limb salvage rate.

Conclusions.—TAEIs can be used successfully to treat patients with critical limb ischemia with acceptable limb salvage rates. Special attention should be given to patients with extensive tissue loss or gangrene because they are at risk for early restenosis and subsequent limb loss. Strict wound and hemodynamic surveillance, wound care, and timely reinterventions are crucial to achieve successful outcomes in this patient population. Amputation or alternative revascularization options, when feasible, should be considered in patients with restenosis and tissue loss given the high rate of limb loss with tibial reinterventions.

► In this article, Dr Saqib and colleagues tackle the subject of tibial artery interventions. Endovascular therapy for lower extremity occlusive disease has matured from a dismissal of restenosis events as clinically irrelevant to "upstaging" of Rutherford class and a cautious examination of potential deleterious effects on runoff. This report parallels the same cautionary clinical tale and indeed suggests that tibial interventions have a narrow safety window. In this regard, we must approach tibial interventions with skepticism because the anticipated high restenosis rates may delay definitive revascularization approaches at the expense of time and amputations. The importance of close surveillance is mentioned, but author recommendations for their protocols based on this experience are not explained. As a greater understanding of tibial interventions is married to anatomy (angiosome) and function of intact feet (healing), the field will march forward.

J. Black, MD

Stent Placement Versus Balloon Angioplasty for the Treatment of Obstructive Lesions of the Popliteal Artery: A Prospective, Multicenter, Randomized Trial

Rastan A, Krankenberg H, Baumgartner I, et al (Universitäts-Herzzentrum Freiburg-Bad Krozingen, Germany; Universitäres Herz-und Gefäszentrum Hamburg, Germany; Universität Bern, Switzerland; et al)

Circulation 127:2535-2541, 2013

Background.—Stenting has been shown to improve patency after femoral artery revascularization compared with balloon angioplasty. Limited data are available evaluating endovascular treatment for obstructive lesions of the popliteal artery.

Methods and Results.—This prospective, randomized, multicenter trial compared primary nitinol stent placement to percutaneous transluminal balloon angioplasty in patients with peripheral artery disease Rutherford-Becker class 2 to 5 who had a de novo lesion in the popliteal artery. The primary study end point was 1-year primary patency, defined as freedom from target-lesion restenosis (luminal narrowing of ≥50%) as detected by duplex ultrasound. Secondary end points included target-lesion revascularization rate and changes in Rutherford-Becker class. Provisional stent placement was considered target-lesion revascularization and loss of primary patency. Two hundred forty-six patients were included in this trial. The mean target-lesion length was 42.3 mm. One hundred ninety-seven patients were available for the 1-year follow-up. The 1-year primary patency rate was significantly higher in the group with primary nitinol stent placement (67.4%) than in the percutaneous transluminal balloon angioplasty group (44.9%, $P = 0.002$). Target-lesion revascularization rates were 14.7% and 44.1%, respectively ($P = 0.0001$); however, when provisional nitinol stent placement was not considered target-lesion revascularization and loss in patency, no significant differences prevailed between the study groups (67.4% versus 65.7%, $P = 0.92$ for primary patency). Approximately 73% of patients in the percutaneous transluminal balloon angioplasty group and 77% in the nitinol stent group showed an improvement of ≥1 Rutherford-Becker class ($P = 0.31$).

Conclusions.—Primary nitinol stent placement for obstructive lesions of the popliteal artery achieves superior acute technical success and higher 1-year primary patency only if provisional stenting is considered target-lesion revascularization. Provisional stenting as part of a percutaneous transluminal balloon angioplasty strategy has equivalent 1-year patency and should be preferred over primary stenting.

Clinical Trial Registration URL.—http://www.clinicaltrials.gov. Unique identifier: NCT00712309.

▶ Isolated popliteal artery disease is uncommon, but the biomechanical forces of knee flexion and artery torsion have implied a hostile environment for endovascular intervention in this territory. The work of Rastan and colleagues informs our decisions with a randomized trial of primary nitinol stenting versus percutaneous transluminal angioplasty (PTA). Of the PTA group, 30% crossed over to stenting for residual stenosis or dissection, and hemodynamic success with a significant increase in ankle-brachial index was achieved. The most interesting finding, and a critical issue in the hostile biomechanical bed of the popliteal fossa, is that optimal angioplasty result (non-crossover) after PTA carried the same success rate at 6 and 12 months as primary stenting. Thus, primary stenting should not be considered over a provisional stenting approach after suboptimal PTA. Our European colleagues are to be congratulated on this thoughtful conclusion, which fits perfectly into the cost-reduction paradigm in which we must engage on this side of the pond.

J. Black, MD

Exercise capacity is the strongest predictor of mortality in patients with peripheral arterial disease

Leeper NJ, Myers J, Zhou M, et al (Stanford Univ School of Medicine, CA; Veterans Affairs Palo Alto Health Care System, Stanford, CA)

J Vasc Surg 57:728-733, 2013

Objective.—The objective of this study was to assess the predictive value of clinical and exercise test variables in patients with peripheral arterial disease (PAD).

Methods.—A customized symptom-limited ramp treadmill protocol was used to assess 725 PAD patients referred for exercise testing at the Palo Alto Veterans Hospital between 1997 and 2011. Detailed clinical and exercise test data were collected at baseline, and patients were followed up for a mean of 11.3 ± 6.3 years.

Results.—During follow-up, there were 364 deaths. Baseline exercise capacity was 7.0 ± 2.6 metabolic equivalents (METs) among survivors and 5.5 ± 2.4 METs in those who died ($P < .001$). Although several physiologic parameters differed between survivors and nonsurvivors, age-adjusted Cox regression revealed that exercise capacity was the strongest independent predictor of death. Each additional MET achieved was associated with age-adjusted 18% and 20% reductions in all-cause and cardiovascular mortality, respectively ($P < .001$ for both). This variable surpassed all classical risk factors (including smoking and history of congestive heart failure) and all measured exercise test responses (including symptoms and electrocardiograph abnormalities).

Conclusions.—Among PAD patients, reduced exercise capacity is the most powerful harbinger of long-term mortality. This factor has predictive power beyond traditional risk factors and confirms the critical importance of fitness in this cohort.

▶ Interventions and medical therapy for peripheral arterial disease (PAD) are under critical examination for clinical effectiveness, and this study provides valuable natural history data. In health care economics, great expenses are incurred at the end of life. This study suggests that among patients with PAD in the Veterans Affairs system, exercise capacity has powerful prognostic power to predict all-cause and cardiovascular mortality (Fig 1 in the original article). This study should be considered in conjunction with the Year Book of Vascular Surgery 2013 review of the study by McDermott et al, which indicated that 6-minute walking distance improvement is closely tied to ankle-brachial index (ABI) improvement. Thus, this study from Leeper and colleagues invites the necessary question: can revascularization lead to ABI increase and concomitant improvement in peak exercise capacity? If so, then vascular intervention can be valuably tied to better overall outcomes for our patients.

J. Black, MD, FACS

Preliminary evidence that low ankle-brachial index is associated with reduced bilateral hip extensor strength and functional mobility in peripheral arterial disease

Parmenter BJ, Raymond J, Dinnen PJ, et al (Univ of Sydney, New South Wales, Australia; Univ of New South Wales, Australia)

J Vasc Surg 57:963-973, 2013

Objective.—Peripheral arterial disease (PAD) has been associated with skeletal muscle pathology, including atrophy of the affected muscles. In addition, oxidative metabolism is impaired, muscle function is reduced, and gait and mobility are restricted. We hypothesized that greater severity of symptomatic PAD would be associated with lower levels of muscle mass, strength, and endurance, and that these musculoskeletal abnormalities in turn would impair functional performance and walking ability in patients with PAD.

Methods.—We assessed 22 persons with intermittent claudication from PAD in this cross-sectional pilot study. Outcome assessments included initial claudication distance and absolute claudication distance via treadmill protocols and outcomes from the 6-minute walk (6MW). Secondary outcomes included one repetition maximum strength/endurance testing of hip extensors, hip abductors, quadriceps, hamstrings, plantar flexors, pectoral, and upper back muscle groups, as well as performance-based tests of function. Univariate and stepwise multiple regression models were constructed to evaluate relationships and are presented.

Results.—Twenty-two participants (63.6% male; mean [standard deviation] age, 73.6 [8.2] years; range, 55-85 years) were studied. Mean (standard deviation) resting ankle-brachial index (ABI) was 0.54 ([0.13]; range, 0.28-0.82), and participants ranged from having mild claudication to rest pain. Lower resting ABI was significantly associated with reduced bilateral hip extensor strength ($r = 0.54$; $P = .007$) and reduced whole body strength ($r = 0.32$; $P = .05$). In addition, lower ABI was associated with a shorter distance to first stop during the 6MW ($r = 0.38$; $P = .05$) and poorer single leg balance ($r = 0.44$; $P = .03$). Reduced bilateral hip extensor strength was also significantly associated with functional outcomes, including reduced 6MW distance to first stop ($r = 0.74$; $P = .001$), reduced 6MW distance ($r = 0.75$; $P < .001$), and reduced total short physical performance battery score (worse function; $r = 0.75$; $P = .003$).

Conclusions.—Our results suggest the existence of a causal pathway from a reduction in ABI to muscle atrophy and weakness, to whole body disability represented by claudication outcomes and performance-based tests of functional mobility in an older cohort with symptomatic PAD. Longitudinal outcomes from this study and future trials are required to investigate the effects of an anabolic intervention targeting the muscles involved in mobility and activities of daily living and whether an increase in muscle strength will improve symptoms of claudication and lead to improvements in other functional outcomes in patients with PAD.

▶ Our understanding of peripheral arterial disease (PAD) continues to evolve from early conventions focused on anatomy and diagnosis to contemporary and more holistic functional processes. The ability of ABI has been called into question for its lack of ability to discriminate patient symptoms, benefits or revascularization, and long-term prognostication. Herein, Parmenter and colleagues suggest a causal link for the aforementioned list unified by whole-body disability incited by loss of walking capacity. The link is intuitive, but more studies such as this one are critically important to support the concept that PAD interventions might have benefit outside the target zone, especially in therapy of claudicant patients who are most often cited for lack of clinical effectiveness.

J. Black, MD

The impact of arterial pedal arch quality and angiosome revascularization on foot tissue loss healing and infrapopliteal bypass outcome

Rashid H, Slim H, Zayed H, et al (Guy's and St Thomas' Hosps, London, UK)

J Vasc Surg 57:1219-1226, 2013

Objective.—This study evaluated the effect of pedal arch quality on the amputation-free survival and patency rates of distal bypass grafts and its direct impact on the rate of healing and time to healing of tissue loss after direct angiosome revascularization in patients with critical limb ischemia (CLI).

Methods.—Between 2004 and 2011, patients undergoing distal bypass for CLI (Rutherford 4-6) were divided in groups taking into consideration the state of the pedal arch and direct angiosome revascularization (DAR) and non-DAR. Angiography was used to divide the pedal arch into three groups: complete pedal arch (CPA), incomplete pedal arch (IPA), and no pedal arch (NPA). The primary end points were patency rates at 12 months, amputation-free survival at 48 months, and the rate of healing and time to healing of foot tissue loss.

Results.—A total of 154 patients (75% men) with CLI underwent 167 infrapopliteal bypasses. Patients were a median age of 75 years (range, 46-96 years). Diabetic mellitus was present in 76%, chronic renal failure in 28%, and ischemic heart disease in 44%. The primary patency rates at 1 year in the CPA, IPA, and NPA groups were 58.4%, 54.6%, and 63.8%, respectively ($P = .5168$), the secondary patency rates were 86.0%, 84.7%, and 88.8%, respectively ($P = .8940$), and the amputation-free survival at 48 months was 67.2%, 69.7%, and 45.9%, respectively ($P = .3883$). Tissue loss was present in 141 of the 167 bypasses. In the CPA group, 83% of tissue loss with DAR healed compared with 92% in the non-DAR (median time to healing, 66 vs 74 days). Similarly in the IPA group, 90% with DAR healed compared with 81% in the non-DAR (median time to healing, 96 vs 86 days). In the NPA group, only 75%

with DAR healed compared with 73% in the non-DAR (median time to healing, 90 vs 135 days). There was a significant difference in healing and time to healing between the CPA/IPA and NPA groups ($P = .0264$).

Conclusions.—The quality of the pedal arch did not influence the patency or the amputation-free survival rates. However, the rates for healing and time to healing were directly influenced by the quality of the pedal arch rather than the angiosome revascularized.

▶ Dr Rashid and colleagues build on the angiosome concept with examination of angiosome revascularization and the status of the pedal arch. Intuitively, those with complete pedal arches can be assumed to contribute collateral flow to the other angiosomes not directly revascularized. Their concept is intriguing and examined vigorously in this study. Whether the surgical bypass directly revascularized the angiosome bore no relevance to patency, wound healing, or amputation-free survival. However, time to heal the wound was significantly reduced if the pedal arch was complete or incomplete, compared with no pedal arch at all. The study may represent a selection bias because more diseased pedal arches involved greater tissue loss. Unfortunately, this bias cannot be rectified given that the natural history of pedal arch disease is not known among the patients with peripheral vascular disease. Nonetheless, the status of the pedal arch may have important prognostic implications if time to wound healing is considered a metric for a viable foot care program.

J. Black, MD

A Prospective Randomized Controlled Clinical Trial on Clopidogrel Combined With Warfarin Versus Clopidogrel Alone in the Prevention of Restenosis After Endovascular Treatment of the Femoropopliteal Artery

Li H, Zhang F, Liang G, et al (Peking Univ Ninth School of Clinical Medicine, Beijing, China)

Ann Vasc Surg 27:627-633, 2013

Background.—We sought to compare the effects of clopidogrel combined with warfarin with clopidogrel alone in the prevention of restenosis after endovascular treatment (EVT) of the femoropopliteal artery.

Methods.—Between June 2008 and May 2009, 88 consecutive patients referred for EVT were randomly divided into a clopidogrel group (42 cases) and a clopidogrel combined with warfarin group (46 cases) before the procedure. Examinations including staging of peripheral arterial disease by Rutherford, ankle-brachial index, and color duplex ultrasonography were performed at baseline, 1 week, 3 months, 6 months, and 12 months after procedure. At the same time, bleeding complications were observed.

Results.—Fifty patients (63 limbs) were included after 12 months of follow-up, in which 25 patients (30 limbs) were from the clopidogrel group and 25 patients (33 limbs) were from the combination group. At 3 months, the rates of restenosis on duplex ultrasonography were 17% in the clopidogrel group and 18% in the combination group ($P = 1.0$). At

6 months, the accumulated restenosis rates were 37% and 36% ($P = 0.98$), respectively. At 12 months, the accumulated restenosis rates were 53% and 42% ($P = 0.523$), respectively. The rate of clinical bleeding events was 21% (6/29) in the combination group compared with 7% (2/27) in the clopidogrel group, and there was no statistical difference ($P = 0.3$).

Conclusions.—The combination of clopidogrel with warfarin was not more effective than clopidogrel alone in restenosis prevention for patients who underwent EVT. Instead, the combination of antiplatelet and anticoagulation therapy was inclined to increase the clinical bleeding events.

► This study seeks to investigate an enhanced strategy of anticoagulation after endovascular therapy of the femoropopliteal territory. In endovascular circles, Plavix administration has assumed primacy, with a variable loading dose and duration of therapy, usually in combination with daily aspirin. In this study, Plavix versus Plavix and daily warfarin were compared after femoropopliteal intervention. Aspirin therapy was not quantified but is assumed to be absent. Unfortunately, the study is underpowered, and the study projection assumed a high (70%) restenosis rate in the Plavix-only group at 12 months. In fact, the study results would require 4 to 5 times the size of the study population to assume statistical significance at the restenosis rates demonstrated. Thus, the finding of a nonstatistically significant increase in bleeding under Plavix and warfarin of 21% versus 7% in Plavix alone is clinically relevant, albeit underpowered and emblematic of the study limitation to derive meaningful answers. For now, the bleeding rate is concerning and should be considered as the "con" of the anticoagulation strategy of warfarin and Plavix.

J. Black, MD

Clinical presentation and outcome after failed infrainguinal endovascular and open revascularization in patients with chronic limb ischemia

Dosluoglu HH, Lall P, Blochle R, et al (VA Western NY Healthcare System, Buffalo; State Univ of New York at Buffalo)

J Vasc Surg 58:98-104.e1, 2013

Objective.—Failure of prior endovascular (EV) interventions for chronic limb ischemia has been reported to negatively affect patency and limb salvage after subsequent revascularization procedures. The goal of our study was to compare the clinical presentation of patients who failed infrainguinal EV and open revascularizations (OR) and the effect of the initial intervention on final outcomes.

Methods.—From June 2001 to October 2010, 216 patients (237 limbs; 66 disabling claudication [DC], 171 critical limb ischemia [CLI]) presented with failed infrainguinal OR or EV revascularization for chronic limb ischemia. Clinical presentation, reinterventions, patency and limb salvage rates, and final outcomes were analyzed.

Results.—The EV group (n = 143) had more diabetes (44% vs 57%; $P = .048$) and ulcers (26% vs 38%; $P = .039$), whereas the OR group (n = 94) had more multilevel revascularizations (59% vs 33%; $P < .001$), rest pain (23% vs 9%; $P = .002$), and infrapopliteal interventions (58% vs 38%; $P = .038$). Presentation at time of failure was non-limb-threatening ischemia in 70% of DC and 16% of CLI patients ($P < .001$), with no difference in those initially treated with EV or OR. In CLI, 23% presented with acute limb ischemia in the OR group vs 10% in the EV group ($P = .024$). Early failure (<3 months) occurred in 15% of DC and in 36% of CLI patients and was more in the OR than in the EV group (30% vs 7% for DC [$P = .011$] and 71% vs 38% for CLI [$P = .024$]). Overall, 195 (82%) had attempted reinterventions (79% in DC and 85% in CLI; $P = .245$). In DC patients, 48% of OR had OR + EV and 26% had EV; 32% of EV had OR + EV and 47% had EV reinterventions. In CLI patients, 40% of OR had OR + EV and 42% had EV; 17% of EV had OR + EV; and 70% had EV reinterventions. A patent revascularized limb was achieved in 66% of OR and in 92% of EV patients ($P < .001$). Patency and limb salvage were significantly better in the EV group, mainly due to the difference in CLI patients, whereas survival was identical.

Conclusions.—Clinical presentation after failed infrainguinal revascularization is determined by the initial indication. CLI patients are more likely to present early with acute limb ischemia, especially after OR. EV reinterventions play a significant role in the management of patients with failed revascularization, and EV failure is associated with better outcomes than those after OR failure, likely due to OR patients having more disadvantaged anatomy and advanced disease at the time of their initial presentation.

▶ Dr Dosluoglu and colleagues have made significant contributions to the arena of clinical research of lower extremity endovascular interventions. Again, the data reporting of open and endovascular procedural data, anatomy classification, and statistical analysis is comprehensively reported. This analysis of outcomes after treatment of primary treatment strategy failure adds to their previous contributions. The essential management paradigm taken from this study is that endovascular management of the failed intervention is associated with better outcomes. As in any retrospective analysis, it is likely those with open surgery initially, and certainly at reintervention, are likely to be more diseased, so some of the reported benefit of endovascular intervention may not be generalizable.

J. Black, MD

Risk factors for readmission after lower extremity procedures for peripheral artery disease

Vogel TR, Kruse RL (Univ of Missouri, Columbia)
J Vasc Surg 58:90-97.e4, 2013

Objective.—As pressure to contain health care costs increases, there has been greater scrutiny of readmissions in the vascular surgery population. The objective of this study was to evaluate postoperative readmissions after open and endovascular lower extremity (LE) procedures for peripheral artery disease (PAD).

Methods.—A retrospective cohort study was performed of elective adult inpatients with PAD and LE procedures which were selected from the Health Facts database (Cerner Corporation, Kansas City, Mo) between October 2008 and December 2010 using International Classification of Disease, 9th Clinical Modification diagnosis codes (claudication, rest pain, and ulceration/gangrene) and procedure codes for LE revascularization (endovascular and open). Multivariable logistic regression and χ^2 were used to compare patients who received endovascular and open procedures. The Charlson Comorbidity Index, comorbid diagnoses, and laboratory results were used to adjust for confounding. The main outcome measure evaluated was readmission ≤30 days of discharge.

Results.—Of 463,362 index admissions, 16,574 patients were identified with a diagnosis of PAD. Combining PAD with elective LE procedures during the index admission, 777 underwent open and 681 underwent endovascular procedures. Unadjusted readmission rates for open and endovascular procedures for claudication, rest pain, and ulceration/gangrene were 10.2% vs 11.3% (P =.69), 14.0% vs 18.2% (P =.43), and 21.1% vs 19.5% (P =.69), respectively. Readmission increased by the severity of the diagnosis for open and endovascular procedures (P =.0006). Men comprised 58% of the cohort; readmission rates were not statistically different by sex (P =.19). Race was not associated with procedure performed (P =.16), but nonwhite race was associated with more severe PAD ($P < .0001$). After adjusting for race, sex, comorbidities, length of stay, and laboratory values outside of normal reference ranges, the association between an endovascular procedure and readmission was not statistically significant (odds ratio, 1.28; 95% confidence interval, 0.94-1.75).

Conclusions.—Less invasive endovascular procedures were not associated with decreased readmission rates compared with open surgery. The overall readmission rate for claudicant patients was 10.7%, which was unexpectedly high. Predictors of readmission included male sex, longer hospital stays, hospital infection, elevated aspartate aminotransferase, and high numbers of medications ordered and dispensed. Further examination exploring reasons for readmission are required to decrease readmission rates in the vascular surgery population.

▶ Drs Vogel and Kruse examine outcomes extracted from the electronic medical record system from Cerner, Inc. The theoretical advantage of such a data set is that it would encompass a wide selection of hospital sizes and private/academic affiliations, as well as a wider range of patient ages. Not surprisingly, among elective vascular procedures, readmission rates paralleled increasing severity. Very surprisingly, endovascular intervention did not protect from readmission, even among claudicant patients who had endovascular versus open surgery. Consequently, the conventional wisdom that less invasive lower extremity intervention is associated with less interruption to the patient is now called into question. Careful analysis of the endovascular paradigm and repeated procedures, readmissions, and facility costs are drawing the attention of payers to cost reduction, so buyer beware.

J. Black, MD

Association of clinical attributes and treadmill walking performance in patients with claudication due to peripheral artery disease

Brass EP, Cooper LT, Hanson P, et al (Harbor-Univ of California Los Angeles (UCLA), Torrance; Mayo Clinic, Rochester, MN; Univ of Colorado School of Medicine, Aurora)

J Vasc Surg 58:396-403, 2013

Background.—Patients with claudication secondary to peripheral artery disease have a substantial impairment in walking capacity. This study evaluated factors suspected to be correlated with treadmill walking performance in an effort to gain insights into the pathophysiology of the impairment.

Methods.—A multivariate model was developed to define the associations between clinical and laboratory biomarkers with treadmill peak walking time (PWT) in patients enrolled in three clinical trials. The model was initially developed in a cohort of 385 patients from one trial using 23 candidate-independent variables and then tested in the combined data from the other two trials (351 patients).

Results.—The final model was built from 14 variables that met the predefined univariate criteria of $P < .15$. Main effects remaining in the model were age, resting ankle-brachial index, smoking status, hypertension, statin use, country (United States vs non-United States countries), and high-sensitivity C-reactive protein. The model was highly statistically significant ($P < .0001$) but explained only a limited portion of the population heterogeneity ($r^2 = 0.173$). The main effects plus interaction terms had an $r^2 = 0.2178$. The main effects model was tested in an independent cohort of 351 patients from two other clinical trials in peripheral arterial disease that did not include high-sensitivity C-reactive protein. The model successfully fit the data set, based on prospectively defined root mean squared error and was statistically significant ($P = .0005$) but had lower overall explanatory power than in the index cohort ($r^2 = 0.0687$).

Conclusions.—As expected, age and ankle-brachial index contributed to exercise limitation among patients with PAD. The association of C-reactive protein, hypertension, and smoking with PWT is consistent with a role for inflammation or oxidative stress in determining treadmill walking performance. In contrast to previous reports from smaller and more homogenous populations, clinical attributes and biomarkers explain only a small portion of PWT heterogeneity.

▶ Vascular and endovascular surgeons are beginning to appreciate the multitude of factors that contribute to functional impairment in peripheral artery disease. Although current TASC II classifications assume the central role of anatomy in treatment selection, the ability for a surgeon to discriminate which patients will benefit most from intervention remains more art than science. This study confirms we are just scratching the surface on the ability to use clinical attributes to determine functional impairment. Indeed, the association of elevated inflammatory markers and smoking only explain 20% of the variability in peak walking time on treadmill testing. The message from this study is clear that clinical assessment is not foolproof, and we should not be surprised when our results fall short of our and our patient's expectations. On the other hand, we are encouraged that there are many more opportunities for research to improve our ability to help our decision making for patients.

J. Black, MD

Drug-coated balloon angioplasty after directional atherectomy improves outcome in restenotic femoropopliteal arteries

Sixt S, Carpio Cancino OG, Treszl A, et al (Heart Ctr, Bad Krozingen, Germany; Univ Med Ctr Hamburg-Eppendorf, Germany)

J Vasc Surg 58:682-686, 2013

Background.—Restenosis remains an unresolved problem despite different treatment modalities and new stent technology in femoropopliteal arteries. No standard therapy has proven to provide acceptable outcome data for this entity. Directional atherectomy alone did not result in satisfactory long-term patency rates. The outcome might be improved in conjunction with drug-coated balloon angioplasty.

Methods.—In this retrospective study, restenotic lesions of the femoropopliteal arteries were treated with directed atherectomy in 89 lesions of consecutive patients (58% male; mean age, 69 ± 11 years). All patients received adjunctive treatment with conventional balloon percutaneous angioplasty (PTA; n = 60) or drug-coated balloon angioplasty (DCB; n = 29).

Results.—Lesion location was in the stent (DCB [n = 27] vs PTA [n = 36]) and in native restenotic vessels (DCB [n = 2] vs PTA [n = 25]). The 1-year Kaplan-Meier freedom from restenosis estimates (95% confidence intervals) in the DCB and PTA groups were 84.7% (70.9%-98.5%) and 43.8% (30.5%-57.1%), respectively. In a multivariable Cox model for restenosis, DCB treatment had a hazard ratio (95% confidence interval) of 0.28 (0.12-0.66; $P = .0036$) compared with the PTA group. In the multivariable model for procedural success, the effect of treatment did not differ between PTA and DCB ($P = .134$).

Conclusions.—The combination of directed atherectomy with adjunctive DCB is associated with a better event-free survival at 12 months of follow-up compared with PTA after directed atherectomy (Fig 1, Table 2).

▶ Restenosis remains a challenging issue that contributes to both treatment failure and repeat intervention rates following endovascular treatment of

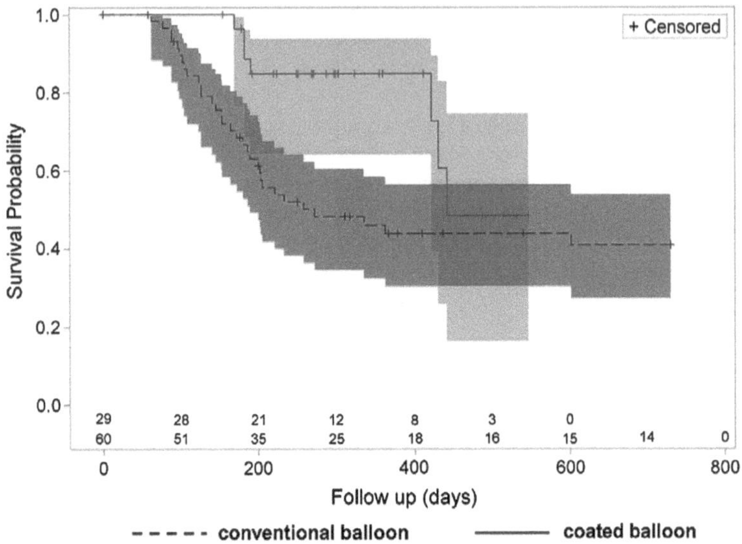

FIGURE.—Probability of being free from restenosis is shown with the 95% confidence interval (*shaded area*). (Reprinted from Sixt S, Carpio Cancino OG, Treszl A, et al. Drug-coated balloon angioplasty after directional atherectomy improves outcome in restenotic femoropopliteal arteries. *J Vasc Surg*. 2013;58:682-686, Copyright 2013, with permission from The Society for Vascular Surgery.)

lower extremity occlusive disease. Although this retrospective study comparing results of regular (percutaneous angioplasty [PTA]) versus drug-coated balloon (DCB) angioplasty following atherectomy for femoropopliteal restenosis suggests that the latter may improve restenosis-free survival, several aspects of the study caution against overenthusiastic interpretation of the findings. Lesion TransAtlantic Inter-Society Consensus classification and postatherectomy stenosis before angioplasty both favored the DCB group (Table 2); given these considerations, it is somewhat surprising that a small but significant difference in stenosis favoring PTA was also observed after angioplasty (9% vs 14%). Additionally, a larger proportion of the treated lesions were located in native arteries within the PTA group (40% vs 2%). Given the increasing body of evidence supporting protective effects of statin medications against restenosis, it is also interesting to note that statin use was significantly lower in the PTA group at baseline (80% vs 97%), with no mention routine postintervention statin administration (a major medical management shortcoming given that all of these patients had restenosis deemed worthy of repeat intervention).

In multivariable models of freedom from restenosis, the authors attempted to adjust for selection bias by using inverse propensity score weighting and adjusting for the year in which the procedure was performed. Although the results were impressive in terms of restenosis-free survival (hazard ratio of 0.28 for DCB compared with PTA; $P < .01$), no corresponding difference in ankle-brachial index or clinical status based on the Rutherford classification was identified. The clinical benefit associated with these differences in imaging findings therefore remains theoretical. Two of the investigators received consulting fees from the atherectomy device manufacturer; oddly, the manufacturer

TABLE 2.—Lesion-Specific Baseline Characteristics

Variable[a]	Entire Cohort (n = 89)	PTA (n = 60)	DCB (n = 29)	Standardized Difference[b]	*P*
Right side	42 (47)	27 (45)	15 (52)	0.135	.652
Common femoral artery	6 (7)	3 (5)	3 (10)	0.202	.387
Deep femoral artery	3 (3)	3 (5)	0	−0.324	.548
Superficial femoral artery	73 (82)	52 (87)	21 (72)	−0.359	.141
Popliteal artery	45 (51)	32 (53)	13 (45)	−0.171	.503
TASC classification				0.262	.808
A	12 (14)	7 (12)	5 (19)		
B	26 (30)	18 (30)	8 (30)		
C	43 (49)	30 (50)	13 (48)		
D	6 (7)	5 (8)	1 (4)		
Reference vessel diameter, mm	5.3 ± 0.8	5.5 ± 0.8	5.0 ± 0.9	−0.555	.013
Lesion length, mm	171 ± 124	180 ± 136	153 ± 93	−0.232	.276
Atherectomy passes	11 ± 6	10 ± 5	13 ± 7	0.431	.094
Vessel runoff				0.458	.132
1 vessel	30 (33)	16 (27)	14 (48)		
2 vessels	39 (43)	29 (48)	10 (34)		
3 vessels	20 (22)	15 (25)	5 (17)		
Additional stenting	11 (12)	8 (13)	3 (10)	−0.093	>.99
Stenosis, %					
Baseline	90 ± 8	90 ± 9	90 ± 7	0.012	.967
After atherectomy	34 ± 17	37 ± 18	28 ± 11	−0.613	.004
Final	11 ± 11	9 ± 12	14 ± 7	0.516	.013
Mean luminal diameter, mm					
Baseline	0.7 ± 0.6	0.7 ± 0.7	0.6 ± 0.5	−0.191	.424
After atherectomy	3.7 ± 1.1	3.8 ± 1.2	3.6 ± 0.7	−0.170	.409
Final	4.9 ± 1.0	5.1 ± 0.9	4.4 ± 0.8	−0.856	<.001

DCB, Drug-coated balloon; *PTA*, balloon percutaneous angioplasty; *TASC*, TransAtlantic Inter-Society Consensus.
[a]Continuous data are presented as means ± standard deviation; categoric data are given as frequency (percentages).
[b]Difference in means or proportions divided by standard error.

of the DCB (which was presumably paclitaxel-coated, although this was not specifically stated within the methods section) was not identified. Despite these shortcomings and potential biases, the study results certainly provide enough benefit to support a prospective randomized trial to further evaluate the benefits of DCB technology for restenosis. Utilization of DCB in combination with atherectomy, as in the current study, would certainly increase both the complexity of a randomized trial and the costs of the intervention.

M. Corriere, MD, MS

Magnetic resonance imaging-based monitoring of collateral artery development in patients with intermittent claudication during supervised exercise therapy

Versluis B, Leiner T, Nelemans PJ, et al (Maastricht Univ Med Ctr, The Netherlands)
J Vasc Surg 58:1236-1243, 2013

Objective.—The purpose of the current study was to determine whether supervised exercise therapy (SET) leads to measurable vascular adaptations in patients with intermittent claudication using contrast-enhanced magnetic resonance angiography and flow measurements.

Methods.—Ten patients with clinical symptoms of intermittent claudication and proven obstructive arterial lesions of the superficial femoral artery were included and underwent SET for a period of 6 months. At baseline, all patients underwent a treadmill test to assess pain free walking distance, ankle brachial index measurement, and magnetic resonance imaging to determine the number of arteries in the upper leg using contrast-enhanced magnetic resonance angiography and arterial peak flow in the popliteal artery using cine phase contrast angiography. All examinations were repeated after 3 and 6 months of SET, respectively, to evaluate vascular responses relative to baseline.

Results.—After 6 months of SET, mean pain free walking distance (395 ± 46 m) was improved by 71% compared with baseline (230 ± 42 m; $P < .01$). No statistically significant changes were found for mean values of ankle brachial index (81 ± 4 and 77 ± 4, respectively, at baseline and after 6 months of SET), number of arteries at the level of the arterial lesion (18 ± 2 and 19 ± 2, respectively) nor arterial peak flow (5.3 ± 0.6 and 5.3 ± 0.8 mL/s, respectively).

Conclusions.—SET in patients with intermittent claudication results in an increase in pain free walking distance, whereas with magnetic resonance imaging no macrovascular adaptations in terms of additional collateral artery formation or flow increases could be observed (Table).

▶ There is no question that supervised exercise therapy (SET) for intermittent claudication is effective; we just aren't sure how it works. In this analysis, anatomic and functional magnetic resonance imaging (MRI)-based assessments were combined with the more familiar ankle-brachial index (ABI) to assess changes in collateral vessels and arterial flow during 6 months of SET for intermittent claudication. The authors observed significant increases in pain-free walking distance but no changes in ABI or MRI-based assessments of collateral

TABLE.—Baseline and Follow-up Results after 3 and 6 Months of SET, Respectively

	Baseline	3 Months	6 Months
SET			
Pain free walking distance (m)	230 ± 42	362 ± 53[a]	395 ± 46[a]
Number of arteries			
5 cm above lesion	23 ± 3	21 ± 3	20 ± 3
At lesion level	18 ± 2	18 ± 3	19 ± 2
5 cm below lesion	12 ± 1	12 ± 1	12 ± 1
APF (mL/s)			
At rest (n = 10)	5.3 ± 0.6	5.5 ± 0.8	5.3 ± 0.8
Maximum hyperemic flow (n = 6)	7.1 ± 3.5	7.8 ± 3.3	7.5 ± 2.4
Ankle-brachial index	81 ± 4	80 ± 4	77 ± 4

APF, Arterial peak flow; *SET,* supervised exercise therapy.
Values are mean ± standard error.
[a] $P < .01$ compared with baseline.

vessel counts and peak arterial flow (Table). Interestingly, 60% of participants (who were newly diagnosed with intermittent claudication) had collateral vessels at baseline before initiation of SET, suggesting that these vessels may form before symptom onset.

The results of this study corroborate previous investigations demonstrating that SET can lead to impressive improvement in pain-free walking distance that occurs in the absence of detectable changes in arterial perfusion. These results provide additional detail to our understanding of how SET works by eliminating macrovascular changes as a likely mechanistic explanation. It would be interesting to see these analyses could be extended with exercise MRI, which would allow direct evaluation of flow under the same conditions that produce symptoms and might result in physiologic circumstances distinct from those that occur during postischemic reactive hyperemia. Further insight is therefore needed to understand whether SET works through changes in microvascular circulation, pain threshold, or other mechanisms; regardless, these results are a reminder that many of the surrogate measures we rely on to assess procedural interventions (such as ABI) often provide an incomplete picture of treatment effect.

M. Corriere, MD, MS

Current efficacy of open and endovascular interventions for advanced superficial femoral artery occlusive disease

Smolock CJ, Anaya-Ayala JE, Kaufman Y, et al (Houston Methodist Hosp, TX)

J Vasc Surg 58:1267-1275, 2013

Background.—There has been a marked paradigm shift in the treatment of symptomatic femoro-popliteal disease with a shift from open to endoluminal therapy. The consequence of this shift in therapy is poorly described. The aim of this study is to examine the clinical efficacy of this shift in treatment strategies.

Methods.—A database of patients undergoing open (OPEN) and endoluminal (ENDO) intervention for TASC II C and D femoro-popliteal lesions between 1990 and 2010 was retrospectively queried. Kaplan-Meier survival analyses were performed to assess time-dependent outcomes. Factor analyses were performed using a multivariant Cox proportional hazard model for time-dependent variables.

Results.—A total of 2593 limbs underwent either OPEN or ENDO treatment for symptomatic and anatomically advanced femoro-popliteal disease over a 20-year period. There was a two-fold rise in endovascular interventions between the first and second decade. In the first decade, 80% of the interventions were OPEN, while in the second decade, 61% of the interventions were ENDO. There were equivalent comorbidities in both groups, and survival was also equivalent. Endoluminal therapy was more commonly performed on claudicants. Thirty-day mortality was equivalent, but major morbidity was higher in OPEN compared with ENDO. Cumulative patency was equivalent in both groups with a similar reintervention rate. In contrast, clinical efficacy (freedom from recurrent symptoms, maintenance of ambulation, and avoidance of major amputation) was significantly higher in the OPEN group ($P = .002$). The presence of critical limb ischemia, diabetes, end-stage renal disease, and poor tibial runoff were predictors of poor anatomic and functional outcomes in both groups.

Conclusions.—There has been a marked shift in treatment modality for advanced femoro-popliteal disease with a lowering of the symptomatic threshold for intervention over 2 decades, likely spurred by the ease of endoluminal interventions. Although peri-procedural and anatomic outcomes for both procedures are equivalent, it appears that open surgery carries a superior long-term clinical efficacy. This superiority is negatively influenced by poor preoperative ambulation status, high modified Cardiac Risk Score, worse presenting symptoms, the occurrence of major adverse cardiovascular events, poor tibial runoff, the absence of hemodynamic success, and occlusion of the original bypass (Figs 1 and 2, Tables 2 and 3).

▶ This retrospective cohort analysis provides a comparison between open and endovascular interventions for superficial femoral artery occlusive disease in a

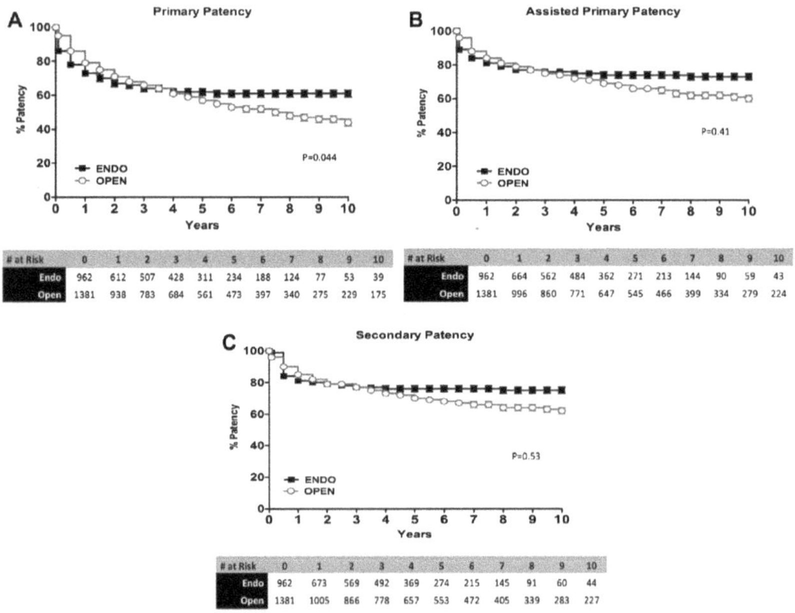

# at Risk	0	1	2	3	4	5	6	7	8	9	10
Endo	962	612	507	428	311	234	188	124	77	53	39
Open	1381	938	783	684	561	473	397	340	275	229	175

# at Risk	0	1	2	3	4	5	6	7	8	9	10
Endo	962	664	562	484	362	271	213	144	90	59	43
Open	1381	996	860	771	647	545	466	399	334	279	224

# at Risk	0	1	2	3	4	5	6	7	8	9	10
Endo	962	673	569	492	369	274	215	145	91	60	44
Open	1381	1005	866	778	657	553	472	405	339	283	227

FIGURE 1.—Anatomic outcomes. Kaplan-Meier analysis of patients with open (*OPEN*) or endovascular (*ENDO*) interventions. Data are the mean ± standard error of the mean and number of limbs at risk shown in the table. No error bars are shown if the standard error of the mean is >10%, and the data set terminates if the number at risk is <10. Log rank sum test was performed for statistical analysis. **A,** Primary patency. **B,** Assisted primary patency. **C,** Secondary patency. (Reprinted from Smolock CJ, Anaya-Ayala JE, Kaufman Y, et al. Current efficacy of open and endovascular interventions for advanced superficial femoral artery occlusive disease. *J Vasc Surg*. 2013;58:1267-1275, with permission from The Society for Vascular Surgery.)

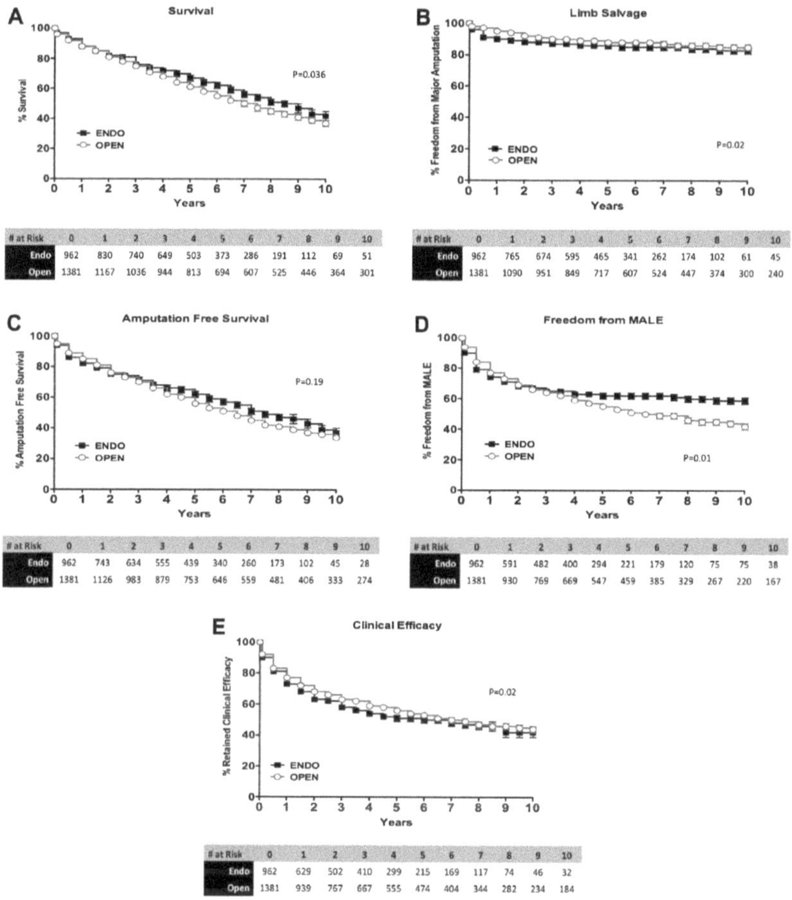

FIGURE 2.—Functional outcomes: Kaplan-Meier analysis of patients with open (*OPEN*) or endovascular (*ENDO*) interventions. Data are the mean ± standard error of the mean and number of patients or limbs at risk shown in the table. No error bars are shown if the standard error of the mean is >10% and the data set terminates if the number at risk is <10. Log rank sum test was performed for statistical analysis. **A**, Survival. **B**, Limb salvage. **C**, Amputation-free survival. **D**, Freedom from MALE. **E**, Clinical efficacy. *MALE*, Major adverse limb event. (Reprinted from Smolock CJ, Anaya-Ayala JE, Kaufman Y, et al. Current efficacy of open and endovascular interventions for advanced superficial femoral artery occlusive disease. *J Vasc Surg*. 2013;58:1267-1275, with permission from The Society for Vascular Surgery.)

single-center institutional cohort over a 20-year period. The authors aimed to examine the clinical efficacy (which they defined based on freedom from recurrent symptoms, maintenance of ambulation, and freedom from major amputation) of the shift from open surgical to endovascular treatment as the predominant method that occurred over the study period. Open surgical revascularization was undertaken most often in the setting of TASC II category D lesions (96% vs 39% for endovascular treatment; Table 2), consistent with the selection bias that would be expected within a nonrandomized study. As might be expected, perioperative rates of major adverse cardiovascular events and morbidity were

TABLE 2.—Runoff and Lesion Characteristics

	ENDO	OPEN	*P* Value
Tibial runoff			
Tibial vessels, No.	2.0 ± 0.8	1.9 ± 0.8	.003[a]
Modified SVS runoff score	5.7 ± 3.4	6.8 ± 4.5	.0001[a]
TASC II category			
C	61	4	.0001[b]
D	39	96	
Amputation risk score			
PREVENT III	2.4 ± 2.3	2.1 ± 1.9	.0004[a]
Low (0-3)	73	78	.0005[b]
Medium (4-7)	22	20	
High (>7)	5	1	

ENDO, Endoluminal intervention; *OPEN*, open intervention; *PREVENT III*, Project of Ex-vivo Vein Graft Engineering via Transfection III; *SVS*, Society for Vascular Surgery; *TASC II*, TransAtlantic Inter-Society Consensus II.
Data are presented as percentages or mean ± standard deviations.
[a]Mann Whitney test.
[b]Fisher exact test.

TABLE 3.—Mortality, Morbidity, and Objective Performance Goals

	ENDO, %	OPEN, %	*P* Value
Mortality and morbidity			
Mortality	1.5	2	.456[a]
Morbidity	3	8	.001[a]
Reintervention rate	27	22	.004[a]
OPG			
30-day MACE	3	7	.001[a]
30-day MALE	11	5	.001[a]
30-day major amputations	4	2	.001[a]

ENDO, Endoluminal intervention; *MACE*, major adverse cardiovascular event; *MALE*, major adverse limb event; *OPEN*, open intervention; *OPG*, objective performance goals.
[a]Fisher exact test.

significantly higher after open revascularization, whereas 30-day risk of major adverse limb events, repeat intervention, and amputation were higher after endovascular treatment (Table 3); no difference in perioperative mortality was noted between groups. Patency outcomes were similar between treatments (Fig 1), but greater clinical efficacy was observed with open versus endovascular treatment (Fig 2), although the magnitude of this difference was small. When considering these findings, it is important to bear in mind that the majority of interventions in both groups were performed for intermittent claudication. Because expected amputation risk would be low among patients with claudication versus patients with critical limb ischemia, combining these patients into a single cohort (a common practice for cohort studies defined by procedural interventions) may have obscured more significant differences in limb salvage and amputation-free survival in the latter group. Unfortunately, subgroup analyses for these end points were not included.

Selecting an approach to lower extremity revascularization requires consideration of a number of factors, including anatomic disease distribution, patient risk and comorbidities, availability of a suitable single-segment vein conduit, and symptom severity. In some instances, anatomic and comorbidity factors align to make the decision easy. Unfortunately, however, these factors are often opposed to each other, such as when patients with significant comorbidities are better anatomic candidates for higher-risk surgical revascularization. In these situations, patients and providers are left to choose which factors to prioritize and which to compromise. Decision making in these situations often comes down to choices between short- and long-term perspectives related to risk versus completeness of revascularization. Along those lines, it is interesting to note that 14% of patients in this study required open bypass within 3 months of their endovascular procedure. This crossover underscores the importance of treatment failure as a consideration during treatment selection, particularly in the setting of intermittent claudication, in which nonoperative treatment options have expanded with availability of cilostazol, and treatment failures may be accompanied by progression to more severe symptoms.

M. Corriere, MD, MS

Atherectomy offers no benefits over balloon angioplasty in tibial interventions for critical limb ischemia

Todd KE Jr, Ahanchi SS, Maurer CA, et al (Eastern Virginia Med School, Norfolk, VA)

J Vasc Surg 58:941-948, 2013

Background.—Endovascular adjuncts, like atherectomy, were developed to improve outcomes of endovascular arterial interventions. The true impact of atherectomy on endovascular outcomes remains to be determined, and little data exist on the influence of atherectomy on tibial interventions. Our study compares early and late outcomes of tibial intervention with angioplasty vs atherectomy-assisted interventions.

Methods.—We completed a retrospective review of all tibial interventions between 2008 and 2010. Outcomes were analyzed using single and multivariate analysis, Cox regression, and Kaplan-Meier curves. Primary outcomes were primary, primary assisted, and secondary patency rates, as well as limb salvage and survival rates.

Results.—Over a 2-year period, 480 tibial interventions were completed for 421 patients. Eighty-seven percent (n = 418) of interventions were performed for critical limb ischemia (CLI) and 13% (n = 62) for claudication. The CLI cohort of 418 interventions was analyzed. These patients had a mean age of 71 years with a mean follow-up time of 16 ± 15 months (range, 0-59 months). Of the 418 interventions, 339 underwent percutaneous transluminal angioplasty (PTA): 333 PTA alone, six PTA + stent. The remaining 79 interventions received atherectomy: 33 laser, 13 directional, and 33 orbital either alone or in conjunction with PTA (11 atherectomy only, 68 atherectomy + PTA). The groups did not differ significantly in terms of demographics, risk factors, or technical success. The atherectomy group had more TASC B lesions (54% vs 38%; $P=.013$), while the PTA-alone group had more TASC D lesions (25% vs 13%; $P=.004$). TASC A and C lesions did not differ significantly between the groups. No significant differences existed with respect to the early (30-day) outcomes of loss of patency (11% vs 13%; $P=.699$), complications (8% vs 13%; $P=.292$), or major amputation (17% vs 13%; $P=.344$) in the PTA-alone group vs the atherectomy-assisted group. Kaplan-Meier analysis revealed no difference for all primary outcomes of PTA alone vs the atherectomy-assisted group at 12 and 36 months: primary patency (69%, 55% vs 61%, 46%; $P=.158$), primary assisted patency (83%, 71% vs 85%, 67%; $P=.801$), secondary patency (94%, 89% vs 95%, 89%; $P=.892$), limb salvage (79%, 70% vs 81%, 77%; $P=.485$), or survival (77%, 56% vs 80%, 50%; $P=.944$).

Conclusions.—The adjunctive use of atherectomy offered no improvement in primary outcomes over PTA alone in either early or late outcomes in CLI patients who underwent endovascular tibial interventions. Considering the additional cost and increased procedural time, these findings put into question the routine use of adjunctive atherectomy (Figs 1 and 4).

▶ The variety of available endovascular treatments for critical limb ischemia (CLI) and their frequent combined use often make it difficult to translate

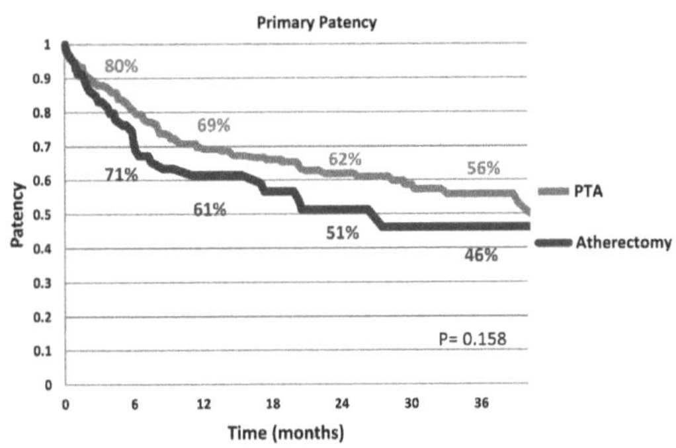

No. At Risk	0 m	6 m	12 m	24 m	36 m
PTA	339	182	123	67	32
Atherectomy	78	63	30	13	3

Standard Error %	0 m	6 m	12 m	24 m	36 m
PTA	0.3	1.3	3.0	3.5	4.1
Atherectomy	0.0	5.8	6.4	7.1	8.0

FIGURE 1.—Primary patency outcomes and Kaplan-Meier life tables for patients with critical limb ischemia (CLI) who underwent either atherectomy (*blue*) or percutaneous transluminal angioplasty (PTA) (*red*). Cox regression analysis revealed no significant difference in primary patency based on treatment method. Results shown at the 6-, 12-, 24-, and 36-month time points. *m*, Months. For interpretation of the references to color in this figure legend, the reader is referred to web version of this article. (Reprinted from Todd KE Jr, Ahanchi SS, Maurer CA, et al. Atherectomy offers no benefits over balloon angioplasty in tibial interventions for critical limb ischemia. *J Vasc Surg*. 2013;58:941-948, Copyright 2013, with permission from The Society for Vascular Surgery.)

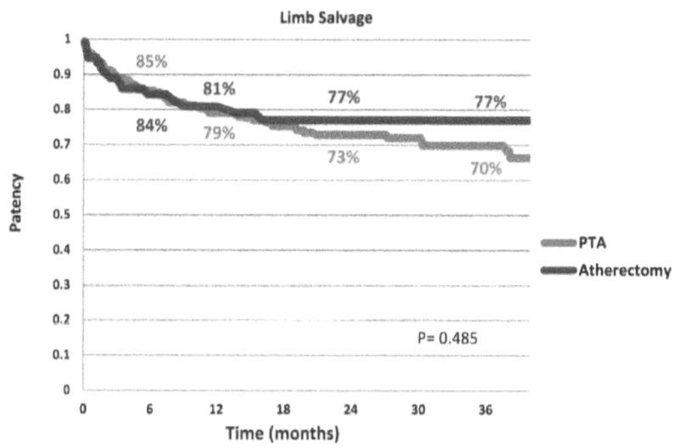

No. At Risk	0 m	6 m	12 m	24 m	36 m
PTA	339	218	168	100	48
Atherectomy	78	54	44	22	6

Standard Error %	0 m	6 m	12 m	24 m	36 m
PTA	0.4	2.0	2.5	2.9	3.3
Atherectomy	1.3	4.4	4.8	5.3	5.3

FIGURE 4.—Limb salvage outcomes and Kaplan-Meier life tables for patients with critical limb ischemia (CLI) who underwent either atherectomy (*blue*) or percutaneous transluminal angioplasty (PTA) (*red*). Cox regression analysis revealed no significant difference in limb salvage based on treatment method. Results shown at the 6-, 12-, 24-, and 36- month time points. *m*, Months. For interpretation of the references to color in this figure legend, the reader is referred to web version of this article. (Reprinted from Todd KE Jr, Ahanchi SS, Maurer CA, et al. Atherectomy offers no benefits over balloon angioplasty in tibial interventions for critical limb ischemia. *J Vasc Surg*. 2013;58:941-948, Copyright 2013, with permission from The Society for Vascular Surgery.)

retrospective cohort study results into evidence-based approaches to procedural management. Although this study was both retrospective and nonrandomized, it nonetheless provides some useful insights into endovascular treatment of CLI. By excluding patients treated for claudication and focusing on a single anatomic location (tibial disease), the results allow assessment of adjunctive atherectomy unencumbered by some confounders that most often limit the conclusions that can be drawn from retrospective analyses. The nonrandomized approach to atherectomy use, however, is a major limitation that may have resulted in a potential selection bias and warrants further consideration when interpreting the results. Presumably, atherectomy was utilized in some scenarios in which transluminal angioplasty (PTA) alone was either technically unsuccessful or might have been avoided because of adverse lesion characteristics (such as significant calcification). In such scenarios, adjunctive atherectomy may have salvaged endovascular interventions that otherwise would have been failures or expanded endovascular treatment options for patients who otherwise might have been limited to surgical revascularization. Interpreted from this perspective, outcomes with adjunctive atherectomy that are equivalent to PTA alone might actually indicate an advantage gained through atherectomy for patients poorly suited to PTA alone. Unfortunately, the report does not provide detailed information regarding the criteria for use of atherectomy beyond surgeon preference. Because several atherectomy devices were utilized (33 laser, 33 orbital, and 13 directional), the results also provide a relatively limited contribution to device-specific outcomes.

Similar outcomes (including primary patency, primary assisted patency, secondary patency, limb salvage, and survival) were observed with PTA versus PTA with adjunctive atherectomy, leading the authors to conclude that the routine use of adjunctive atherectomy has questionable benefit, particularly when the increased costs and procedure durations versus PTA alone are taken into account. Whether these disadvantages are partially mitigated by expansion of endovascular treatment options through use of atherectomy remains to be determined, and randomized comparisons with specific anatomic inclusion criteria may be necessary to definitively answer these questions and define the role of atherectomy for CLI.

M. Corriere, MD, MS

Patient radiation exposure during percutaneous endovascular revascularization of the lower extremity

Segal E, Weinberg I, Leichter I, et al (Hadassah Hebrew Univ Med Ctr, Jerusalem, Israel; et al)

J Vasc Surg 58:1556-1562, 2013

Background.—Percutaneous endovascular revascularization is emerging as the first line treatment for peripheral artery disease for both intermittent claudication and chronic critical limb ischemia. Radiation doses for these interventions have not been well documented.

Methods.—A single center retrospective study of therapeutic endovascular lower extremity interventions performed between September 2006 and December 2011 was undertaken. Collected data included patient demographics, procedure indication, procedural access, anatomic location of occlusive disease (pelvis, thigh, below-knee, or multilevel), and radiation exposure parameters including dose area product (DAP) and fluoroscopy time.

Results.—Data was available for 382 procedures performed in 313 patients. Eighteen procedures bilateral procedures were excluded. Access site and complete anatomic data were available for 346 procedures. DAP was significantly higher for procedures performed in the pelvis compared with thigh procedures (179.6 vs 63.2 Gy*cm^2; $P < .0001$) and below-knee procedures (179.6 vs 28.9 Gy*cm^2; $P < .0001$), despite shorter fluoroscopy times (11.8 vs 16.4 minutes; $P < .0001$ and 11.1 vs 31.06 minutes; $P < .0001$, respectively). Procedure access-site affected radiation dose as well; contralateral up-and-over access resulted in a higher DAP than antegrade access (112.2 vs 42.6 Gy*cm^2; $P < .0001$). In a multivariable analysis, anatomic location of the procedure showed the strongest association with radiation dose ($P < .0001$).

Conclusions.—Percutaneous endovascular revascularization for lower extremity peripheral artery disease involves a substantial radiation dose, comparable, on average, to a computed tomography scan of the abdomen and pelvis. Procedures performed in the pelvis for intermittent claudication involve more radiation than thigh or below-knee procedures for chronic critical limb ischemia. Radiation dose should be considered when planning these procedures (Figs 1 and 2, Table 3).

▶ Procedure-related radiation exposure is seldom the emphasis of routine preoperative counseling, but increasing emphasis is being placed on the associated risks (particularly related to cumulative effects of repeated exposures) for both patients and providers, especially given the increasingly common use of diagnostic computed tomography scans for both vascular and nonvascular indications. Although this retrospective study did not include skin dose measurement and was unable to account for patient body mass index in dose calculations, it nonetheless provides useful data on an important topic that is understudied. The retrospective design may also offer a more genuine approximation of "real-world" radiation doses associated with lower extremity endovascular procedures by minimizing potential effects of study observation on provider behavior (commonly known as the Hawthorne effect).

In their multivariate analysis, the authors identified anatomic imaging location (Table 3) and arterial access site as the primary factors associated with radiation dose (calculated as the dose area product [DAP]). Fluoroscopy time, one of the variables that operators may often rely on to gauge when a radiation exposure is approaching potentially hazardous levels, was not a significant predictor of DAP;

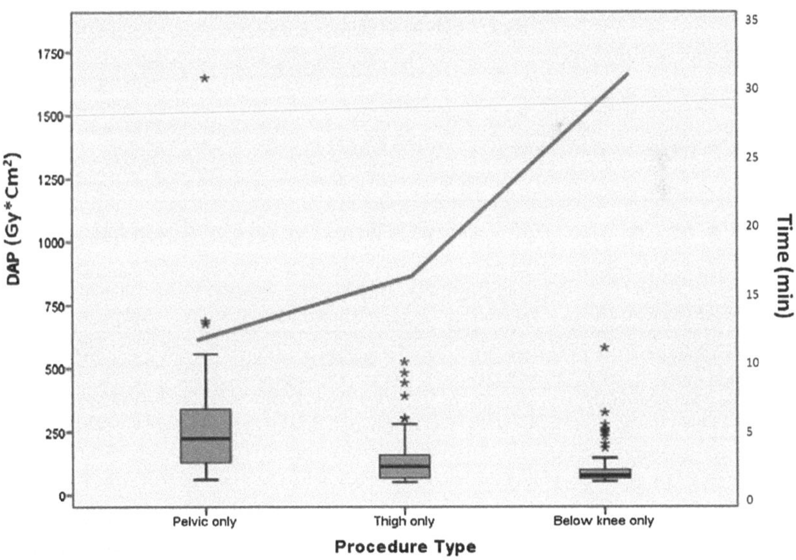

FIGURE 1.—Dose area product (*DAP*) (*Gy***cm*^{2}, *box plots*) and fluoroscopy time (*blue line*) in respect to anatomic location of the procedure. *Extreme outliers: [interquartile 75 + 1.5 *(interquartile range, 75-25)]. For interpretation of the references to color in this figure legend, the reader is referred to web version of this article. (Reprinted from Segal E, Weinberg I, Leichter I, et al. Patient radiation exposure during percutaneous endovascular revascularization of the lower extremity. *J Vasc Surg*. 2013;58:1556-1562, Copyright 2013, with permission from The Society for Vascular Surgery.)

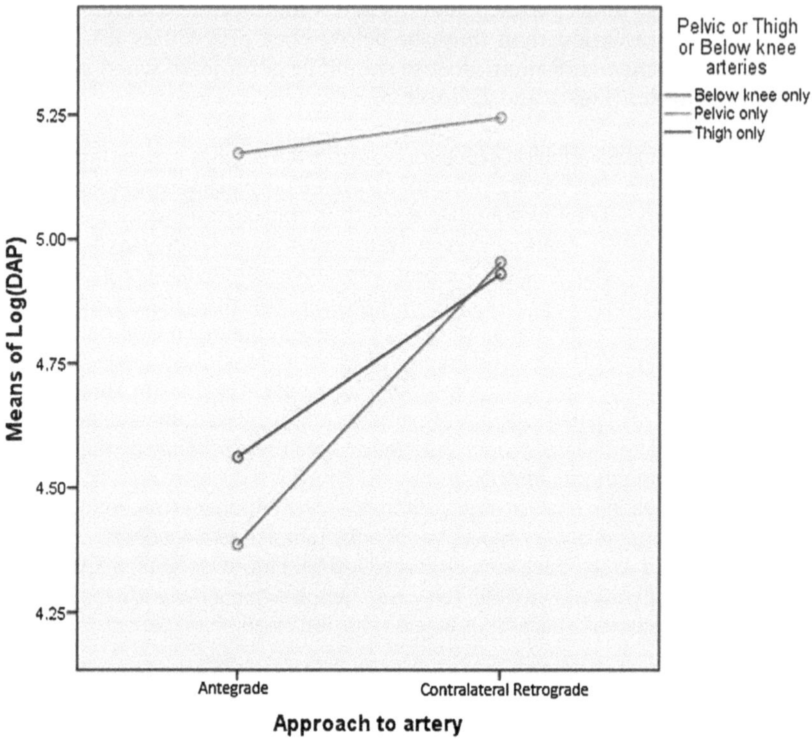

FIGURE 2.—Relative influences of anatomic location and access. The statistically dominant factors impacting the dose area product (*DAP*), calculated by multivariate analysis (log DAP). (Reprinted from Segal E, Weinberg I, Leichter I, et al. Patient radiation exposure during percutaneous endovascular revascularization of the lower extremity. *J Vasc Surg*. 2013;58:1556-1562, Copyright 2013, with permission from The Society for Vascular Surgery.)

TABLE 3.—Group size, DAP Values, and Fluoroscopy Time by Type of Intervention

Type of Intervention	Group Size, No. (%)[a]	DAP, Gy*cm^2, Median [Interquartile Range]	Fluoroscopy Time, Minutes, Median [Interquartile Range]
Pelvic intervention	98 (27)	179.6 [81.2-343.2][b]	11 [8-20][b]
Thigh intervention	95 (26)	63.2 [18.9-109.6]	16 [10-31]
Below-knee intervention	62 (17)	28.9 [16.6-72.9]	31 [20-51]
Multilevel intervention	109 (30)	49.5 [24.7-119.1]	36.1 [21.8-48.5]

DAP, Dose area product.
[a]Percentages for patient and procedure characteristics were calculated from the total number of available data for any respective dataset.
[b]Statistically higher when compared with the thigh, below-knee, and multilevel intervention group ($P < .0001$).

indeed, the anatomic procedure categories with the lowest DAP tended to have the highest fluoroscopy times (Fig 1). Although the anatomic procedure category is not a modifiable risk factor, it is interesting to consider the implications of the association between greater DAP and contralateral retrograde versus antegrade access. Based on these findings, procedure-related radiation exposure could potentially be reduced through preferential use of antegrade arterial access. Because providers may often base access location on anatomic considerations that may influence both technical success and complication risk, these issues must be weighed against radiation exposure when choosing an access site. For procedures in which antegrade arterial access does not compromise risk or create technical issues, this approach may allow reduction in radiation exposure, particularly for patients undergoing thigh or below-knee interventions associated with the greatest access-related increases in exposure (Fig 2).

M. Corriere, MD, MS

Percutaneous transluminal angioplasty results in improved physical function but not balance in patients with intermittent claudication

Gohil RA, Mockford KA, Mazari FA, et al (Univ of Hull, UK)

J Vasc Surg 58:1533-1539, 2013

Objective.—The aim of this study was to identify whether revascularization by percutaneous transluminal angioplasty (PTA) for patients with intermittent claudication improved measures of functional performance including balance.

Methods.—A prospective observational study was performed at a single tertiary vascular center. Patients with symptomatic intermittent claudication (Rutherford grades 1-3) were recruited to the study. Participants were assessed at baseline (pre-PTA) and then 3, 6, and 12 months post-PTA for markers of (1) lower limb ischemia (treadmill walking distances and ankle-brachial pressure index), (2) physical function (6-minute walk, Timed Up and Go, and chair stand time), (3) balance impairment using computerized dynamic posturography with the Sensory Organization Test, and (4) quality of life (VascuQoL and Short Form Health Survey [SF-36]).

Results.—Forty-three participants underwent PTA. Over 12 months, a significant improvement was demonstrated in initial ($P = .04$) and maximum treadmill walking distance ($P = .019$). Physical functional ability improved across all outcome measures ($P < .02$), and some domains of both generic ($P < .03$) and disease-specific quality of life ($P < .01$). No significant improvement in balance was demonstrated by the Sensory Organization Test ($P = .24$).

Conclusions.—Balance impairment is common in claudicants and does not improve with revascularization. Further research regarding effective treatment of balance impairment is required in this specific group of patients (Tables 1-5).

▶ Walking impairment among patients with peripheral arterial disease (PAD) is often a manifestation of several contributing factors, particularly among elderly people with a high prevalence of neuropathy, osteoarthritis, dementia, and cerebrovascular disease. Although treatment decision making can be relatively

TABLE 1.—Patient Demographics at Baseline for all PTA Patients

Demographics	Angioplasty, No. (%)
Number	43
Bilateral symptoms	23 (55)
Level of lesion treated by PTA	
Suprainguinal	11 (26)
Infrainguinal	12 (28)
Combined	20 (46)
Rutherford grade[14]	
2	4 (9)
2	27 (63)
3	12 (28)
Comorbidity	
Ischemic heart disease	20 (47)
Hypertension	29 (67)
On statin therapy	32 (74)
Cerebrovascular disease	9 (21)
Diabetes	7 (16)
Smoker (current/ex)	9 (21)/28 (65)
Osteoarthritis lower limb	18 (42)

PTA, Percutaneous transluminal angioplasty.

Ischemic heart disease was defined as a previous cardiac event (myocardial infarction, angina, or coronary artery bypass graft), and hypertension was defined as a systolic blood pressure greater than 140 mm Hg (in diabetics, it was lowered to 130 mm Hg), or the requirement of antihypertensives. Cerebrovascular disease was defined as having had a previous stroke, transient ischemic attack, or previous carotid endarterectomy.

Editor's Note: Please refer to original journal article for full references.

TABLE 2.—Changes in Markers of Lower Limb Ischemia and Physical Function Over 12 Months Post-PTA

	Baseline	3 Months	6 Months	12 Months	Friedman Analysis of Variance
Pre-exercise ABPI	.80 (.66-.93)	.92 (.86-1.03)	.86 (.77-1.09)	.90 (.83-1.01)	<.01
Postexercise ABPI	.52 (.31-.76)	.77 (.53-.87)	.60 (.44-1.00)	.69 (.49-.94)	.12
Treadmill ICD, m	28.6 (16.1-40.2)	41.0 (35.5-87.5)	55.0 (30.5-123.5)	61.0 (25.1-110.5)	.04
Treadmill MWD, m	60.8 (49.0-125.0)	82.0 (65.0-125.5)	86.0 (64.5-215.0)	105.0 (64.0-215.0)	.02
6-minute ICD, m	120 (50-135)	200 (120-260)	325 (190-367.5)	220 (120-385)	.01
6-minute MWD, m	315 (185-400)	360 (280-440)	380 (340-450)	300 (290-360)	.02
SPPB	8 (6-10)	10 (8-12)	10 (8-11)	11 (8-11)	<.01
4-meter usual walk, seconds	3.9 (3.6-6.3)	4.1 (3.6-5.1)	3.9 (3.5-4.9)	3.7 (3.3-5.3)	.03
4-meter fast walk, seconds	3.3 (2.9-4.1)	3.3 (2.6-4.1)	2.9 (2.7-3.6)	2.9 (2.4-3.8)	.04
Mean chair stand time, seconds	17.2 (12.4-20.0)	13.3 (11.4-16.3)	12.7 (10.5-16.3)	13.1 (11.9-19.5)	.02
TUG, seconds	10.0 (9.3-13.4)	9.2 (7.9-12.0)	8.4 (7.3-10.9)	8.6 (7.4-11.2)	<.01

ABPI, Ankle-brachial pressure index; ICD, initial claudication distance; MWD, maximal walking distance; PTA, percutaneous transluminal angioplasty; SBBP, short physical performance battery; TUG, timed up and go test.

Data are presented as median and interquartile range values.

TABLE 3.—Changes in Generic (SF-36) QOL Over Time Post-PTA Over 12 Months

SF-36 Domain	Baseline	3 Months	6 Months	12 Months	Friedman Analysis of Variance
Physical functioning	35.0 (25.0-50.0)	55.0 (40.0-80.0)	52.5 (37.5-72.5)	60.0 (35.5-80.0)	<.01
Role physical	25.0 (0.0-50.0)	50.0 (0.0-100.0)	25.0 (0.0-100.0)	12.5 (0.0-100.0)	.03
Bodily pain	41.0 (31.0-51.0)	62.0 (41.0-74.0)	41.0 (31.0-92.0)	52.0 (31.0-62.0)	.08
General health	50.0 (40.0-72.0)	57.0 (40.0-72.0)	47.0 (40.0-67.0)	45.0 (35.0-72.0)	.34
Vitality	50.0 (30.0-65.0)	60.0 (45.0-75.0)	57.5 (42.5-70.0)	50.0 (43.9-75.0)	.03
Role emotional	56.3 (33.3-87.5)	100.0 (33.3-100.0)	96.0 (0.0-100.0)	66.7 (0.0-100.0)	.17
Social functioning	75.0 (50.0-88.0)	81.3 (50.0-100.0)	75.0 (50.0-100.0)	62.5 (56.8-87.5)	.27
Mental health	70.0 (52.0-100.0)	76.0 (64.0-88.0)	80.0 (56.0-92.0)	74.0 (56.0-84.0)	.40
Physical summary score	30.3 (25.3-34.5)	42.6 (28.2-48.9)	33.0 (27.1-49.6)	36.5 (24.5-49.3)	.01
Mental summary score	52.3 (41.1-61.2)	53.9 (44.4-60.8)	53.5 (40.5-59.9)	51.4 (43.1-58.2)	.62

SF-36, Short Form Health Survey; *PTA*, percutaneous transluminal angioplasty; *QOL*, quality of life.
Data are presented as median and interquartile range values.

TABLE 4.—Changes in Disease-Specific (VascuQol) QOL Over Time Post-PTA Over 12 Months

VascuQol Domain	Baseline	3 Months	6 Months	12 Months	Friedman Analysis of Variance
Pain	3.0 (4.6-2.6)	5.0 (3.9-6.1)	5.3 (4.0-6.4)	5.8 (5.1-6.3)	<.01
Social	4.5 (3.3-6.3)	6.5 (5.3-7.0)	6.5 (4.3-7.0)	6.0 (5.3-7.0)	.11
Activities	3.6 (3.3-4.1)	5.5 (4.5-6.5)	5.6 (3.9-6.6)	5.6 (4.1-6.1)	.02
Symptoms	4.8 (3.8-5.6)	5.8 (5.5-6.6)	6.0 (5.1-6.5)	6.3 (5.6-6.8)	.01
Emotions	4.4 (3.6-5.4)	6.6 (5.5-6.9)	6.3 (5.4-6.9)	6.6 (5.8-7.0)	<.01
Total	4.2 (3.3-4.8)	5.8 (5.2-6.4)	6.1 (4.6-6.4)	6.0 (5.1-6.5)	<.01

PTA, Percutaneous transluminal angioplasty; *QOL*, quality of life.
Data are presented as median and interquartile range values.

TABLE 5.—Changes in Markers of Objective Balance Post-PTA Over 12 Months

	Baseline	3 Months	6 Months	12 Months	*P*
N (missing)	43	39 (4)	22 (21)	28 (15)	
Semi-tandem stance, seconds	30.0 (11.7-30.0)	30.00 (30.00-30.00)	30.00 (30.00-30.00)	30.00 (30.00-30.00)	.05[a]
Full tandem stance, seconds	29.5 (7.6-30.0)	30.0 (15.0-30.0)	30.0 (19.0-30.0)	30.0 (20.4-30.0)	.41[a]
Composite SOT score	65.0 (57.8-70.5)	70.0 (63.0-75.5)	69.5 (57.0-77.0)	68.0 (63.3-74.8)	.24[a]

PTA, Percutaneous transluminal angioplasty; *QOL*, quality of life; *SOT*, Sensory Organization Test.
Data are presented as median and interquartile range values.
[a]Friedman analysis of variance.

straightforward when symptoms are limited to claudication alone, the potential benefit of revascularization becomes more difficult to predict when patients also have gait instability related to factors other than PAD. This study gives us a valuable characterization of the complex associations among limb ischemia, physical ability, balance, and quality of life (QOL) and provides some insight into which of these domains respond to endovascular treatment.

Sample size calculation for this prospective study was based on a balance end point (the composite equilibrium score from the sensory organization test), with assessment of multiple domains before percutaneous transluminal angioplasty for intermittent claudication and at 3, 6, and 12 months postprocedure. Although study participants had a median age of 69 years and several comorbidities other than PAD that might contribute to walking impairment (Table 1), it is important to note that patients with neuropathy, dementia, or significant systemic disease that would impair ability to participate in balance testing were excluded. The study therefore excluded some of the clinical scenarios in which treatment decision making is most challenging, although this approach likely increased the sensitivity to detect balance improvement. The results demonstrated improvement in walking distances and resting ankle brachial index (Table 2), 4 of 10 generic QOL domains (Table 3), and 5 of 6 disease-specific QOL domains (Table 4) over 12 months, but there was no change in objective balance assessments (Table 5).

These results confirm that balance impairment should not be presumed to be a direct consequence of limb ischemia and that balance improvement should not be an expected symptomatic response after revascularization for intermittent claudication. These observations may support a more conservative approach when walking impairment symptoms include falls and/or balance impairment and may also help providers and patients establish reasonable expectations regarding treatment outcomes when revascularization is undertaken in these complex scenarios.

M. Corriere, MD, MS

External Support of a Polytetrafluoroethylene Graft Improves Patency for Bypass to Below-Knee Arteries

Lundgren F, on behalf of the Swedish External Support Study (SWEXSUS) (Univ Hosp, Linköping, Sweden)
Ann Vasc Surg 27:1124-1133, 2013

Background.—Patency and limb salvage after synthetic bypass to the arteries below the knee are inferior to that which can be achieved with autologous vein. The use of external support of synthetic polytetrafluoroethylene (PTFE) grafts to the below-knee position has been suggested to improve patency and limb salvage, a problem analyzed in this randomized clinical trial. We examined whether external graft support improves patency and/or limb salvage in patients undergoing reconstruction with synthetic PTFE grafts to the below-knee arteries.

Methods.—Three hundred thirty-four patients with critical limb ischemia undergoing PTFE bypass to below-knee arteries were randomly assigned to have an ordinary PTFE graft or one with external support. Follow-up was scheduled until amputation, death, or at most 5 years, whichever event occurred first.

Results.—Patients in both the femoropopliteal and femorodistal groups were randomized to have an externally supported PTFE graft (101/195 patients in the femoropopliteal group and 72/139 patients in the femorodistal group). Follow-up information was available for 329 of 334 randomized patients (99%). At 1 year postprocedure, primary patency for below-knee bypass was 0.55 (95% confidence interval [CI], 0.47–0.64) with and 0.42 (95% CI, 0.34–0.50) without externally supported PTFE grafts, and secondary patency was 0.58 (95% CI, 0.51–0.67) and 0.47 (95% CI, 0.39–0.56), respectively. The corresponding figures for limb salvage were 0.75 (95% CI, 0.68–0.82) and 0.69 (95% CI, 0.62–0.77), respectively. The log rank test revealed statistically significant differences between patients with or without externally supported grafts for patency (primary patency: $\chi^2 = 4.2$ [degrees of freedom = 1; $P = 0.041$]; secondary patency: $\chi^2 = 4.3$ [degrees of freedom = 1; $P = 0.037$]) but not for limb salvage (limb salvage: $\chi^2 = 0.2$ [degrees of freedom = 1; $P = 0.657$]).

Conclusions.—External support to a PTFE graft used for bypass to below-knee arteries improves primary and secondary patency but not limb salvage (Figs 2-4, Table 1).

▶ This prospective trial randomized 335 patients to externally supported versus unsupported polytetrafluoroethylene (PTFE) grafts for below-knee bypass.

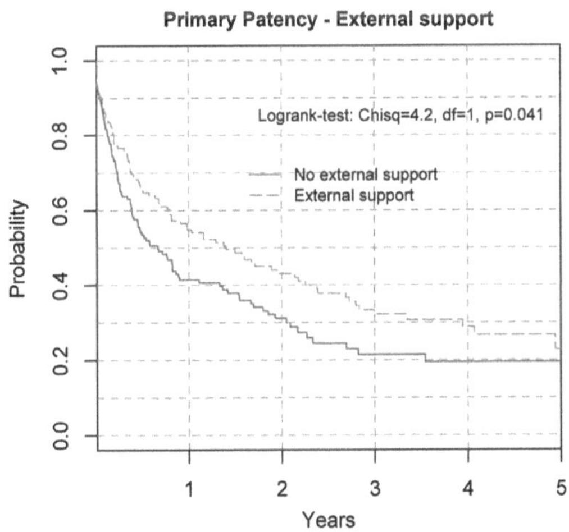

FIGURE 2.—Primary patency for femoropopliteal below-knee bypass to the popliteal or crural arteries with and without an externally supported polytetrafluoroethylene graft. In the log rank test, stratification was used for "vein collar" as explained in the text. The standard error of the Kaplan–Meier curves did not exceed 10%. (Reprinted from Lundgren F, on behalf of the Swedish External Support Study (SWEXSUS). External support of a polytetrafluoroethylene graft improves patency for bypass to below-knee arteries. *Ann Vasc Surg*. 2013;27:1124-1133, Copyright, with permission from Annals of Vascular Surgery, Inc.)

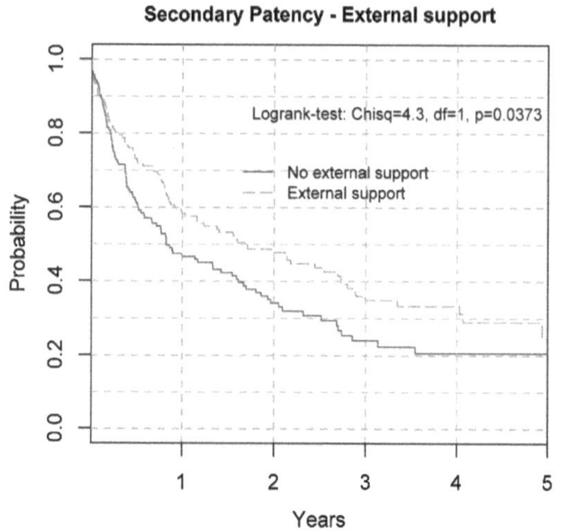

FIGURE 3.—Secondary patency for below-knee bypass to the popliteal or crural arteries with and without an externally supported polytetrafluoroethylene graft. In the log rank test, stratification was used for "vein collar" as explained in the text. The standard error of the Kaplan–Meier curves did not exceed 10%. (Reprinted from Lundgren F, on behalf of the Swedish External Support Study (SWEXSUS). External support of a polytetrafluoroethylene graft improves patency for bypass to below-knee arteries. *Ann Vasc Surg*. 2013;27:1124-1133, Copyright, with permission from Annals of Vascular Surgery, Inc.)

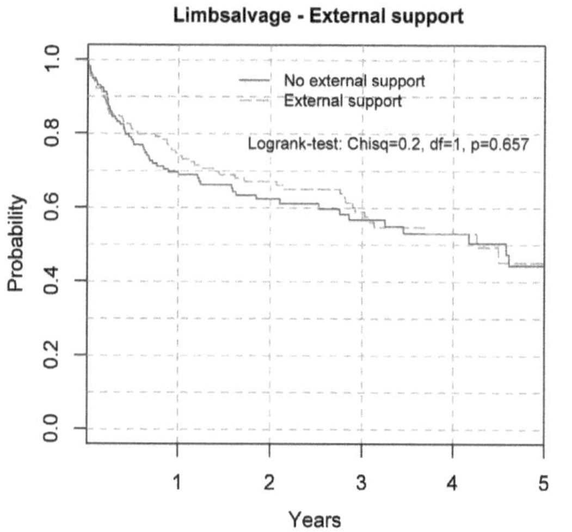

FIGURE 4.—Limb salvage for femoropopliteal below-knee bypass to the popliteal or crural arteries with and without an externally supported polytetrafluoroethylene graft. In the log rank test, stratification was used for "vein collar" as explained in the text. The standard error of the Kaplan–Meier curves did not exceed 10%. (Reprinted from Lundgren F, on behalf of the Swedish External Support Study (SWEXSUS). External support of a polytetrafluoroethylene graft improves patency for bypass to below-knee arteries. *Ann Vasc Surg*. 2013;27:1124-1133, Copyright, with permission from Annals of Vascular Surgery, Inc.)

TABLE 1.—Baseline Data of Randomized and Finally Analyzed Patients with Polytetrafluoroethylene Bypass to the Popliteal Below-Knee or Crural Arteries with and without Externally Supported Grafts[a]

	External Support	No External Support	All
N	172	157	329
Male sex	64/167 (38%)	68/162 (42%)	132/329 (40%)
Age (yr)	78 (71 83)	79 (72 83.75)	79 (72 83)
Rest pain/arterial ulcer/gangrene	158/167 (95%)	151/162 (93%)	309/329 (94%)
Acute ischemia or severe intermittent claudication	9/167 (5%)	11/162 (7%)	20/329 (6%)
Diabetes	66/162 (41%)	53/158 (34%)	149/320 (37%)
Cardiac disease	106/164 (65%)	95/158 (60%)	201/320 (63%)
Previous vascular or cardiac surgery or amputation	88/163 (54%)	90/159 (57%)	178/322 (55%)
Pulmonary disease	14/162 (9%)	16/157 (10%)	30/319 (9%)
Renal disease	14/161 (9%)	20/155 (13%)	34/316 (11%)
Smokers[b]	49/145 (34%)	41/142 (29%)	90/287 (32%)

[a]Categorical data are presented as *n*/N. Median (1st–3rd quartile) is used for age. The numbers do not necessarily add up to the total number of patients because full information was not available for all patients.
[b]Any regular smoking during the last 5 years.

Participants were also part of the Scandinavian Miller Collar Study[1] within a factorial randomization design, and the treatment groups were stratified by vein cuff randomization to control for this variable. It is interesting to note that lack of a suitable single-segment saphenous vein conduit was not a consideration for study inclusion or exclusion. Presumably, many of these participants had no suitable autogenous conduit; otherwise, the lack of provider equipoise would likely represent a major recruitment barrier. Compared with unsupported grafts, use of supported grafts for below-knee bypass was associated with improved primary and secondary patency (Figs 2 and 3); limb salvage, however, was similar between groups (Fig 4).

The trial results certainly suggest a significant (albeit modest) patency advantage associated with the use of supported PTFE grafts, but several design limitations potentially predisposed the study to bias and/or confounding. First, the lack of standardized medical management potentially permitted use of different approaches by providers who were not blinded. The authors correctly assert that treatment randomization accounts for both known and unknown differences between groups at baseline, but postrandomization use of medications that influence patency (including statins, clopidogrel, and/or cilostazol) was unaccounted for and could have had an impact on the results. Second, it is unclear why 20 participants with severe claudication or acute ischemia were enrolled and randomized given that the methods state that all participants had bypass for critical limb ischemia (defined as rest pain, arterial ulcers, or gangrene; Table 1). Third, the use of more than 1 graft product (providers were permitted to use grafts from different manufacturers based on their preference) and lack of a standardized approach to graft diameter selection (graft diameter was not recorded for 21 participants) introduced additional graft-specific factors (apart from external reinforcement) that may have influenced patency outcomes but could not be accounted for.

Fourth, detailed anatomic criteria (such as TransAtlantic Inter-Society Consensus classification or runoff score) were not provided or used to stratify randomization. Finally, the lack of a standardized approach to graft surveillance (with pulse examinations accepted as an alternative to imaging based on the unblinded provider's inclination) may have resulted in incorrect patency assessments or differing levels of sensitivity for detecting graft occlusion. Although randomized trials often provide us with the best evidence-based comparisons between treatments, it is disappointing that several important details omitted from the study design limit the conclusions that can be made from this analysis.

M. Corriere, MD, MS

Reference

1. SCAMICOS. PTFE bypass to below-knee arteries: distal vein collar or not? A prospective randomised multicentre study. *Eur J Vasc Endovasc Surg*. 2010; 39:747-754.

Heparin-Bonded Covered Stents Versus Bare-Metal Stents for Complex Femoropopliteal Artery Lesions: The Randomized VIASTAR Trial (Viabahn Endoprosthesis With PROPATEN Bioactive Surface [VIA] Versus Bare Nitinol Stent in the Treatment of Long Lesions in Superficial Femoral Artery Occlusive Disease)

Lammer J, Zeller T, Hausegger KA, et al (Med Univ Vienna, Austria; Universitaets-Herzzentrum Freiburg-Bad Krozingen, Germany; Klinikum Klagenfurt, Austria; et al)

J Am Coll Cardiol 62:1320-1327, 2013

Objectives.—The hypothesis that endovascular treatment with covered stents has equal risks but higher efficacy than bare-metal stents (BMS) in long femoropopliteal artery disease was tested.

Background.—Although endovascular treatment of short superficial femoral artery lesions revealed excellent results, efficacy in long lesions remains unsatisfactory.

Methods.—In a prospective, randomized, single-blind, multicenter study, 141 patients with symptomatic peripheral arterial disease were assigned to treatment with heparin-bonded, covered stents (Viabahn 72 patients) or BMS (69 patients). Clinical outcomes and patency rates were assessed at 1, 6, and 12 months.

Results.—Mean ± SD lesion length was 19.0 ± 6.3 cm in the Viabahn group and 17.3 ± 6.6 cm in the BMS group. Major complications within 30 days were observed in 1.4%. The 12-month primary patency rates in the Viabahn and BMS groups were: intention-to-treat (ITT) 70.9% (95% confidence interval [CI]: 0.58 to 0.80) and 55.1% (95% CI: 0.41 to 0.67) (log-rank test $p = 0.11$); treatment per-protocol (TPP) 78.1% (95% CI: 0.65 to 0.86) and 53.5% (95% CI: 0.39 to 0.65) (hazard ratio: 2.23 [95% CI: 1.14 to 4.34) (log-rank test $p = 0.009$). In lesions

≥20 cm, (TransAtlantic Inter-Society Consensus class D), the 12-month patency rate was significantly longer in VIA patients in the ITT analysis (VIA 71.3% vs. BMS 36.8%; $p = 0.01$) and the TPP analysis (VIA 73.3% vs. BMS 33.3%; $p = 0.004$). Freedom from target lesion revascularization was 84.6% for Viabahn (95% CI: 0.72 to 0.91) versus 77.0% for BMS (95% CI: 0.63 to 0.85; $p = 0.37$). The ankle-brachial index in the Viabahn group significantly increased to 0.94 ± 0.23 compared with the BMS group (0.85 ± 0.23; $p < 0.05$) at 12 months.

Conclusions.—This randomized trial in symptomatic patients with peripheral arterial disease who underwent endovascular treatment for long femoropopliteal lesions demonstrated significant clinical and patency benefits for heparin-bonded covered stents compared with BMS in lesions ≥20 cm and for all lesions in the TPP analysis. In the ITT analysis for all lesions, which was flawed by major protocol deviations in 8.5% of the patients, the difference was not significant. (GORE VIABAHN® endoprosthesis with bioactive propaten surface versus bare nitinol stent in the treatment of TASC B, C and D lesions in superficial femoral artery occlusive disease; ISRCTN48164244) (Figs 2 and 3, Table 2).

▶ Endovascular treatment of long-segment occlusive lesions are often challenging in terms of both procedural technical success and long-term patency. This randomized trial compared bare metal stents (BMS) and covered, heparin-bonded Viabahn stents (VIA) for percutaneous treatment of long femoropopliteal occlusive lesions (defined based on a length of 10–35 cm). The authors hypothesized that the heparin-bonded covering might prevent ingrowth of neointimal hyperplasia through the stent interstices, whereas the heparin bonding might inhibit both intimal hyperplasia and thrombosis. Medical therapy was standardized (although statin medication use was conspicuously absent), successful wire crossing of target lesion was randomization entry criterion, and the primary clinical endpoint was primary patency at 1 year. Three different bare metal stents were used in the trial at the discretion of the operator. Although target lesion lengths were similar between treatment groups, stented segment lengths were significantly longer in the VIA group (Table 2), perhaps reflecting either a more aggressive approach or more conservative attitude regarding stent overlap with covered devices.

Although presentation of both intention-to-treat (ITT) and treatment-per-protocol (TPP) analyses often indicates high rates of crossover between treatment groups, none of the exclusions in this study were related to this issue. Of the 12 participants excluded from the ITT but included in the TPP analysis, 6 did not meet anatomic inclusion criteria, 4 had either PTA alone or incomplete stenting after PTA, 1 did not take protocol medications, and 1 withdrew consent. Although no difference in primary patency was noted within the ITT analysis, a small but significant primary patency advantage at 12 months was observed in the VIA group (Fig 2). A subgroup analysis restricted to lesions ≥20 cm in length showed a primary patency benefit within both ITT and TPP analyses. This subgroup analysis of ≥20-cm lesions was not prespecified, and subgroup analyses for the shorter-length lesions (where it is likely that

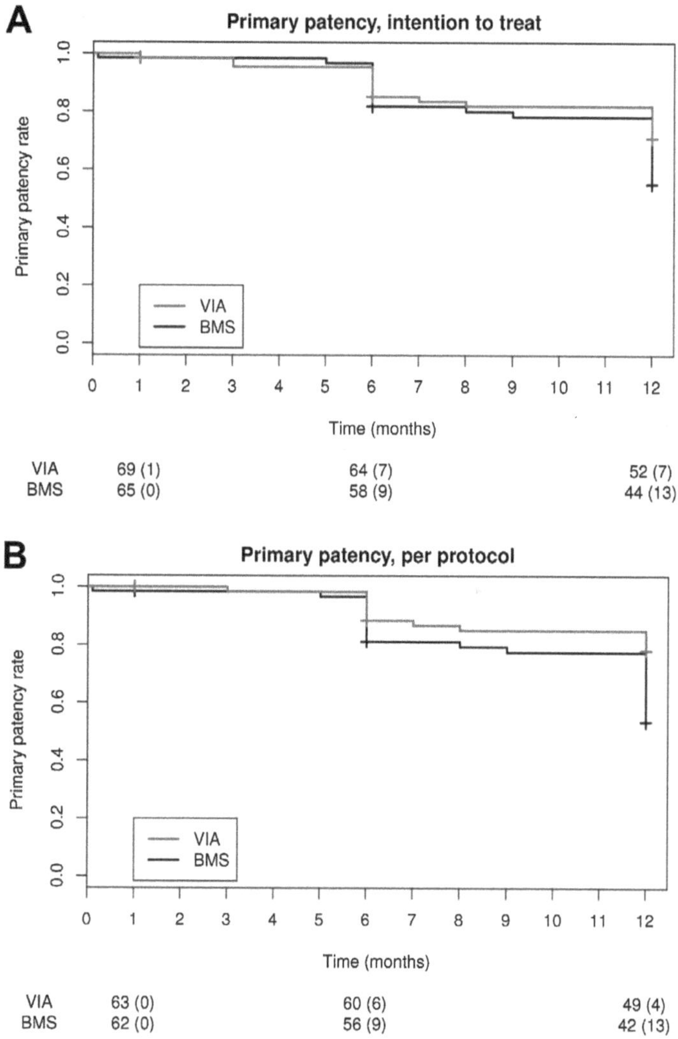

FIGURE 2.—Patency rate of all lesions. Primary patency of Viabahn endoprosthesis (VIA) (**red**) versus bare-metal stent (BMS) (**black**) in the superficial femoral artery lesions of patients with symptomatic peripheral arterial disease. (**A**) ITT: at 12 months VIA 70.9% (95% confidence interval [CI]: 0.58 to 0.80) versus BMS 55.1% (95% CI: 0.41 to 0.67; log-rank test $p = 0.11$). (**B**) TPP: at 12 months VIA 78.1% (95% CI: 0.65 to 0.86) versus BMS 53.5% (95% CI: 0.39 to 0.65) (hazard ratio 2.23 [95% CI: 1.14 to 4.34]; log-rank test $p = 0.009$). Abbreviations as in Figure 1. For interpretation of the references to color in this figure legend, the reader is referred to web version of this article. (Reprinted from the Journal of the American College of Cardiology. Lammer J, Zeller T, Hausegger KA, et al. Heparin-bonded covered stents versus bare-metal stents for complex femoropopliteal artery lesions: the randomized VIASTAR trial (viabahn endoprosthesis with PROPATEN bioactive surface [VIA] versus bare nitinol stent in the treatment of long lesions in superficial femoral artery occlusive disease). *J Am Coll Cardiol.* 2013;62:1320-1327, Copyright 2013, with permission from the American College of Cardiology.)

no patency difference was observed) were also not included. Despite the reported differences in patency, clinical improvement (based on Rutherford category and mean walking distance) was similar between groups.

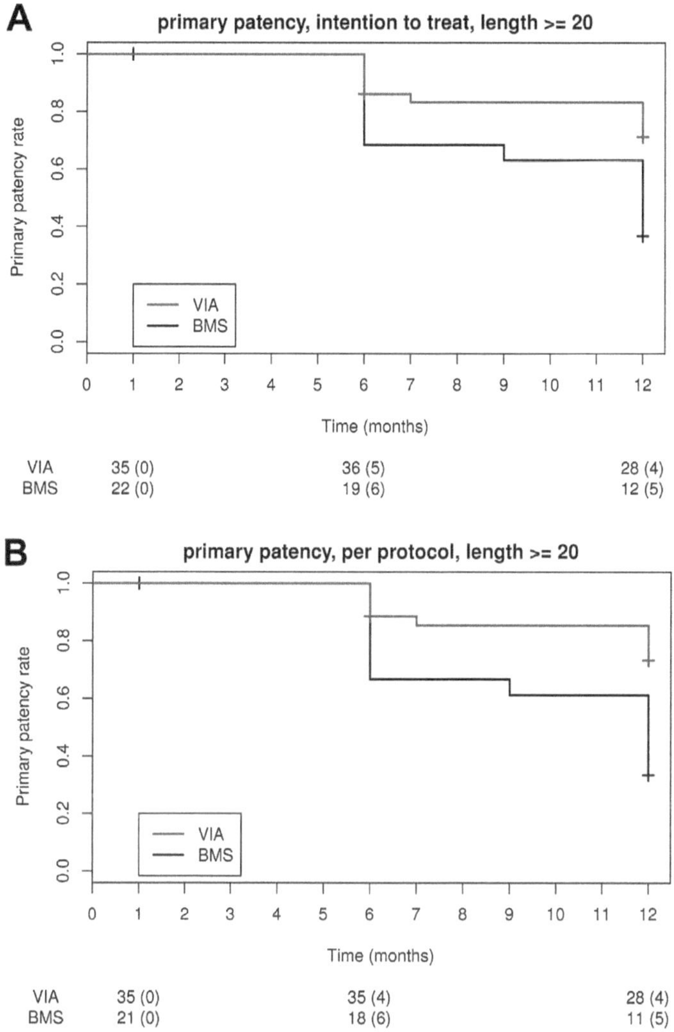

FIGURE 3.—Patency Rate of Lesions ≥20 cm. Primary patency of VIA (**red**) versus BMS (**black**) in superficial femoral artery lesions of patients with symptomatic peripheral arterial disease and lesions ≥20 cm. (**A**) ITT: at 12 months VIA: 71.3% (95% CI: 0.53 to 0.83) versus BMS: 36.8% (95% CI: 0.17 to 0.57; log-rank test $p = 0.01$). (**B**) TPP: at 12 months VIA: 73.3% (95% CI: 0.54 to 0.85) versus BMS: 33.3% (95% CI: 0.13 to 0.54; log-rank test $p = 0.004$). Abbreviations as in Figures 1 and 2. For interpretation of the references to color in this figure legend, the reader is referred to web version of this article. (Reprinted from the Journal of the American College of Cardiology. Lammer J, Zeller T, Hausegger KA, et al. Heparin-bonded covered stents versus bare-metal stents for complex femoropopliteal artery lesions: the randomized VIASTAR trial (viabahn endoprosthesis with PROPATEN bioactive surface [VIA] versus bare nitinol stent in the treatment of long lesions in superficial femoral artery occlusive disease). *J Am Coll Cardiol*. 2013;62:1320-1327, Copyright 2013, with permission from the American College of Cardiology.)

No significant differences in rates of occlusion between groups were identified (6 for VIA vs 4 for BMS), but it appears that VIA occlusions had more drastic clinical consequences. Although half of the BMS occlusions were left untreated, all

TABLE 2.—Baseline Angiographic and Interventional Data

	VIA (n = 72)	BMS (n = 69)	*p* Value
Length of target lesion (mm)	189.8 ± 63	173.2 ± 66	0.13
Length of stented segment (mm)	236.8 ± 77	203.1 ± 77	0.01
Target vessel diameter (mm)	6.08 ± 0.6	6.25 ± 0.7	0.88
Target vessel diameter (mm)	6.08 ± 0.6	6.25 ± 0.7	0.88
Occlusion	56 (79)	46 (70)	0.21
Target-lesion calcification*			0.15
None or mild	16 (23)	12 (17)	
Moderate	44 (62)	34 (49)	
Severe	11 (15)	19 (28)	
Not applicable		4 (6)	
TASC II class†			0.09
TASC A	0	2 (3)	
TASC B >10 cm	20 (28)	29 (42)	
TASC C	18 (25)	16 (23)	
TASC D	34 (47)	22 (32)	
No. of crural runoff vessels			0.96
3	32 (44)	29 (42)	
2	28 (39)	27 (40)	
1	10 (14)	10 (14)	
0	2 (3)	3 (4)	
No. of implants			0.04
0	2 (3)	0 (0)	
1	18 (26)	29 (42)	
2	41 (57)	36 (52)	
≥3	11 (15)	4 (6)	
Adverse events	11 (15)	9 (13)	0.77
Peripheral embolization	4	1	
Hematoma	2	2	
Pseudoaneurysm	1	0	
Other	3	2	
Death	0	0	
Study limb amputation	0	0	
Severe adverse events	1 (1.4)	1 (1.4)	1.0
ABI before discharge	0.93 ± 0.18	0.96 ± 0.14	0.24

Values are mean ± SD or n (%).
Abbreviations as in Table 1.
*Calcification was assessed by the investigator.
†TransAtlantic. Inter-Society Consensus (TASC) II classification is a lesion classification according to the Inter-Society Consensus for the Management of Peripheral Arterial Disease.

of the VIA occlusions were managed with either thrombolysis or bypass. It is unclear whether these patients had more severe symptoms because of occlusion of side branches (which might serve as collaterals) by the covered device, distal embolization at the time of occlusion (which is often observed with prosthetic bypass graft occlusions), or other factors. The decision to use a covered versus a bare metal stent may then come down to considering the patency advantages (which appear limited to longer lesions) versus the more severe presentations associated with occlusion. In the absence of a direct comparison, providers trying to decide whether to use a heparin-bonded device (which is presumably more expensive) will have to speculate on whether the patency advantages reported in the VIA group were associated with the covered stent design, the heparin bonding, or both.

M. Corriere, MD, MS

Outcomes of lower extremity bypass performed for acute limb ischemia

Baril DT, for the Vascular Study Group of New England (Univ of Massachusetts Med School, Worcester; et al)

J Vasc Surg 58:949-956, 2013

Objective.—Acute limb ischemia remains one of the most challenging emergencies in vascular surgery. Historically, outcomes following interventions for acute limb ischemia have been associated with high rates of morbidity and mortality. The purpose of this study was to determine contemporary outcomes following lower extremity bypass performed for acute limb ischemia.

Methods.—All patients undergoing infrainguinal lower extremity bypass between 2003 and 2011 within hospitals comprising the Vascular Study Group of New England were identified. Patients were stratified according to whether or not the indication for lower extremity bypass was acute limb ischemia. Primary end points included bypass graft occlusion, major amputation, and mortality at 1 year postoperatively as determined by Kaplan-Meier life table analysis. Multivariable Cox proportional hazards models were constructed to evaluate independent predictors of mortality and major amputation at 1 year.

Results.—Of 5712 lower extremity bypass procedures, 323 (5.7%) were performed for acute limb ischemia. Patients undergoing lower extremity bypass for acute limb ischemia were similar in age (66 vs 67; $P = .084$) and sex (68% male vs 69% male; $P = .617$) compared with chronic ischemia patients, but were less likely to be on aspirin (63% vs 75%; $P < .0001$) or a statin (55% vs 68%; $P < .0001$). Patients with acute limb ischemia were more likely to be current smokers (49% vs 39%; $P < .0001$), to have had a prior ipsilateral bypass (33% vs 24%; $P = .004$) or a prior ipsilateral percutaneous intervention (41% vs 29%; $P = .001$). Bypasses performed for acute limb ischemia were longer in duration (270 vs 244 minutes; $P = .007$), had greater blood loss (363 vs 272 mL; $P < .0001$), and more commonly utilized prosthetic conduits (41% vs 33%; $P = .003$). Acute limb ischemia patients experienced increased in-hospital major adverse events (20% vs 12%; $P < .0001$) including myocardial infarction, congestive heart failure exacerbation, deterioration in renal function, and respiratory complications. Patients who underwent lower extremity bypass for acute limb ischemia had no difference in rates of graft occlusion (18.1% vs 18.5%; $P = .77$), but did have significantly higher rates of limb loss (22.4% vs 9.7%; $P < .0001$) and mortality (20.9% vs 13.1%; $P < .0001$) at 1 year. On multivariable analysis, acute limb ischemia was an independent predictor of both major amputation (hazard ratio, 2.16; confidence interval, 1.38-3.40; $P = .001$) and mortality (hazard ratio, 1.41; confidence interval, 1.09-1.83; $P = .009$) at 1 year.

Conclusions.—Patients who present with acute limb ischemia represent a less medically optimized subgroup within the population of patients undergoing lower extremity bypass. These patients may be expected to have more complex operations followed by increased rates of perioperative

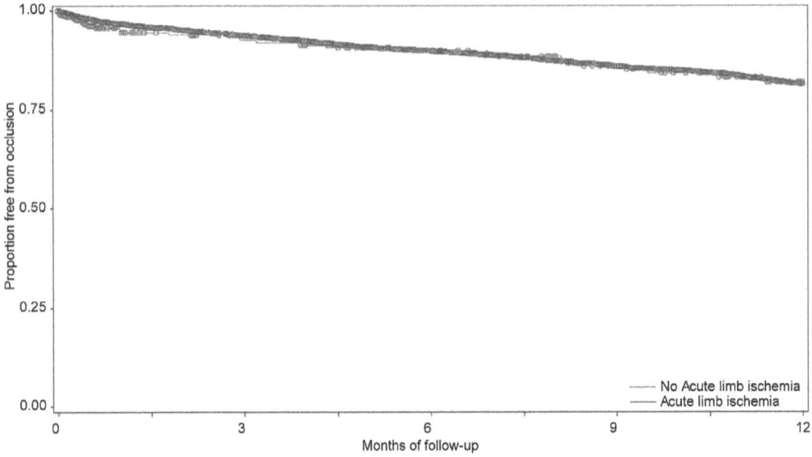

Number at risk:				
No ALI: 5363	3216	2784	2265	1252
ALI: 312	143	128	103	64

FIGURE 1.—Freedom from graft occlusion. (Reprinted from Baril DT, for the Vascular Study Group of New England. Outcomes of lower extremity bypass performed for acute limb ischemia. *J Vasc Surg.* 2013;58:949-956, Copyright 2013, with permission from The Society for Vascular Surgery.)

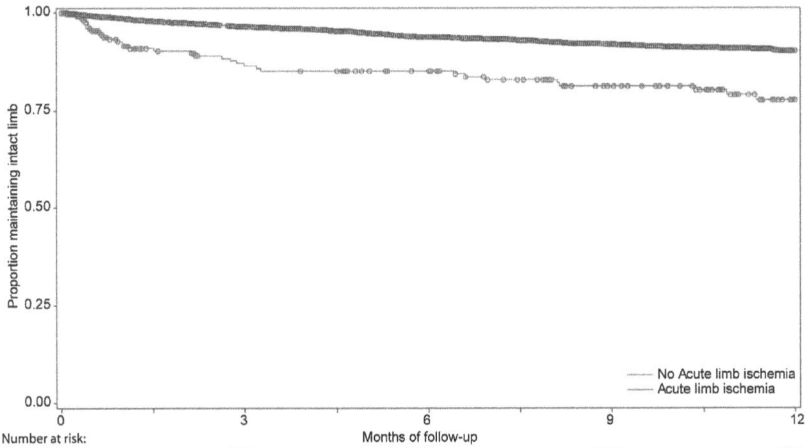

Number at risk:				
No ALI: 4951	3114	2739	2237	1214
ALI: 297	132	130	98	57

FIGURE 2.—Freedom from major amputation. (Reprinted from Baril DT, for the Vascular Study Group of New England. Outcomes of lower extremity bypass performed for acute limb ischemia. *J Vasc Surg.* 2013;58:949-956, Copyright 2013, with permission from The Society for Vascular Surgery.)

adverse events. Additionally, despite equivalent graft patency rates, patients undergoing lower extremity bypass for acute ischemia have significantly higher rates of major amputation and mortality at 1 year (Figs 1-4, Tables 1-4).

▶ Several of the findings of this retrospective analysis from the Vascular Study Group of New England should come as no surprise to any provider who takes

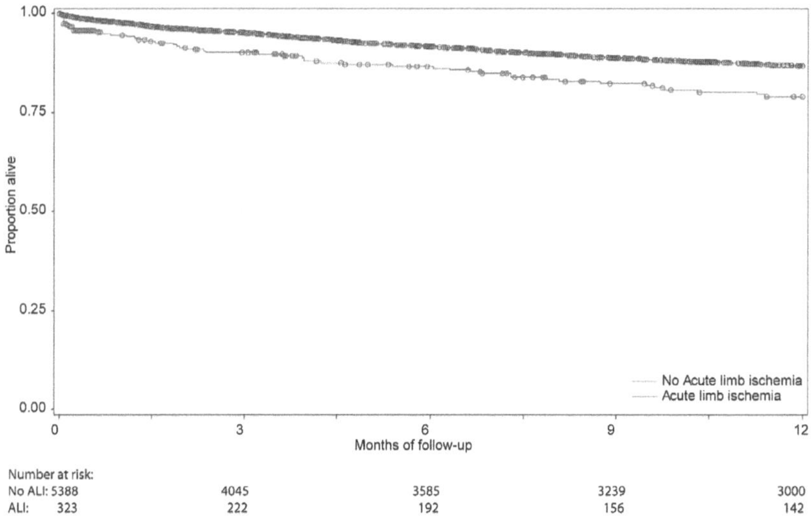

FIGURE 3.—Survival. (Reprinted from Baril DT, for the Vascular Study Group of New England. Outcomes of lower extremity bypass performed for acute limb ischemia. *J Vasc Surg*. 2013;58:949-956, Copyright 2013, with permission from The Society for Vascular Surgery.)

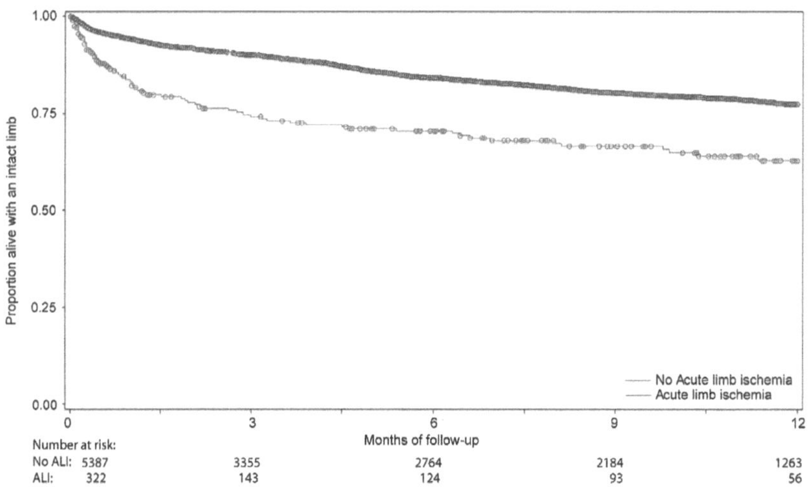

FIGURE 4.—Amputation-free survival. (Reprinted from Baril DT, for the Vascular Study Group of New England. Outcomes of lower extremity bypass performed for acute limb ischemia. *J Vasc Surg*. 2013;58:949-956, Copyright 2013, with permission from The Society for Vascular Surgery.)

care of patients with acute limb ischemia. Compared with patients undergoing elective lower-extremity bypass, patients who underwent urgent or emergent lower-extremity bypass for acute limb ischemia had a higher risk of perioperative adverse events (Table 2) and increased rates of major amputation and mortality at 1 year (Figs 2-4). Freedom from graft occlusion, however, was the same

TABLE 1.—Patient Demographics

Variable	Bypass Performed for Acute Limb Ischemia (n = 323)	All Other Bypasses (n = 5389)	*P* Value
Age, mean, years	66.3	67.4	.084
Male sex, %	67.8	69.1	.617
CAD, %	30.3	35.7	.051
CHF, %	13.9	15.7	.393
COPD, %	32.2	26.2	.017
Diabetes, %			
NIDDM	18.0	25.3	<.001
IDDM	18.9	25.2	<.001
Hypertension, %	81.4	86.5	.010
Renal insufficiency, %	13.9	13.1	.687
Hemodialysis, %	5.3	6.0	.193
Current tobacco use, %	48.5	39.4	<.001
Beta-blocker usage, %	71.1	76.7	.023
Aspirin usage, %	62.5	74.8	<.001
Statin usage, %	54.8	68.1	<.001
Prior ipsilateral bypass, %	32.8	23.5	.004
Prior ipsilateral percutaneous intervention, %	41.1	28.8	<.001
Aneurysm as indication, %	14.0	6.8	<.001

CAD, Coronary artery disease; *CHF*, congestive heart failure; *COPD*, chronic obstructive pulmonary disease; *IDDM*, insulin-dependent diabetes mellitus; *NIDDM*, noninsulin-dependent diabetes mellitus.

TABLE 2.—Perioperative Major Adverse Events

Variable	Bypass Performed for Acute Limb Ischemia (n = 323)	All Other Bypasses (n = 5389)	*P* Value
Any in-hospital major adverse event, %	19.8	11.6	<.0001
Myocardial infarction, %	7.5	3.6	.001
Dysrhythmia, %	4.4	4.0	.727
CHF, %	5.6	3.3	.028
Deterioration in renal function, %	6.6	4.4	.001
Respiratory, %	3.7	1.4	.004

CHF, Congestive heart failure.

between groups at 1 year (Fig 1); this finding is somewhat unexpected, particularly given that patients undergoing bypass for acute ischemia had a higher prevalence of tobacco use, prior ipsilateral bypass, and suboptimal medical management (Table 1). Patients with acute ischemia also had a higher rate of prosthetic conduit utilization (41% vs 33%) but still had longer procedures with greater blood loss than patients undergoing elective bypass. In multivariable modeling, both acute ischemia and prosthetic conduit use were associated with both amputation (Table 3) and 1-year mortality (Table 4).

Several factors that might affect perioperative adverse events, patency, and amputation-free survival were not included in the analysis, presumably because of lack of availability within the dataset. First, the rate of fasciotomy use (either

TABLE 3.—Independent Predictors of Amputation at 1 Year

	HR	95% CI	*P* Value
NIDDM	1.56	1.09-2.24	.016
IDDM	1.98	1.44-2.74	<.0001
Prosthetic conduit	2.03	1.51-2.72	<.0001
Prior ipsilateral percutaneous intervention	2.08	1.23-3.53	.007
Acute ischemia	2.16	1.38-3.40	<.0001
Tibial target vessel	2.75	2.05-3.69	<.0001

CI, Confidence interval; *HR*, hazard ratio; *IDDM*, insulin-dependent diabetes mellitus; *NIDDM*, noninsulin-dependent diabetes mellitus.

TABLE 4.—Independent Predictors of Mortality at 1 Year

	HR	95% CI	*P* Value
Statin therapy	0.80	0.71-0.91	.0007
Tibial target	1.15	1.01-1.32	.036
CAD	1.19	1.05-1.36	.009
IDDM	1.26	1.08-1.48	.004
NIDDM	1.29	1.10-1.51	.029
Prosthetic conduit	1.30	1.13-1.49	.0002
Acute ischemia	1.41	1.09-1.83	.009
COPD	1.46	1.28-1.67	<.0001
Renal insufficiency	1.58	1.36-1.83	<.0001
CHF	1.63	1.41-1.89	<.0001
Perioperative major adverse event	1.73	1.48-2.02	<.0001

CAD, Coronary artery disease; *CHF*, congestive heart failure; *CI*, confidence interval; *COPD*, chronic obstructive pulmonary disease; *HR*, hazard ratio; *IDDM*, insulin-dependent diabetes mellitus; *NIDDM*, noninsulindependent diabetes mellitus.

during the same anesthetic or as a separate procedure) was not included, but might have provided valuable insight into how compartment syndrome and open fasciotomy wounds influence outcomes. The former would presumably affect perioperative risk of both mortality and renal failure (which was higher in the acute ischemia group [Table 2]), whereas the latter might affect rates of graft loss caused by prosthetic graft infections. Second, it is unclear that use of thrombolysis before lower extremity bypass was accounted for in this analysis. For certain indications (such as thrombosed popliteal aneurysm or bypass graft thrombosis, both of which were likely more common in the acute limb ischemia group [Table 1]), one might expect a higher incidence of preoperative thrombolysis to improve distal runoff or attempt graft salvage. It therefore would have been interesting to see whether thrombolysis before bypass affected procedure-associated blood loss, risk of reoperation, or long-term patency (particularly among bypasses performed for aneurysms). Finally, it would have been interesting to compare amputation levels between groups to see if above-knee amputations were more common in the acute ischemia group. Despite these limitations, this analysis provides valuable information related to the risk associated with acute limb ischemia that may provide valuable information for both patient counseling and risk adjustment.

M. Corriere, MD, MS

Comparison of surgical bypass with angioplasty and stenting of superficial femoral artery disease

Malas MB, Enwerem N, Qazi U, et al (Johns Hopkins Bayview Med Ctr and Johns Hopkins Hosp, Baltimore, MD)

J Vasc Surg 59:129-135, 2014

Objective.—To evaluate the contemporary outcome of femoral-popliteal bypass compared with angioplasty and stenting in patients with symptomatic peripheral arterial disease (PAD) in terms of patency and reintervention rates.

Methods.—We identified all patients evaluated at the Johns Hopkins Bayview Medical Center with the presumptive diagnosis of PAD from September 2005 to September 2010. In this group, we selected all symptomatic patients after failing medical management who received percutaneous transluminal angioplasty/stenting of the superficial femoral artery or femoral-popliteal bypass. We compared the overall patency and reintervention rates between the two groups as well as patency within TransAtlantic Inter-Society Consensus (TASC) II subgroups. Descriptive analyses were performed using χ^2 and two-sided *t*-tests. The Mann-Whitney *U* test was used to compare distributions of continuous variables and the Fisher exact test for categorical variables. Cox proportional hazard model was used to examine the treatment effect within each lesion type, using bypass as the reference group.

Results.—Out of 1237 patients evaluated at Johns Hopkins Bayview Medical Center for PAD from September 2005 to September 2010, we identified 104 symptomatic patients who received percutaneous transluminal angioplasty/stenting of the superficial femoral artery or femoral-popliteal bypass after failing medical management. There were 61 male patients (56%), and the mean age was 68 years in both groups. Both treatment groups had similar risk factors. Overall, 77% of patients with TASC II A and B lesions underwent angioplasty and stenting, whereas 73% of patients with TASC C and D lesions underwent bypass ($P < .01$). The primary patency at 24 months was better for the stent group 67% (95% confidence interval [CI], 0.52-0.78) vs bypass group 49% (95% CI, 0.32-0.64; $P = .05$). The rate of reintervention within the 2-year period was higher in the bypass group compared with the stent group (54% vs 31%; $P = .02$). TASC A and B lesions combined demonstrated a reduced hazard of patency failure compared with TASC C or D lesions combined (hazard ratio, 2.42; 95% CI, 1.26, 4.65; $P < .01$).

Conclusions.—This is the first study that documents higher reintervention rates for femoral-popliteal bypass compared with angioplasty and stenting. We believe that the main reason for this finding is the fact that the bypass patients had significantly more advanced disease. This, emphasizes that one must consider the patient population undergoing intervention when comparing revascularization procedures. A prospective randomized trial is needed to determine the overall better treatment option.

▶ I thought this retrospective review of treatment options for the superficial femoral artery (SFA) presented valuable insight into the results a surgeon can expect from a real-life vascular surgery practice. The conservative approach with an emphasis on exercise and ambulation, risk reduction, and the reservation of angiography to a strictly preoperative planning tool was commendable. The authors found that the majority of TransAtlantic Inter-Society Consensus (TASC) II A and B lesions were treated endovascularly, whereas the majority of TASC II C and D lesions required bypass; I suspect this mirrors closely the current practice of many vascular surgeons. In particular, I thought this article offered insights that will help me counsel patients regarding the reasons for choosing open or endovascular options and the results one can expect in various circumstances. As the authors state, these results might more accurately reflect current results than patency rates from studies when endovascular therapy was not an option at all.

P. White, MD, FACS

Toward a mouse model of hind limb ischemia to test therapeutic angiogenesis

Brenes RA, Jadlowiec CC, Bear M, et al (Yale Univ School of Medicine, New Haven, CT)

J Vasc Surg 56:1669-1679, 2012

Introduction.—Several clinical trials are currently evaluating stem cell therapy for patients with critical limb ischemia that have no other surgical or endovascular options for revascularization. However, these trials are conducted with different protocols, including use of different stem cell populations and different injection protocols, providing little means to compare trials and guide therapy. Accordingly, we developed a murine model of severe ischemia to allow methodic testing of relevant clinical parameters.

Methods.—High femoral artery ligation and total excision of the superficial femoral artery was performed on C57BL/6 mice. Mononuclear cells (MNCs) were isolated from the bone marrow of donor mice, characterized using fluorescence-activated cell sorting, and injected (5×10^5 to 2×10^6) into the semimembranosus (proximal) or gastrocnemius (distal) muscle. Vascular and functional outcomes were measured using invasive Doppler imaging, laser Doppler perfusion imaging, and the Tarlov and ischemia scores. Histologic analysis included quantification of muscle fiber area and number as well as capillary density.

Results.—Blood flow and functional outcomes were improved in MNC-treated mice compared with controls over 28 days (flow: $P < .0001$; Tarlov: $P = .0004$; ischemia score: $P = .0002$). MNC-treated mice also showed greater gastrocnemius fiber area ($P = .0053$) and increased capillary density ($P = .0004$). Dose–response analysis showed increased angiogenesis and gastrocnemius fiber area but no changes in macroscopic vascular flow or functional scores. Overall functional outcomes in mice injected proximally to the ischemic area were similar to mice injected more distally, but muscle flow, capillary density, and gastrocnemius fiber area were increased ($P < .05$).

Conclusions.—High femoral ligation with complete excision of the superficial femoral artery is a reliable model of severe hind limb ischemia in C57BL/6 mice that shows a response to MNC treatment for functional and vascular outcomes. A dose response to the injection of MNCs appears to be present, at least microscopically, suggesting that an optimal cell number for stem cell therapy exists and that preclinical testing needs to be performed to optimally guide human trials. Injection of MNCs proximal to the site of ischemia may provide different outcomes compared with distal injection and warrants additional study.

▶ Limb ischemia, which is characterized by markedly reduced blood flow, is a serious form of peripheral arterial disease and can result in limb loss within 6 months of diagnosis in 25% to 40% of patients who present with nonreconstructable disease. At present, no standard effective treatment strategies are available for patients who are not candidates for surgical or endovascular treatment. The best end result for all patients with limb ischemia is neovascularization. Studies have demonstrated that using bone marrow–derived stem cells is a potential method for inducing therapeutic angiogenesis, and recent publications have been generally positive with regard to improvements in extremity perfusion and motor function when using mononuclear cells (MNCs) in humans for the treatment of critical limb ischemia. However, some inconsistencies in these reports due to variability in cell preparation, culture, and injection site, as well as small patient numbers with variable degrees of ischemia, still leave many questions unanswered and highlight the importance of having a reproducible animal model to investigate therapeutic angiogenesis. In this article, the authors establish an acute but reproducible murine model of severe ischemia that would allow methodic testing of such parameters. They describe an easy-to-perform preclinical model to test different parameters of stem cell therapy and show that MNC treatment provides a more rapid improvement in perfusion in this ischemic model, that a dose–response curve is likely to exist for stem cells, and that the site of stem cell injection may have functional consequences. This is an interesting and reproducible preclinical model that should yield important results in the study of therapeutic angiogenesis.

J. Cullen, PhD

Angiosome-targeted infrapopliteal endovascular revascularization for treatment of diabetic foot ulcers

Söderström M, Albäck A, Biancari F, et al (Helsinki Univ Central Hosp, Finland; Oulu Univ Hosp, Finland)

J Vasc Surg 57:427-435, 2013

Objective.—Because of the prolonged healing time of diabetic foot ulcers, methods for identifying ways to expedite the ulcer healing process are needed. The angiosome concept delineates the body into three-dimensional blocks of tissue fed by specific source arteries. The aim of this study was to evaluate the benefit of infrapopliteal endovascular revascularization guided by an angiosome model of perfusion in the healing process of diabetic foot ulcers.

Methods.—A total of 250 consecutive legs with diabetic foot ulcers in 226 patients who had undergone infrapopliteal endovascular revascularization in a single center were evaluated. Patient records and periprocedural leg angiograms were reviewed. The legs were divided into two groups depending on whether direct arterial flow to the site of the foot ulcer based on the angiosome concept was achieved (direct group) or not achieved (indirect group). Ulcer healing time was compared between the two groups. A propensity score was used for adjustment of differences in pretreatment covariables in multivariate analysis and for 1:1 matching.

Results.—Direct flow to the angiosome feeding the ulcer area was achieved in 121 legs (48%) compared with indirect revascularization in 129 legs. Foot ulcers treated with angiosome-targeted infrapopliteal percutaneous transluminal angioplasty healed better. The ulcer healing rate was mean (standard deviation) 72% (5%) at 12 months for the direct group compared with 45% (6%) for the indirect group ($P < .001$). When adjusted for propensity score, the direct group still had a significantly better ulcer healing rate than the indirect group (hazard ratio, 1.97; 95% confidence interval, 1.34-2.90; $P = .001$).

Conclusions.—Attaining a direct arterial flow based on the angiosome model of perfusion to the foot ulcer appears to be important for ulcer healing in diabetic patients.

► Diabetic foot ulcers in dysvascular limbs remain one of the most vexing problems facing vascular surgeons. Patients with diabetic foot ulcers suffer significantly and are at great risk of losing their limb. The angiosome concept, introduced by Ian Taylor in 1987, held the first promise to improve the outcomes of revascularization in these patients. The current article compared "direct" revascularization of the angiosome containing a diabetic ulcer to "indirect" revascularization of the angiosome. With a large cohort, this retrospective study offers further confirmation that wound healing rates might be improved by treating the artery supplying the angiosome in which the ulcer has occurred. This study revealed a significant benefit in terms of ulcer healing rate at 12 months to directly revascularizing the angiosome in question. It was interesting that limb-salvage and amputation-free survival rates were not disparate in the 2 groups. This might be the result of the close follow-up and concomitant to wound care that patients received during the course of the study period. It would be interesting to learn if patients received additional follow-up for wound care apart from the follow-up described in the study.

Because this article is retrospective, several questions remain unanswered. Patients in whom direct revascularization could not be achieved had more severe atherosclerotic disease than those in whom direct revascularization was achieved. Could this account for the difference in healing rate? Is it an indication of more severe microvascular angiopathy in the affected limb? This article did attempt to address some of these issues by looking at propensity-matched pairs, but clearly prospective analysis must still be done. Prospective studies would also help answer questions such as whether a surgeon should eschew a more appealing distal target for a less appealing target that supplies the wounded angiosome. Should endovascular revascularization to the wounded angiosome be pursued over open bypass to an artery not supplying the wounded angiosome? Nonetheless, this article compellingly adds to the growing body of evidence that the angiosome concept is useful and that, whenever possible, direct revascularization is preferable. Endovascular therapy is also supported as an effective modality even for difficult infrageniculate lesions.

P. White, MD, FACS

The prognosis of patients on hemodialysis with foot lesions

Orimoto Y, Ohta T, Ishibashi H, et al (Aichi Med Univ, Nagakute, Japan)
J Vasc Surg 58:1291-1299, 2013

Objective.—Many studies have shown the high prevalence and incidence of peripheral arterial disease and the marked morbidity and mortality associated with peripheral arterial disease in hemodialysis patients. The purpose of this retrospective study was to clarify the probability of survival and limb salvage in patients with foot lesions and how to manage these patients.

Methods.—Data were collected in a retrospectively maintained database for 319 lower limbs with foot lesions in 234 hemodialysis patients treated in a university hospital between 1980 and 2011. Variances influencing survival and limb salvage were compared using log-rank tests and Cox regression analysis. These variables were examined using Kaplan-Meier analysis. Significant factors in bivariate analysis were included in a logistic regression model to determine independent predictors and the probability of failure.

Results.—The 234 patients (72% men) were a mean age of 65.4 years on admission, and 84% had diabetes. The mean duration of hemodialysis was 6.8 years. During the follow-up period, 171 patients (73%) died. The 1-, 3-, 5-, and 7-year survival rates were 65.2%, 35.5%, 23.4%, and 12.8%, respectively. According to Cox multivariate models, age at admission and ischemic changes on an electrocardiogram independently increased the risk of death (hazard ratios, 1.02 and 1.48, respectively). Conversely, hyperlipidemia independently decreased the risk of death (hazard ratio, 0.56).

Critical limb ischemia was present in 247 limbs (77%). Arterial reconstruction was done in 88 limbs (28%), and 119 limbs (37%) required major amputation. The overall 1-, 3-, 5- and 7-year limb salvage rates were 68.9%, 57.2%, 53.8%, and 51.7 %, respectively. According to Cox multivariate models, patent arterial reconstruction and albumin independently decreased the risk of major amputation (hazard ratios, 0.265 and 0.392, respectively).

Conclusions.—Hemodialysis patients with foot lesions have a poor prognosis, with high rates of mortality and amputation. Prompt assessments of the severity of systemic conditions, such as cardiac ischemia, and focal wound conditions, such as ischemia and infection, are necessary to treat hemodialysis patients with foot lesions.

▶ This article is a must read, as all vascular surgeons at some point take care of multiple patients who present with critical limb ischemia and have concomitant end-stage renal disease necessitating hemodialysis. This group of patients has multiple medical comorbidities, worse outcomes with interventions, and high rates of amputation and death. As seen in this study, this unfortunate cohort is younger and diabetic, thus, predisposed to severe cardiac disease and infections. As the country's population is aging, this will be a growing population of patients who will present ongoing challenges to the surgeon. Finding the balance between maintaining independent living of a patient versus maintaining a limb versus maintaining a life may become a difficult choice for some physicians and patients to be a difficult choice. The survival rates of patients in this Japanese cohort were incredibly poor, 23% alive at 5 years with an average survival of only 1.8 years. Recommendations made by the authors to improve outcomes, including survival include nutrition maximization, glucose control, and judicious use of revascularization in those patients that will tolerate the stress of an operation. Overall, we all recognize this challenging, and expanding, population of patients as life expectancy improves. It is imperative to be selective with interventions and maintain quality of life.

R. L. Bush, MD, JD, MPH

10 Upper Extremity Ischemia/Dialysis Access

A comparison of the outcomes of one-stage and two-stage brachiobasilic arteriovenous fistulas

Vrakas G, Defigueiredo F, Turner S, et al (King's College Hosp, London, UK)

J Vasc Surg 58:1300-1304, 2013

Objective.—The brachiobasilic arteriovenous fistula (BBAVF) can be formed in one or two stages. This study examined the failure rates and functional patencies of one-stage vs two-stage brachiobasilic transposition fistulas to compare the two surgical techniques.

Methods.—We retrospectively identified all the patients who underwent BBAVF access surgery at King's College Hospital between January 1, 2009, and December 31, 2011 (3 years). Patients were divided into two groups according to one-stage or two-stage procedure. All patients were seen in the access clinic 4 to 6 weeks postoperatively, and their fistulas were scanned (duplex). The surveillance of fistulas consists of duplex scans every 6 months to assess volume flow.

Results.—During the study interval, 149 brachiobasilic transpositions (65 one-stage and 84 two-stage) were performed in 141 patients. Patients undergoing the two-stage procedure had a smaller mean preoperative vein diameter (4.0 ± 1.1 vs 3.6 ± 1.3 mm; $P = .041$) and tended to be older (58 ± 15 vs 63 ± 15 years; $P = .062$). Mean overall follow-up was 559 ± 333 days. There was no difference in primary failure between the two groups (45% vs 42%; $P = .718$). At 1 year, the two-stage BBAVFs had significantly better primary (71% vs 87%; $P = .034$), assisted primary (77% vs 95%; $P = .017$), and secondary functional (79% vs 95%; $P = .026$) patencies. The same applied to 2-year primary (53% vs 75%; $P = .034$), assisted primary (57% vs 77%; $P = .017$), and secondary functional (57% vs 77%; $P = .026$) patencies. Multivariate Cox regression showed that the one-stage procedure was 3.2 times more likely to fail ($P = .028$). Men were 2.7 times more likely to lose their access ($P = .054$).

Conclusions.—This study describes a large series of BBAVFs and makes an extensive comparison between the one-stage and two-stage operations.

Significantly improved overall functional patency is demonstrated for the two-stage operation.

▶ The need for reliable dialysis access, the advantages of autologous accesses, and the difficulty in maintaining reliably functioning fistulas and grafts will all contribute to the increasing need for basilic vein transpositions (BVTs). This article provides an interesting analysis of the use of 1- and 2-stage BVTs in a single practice. Our practice is similar with some surgeons preferring 2-stage procedures in all patients and others preferring a single-stage BVT if the vein is judged to be of adequate caliber. The authors lay out the advantages of each decision, but their results indicate a clear superiority of the 2-stage procedure over the 1-stage. This article and others indicate the need for a large, prospective examination of these 2 procedures to elucidate which BVT should be the choice in the future. If the superiority in patency for the 2-stage procedure found in this article holds up, it would more than outweigh the proposed advantages of the 1-stage procedures.

P. White, MD, FACS

Temporal Risk Profile for Infectious and Noninfectious Complications of Hemodialysis Access

Ravani P, Gillespie BW, Quinn RR, et al (Univ of Calgary, Alberta, Canada; Univ of Michigan, Ann Arbor; et al)

J Am Soc Nephrol 24:1668-1677, 2013

Vascular access complications are a major cause of morbidity in patients undergoing hemodialysis, and determining how the risks of different complications vary over the life of an access may benefit the design of prevention strategies. We used data from the Dialysis Outcomes and Practice Patterns Study (DOPPS) to assess the temporal profiles of risks for infectious and noninfectious complications of fistulas, grafts, and tunneled catheters in incident hemodialysis patients. Weused longitudinal data to model time from access placement or successful treatment of a previous complication to subsequent complication and considered multiple accesses per patient and repeated access complications using baseline and time-varying covariates to obtain adjusted estimates. Of the 7769 incident patients identified, 7140 received at least one permanent access. During a median follow-up of 14 months (interquartile range, 7–22 months), 10, 452 noninfectious and 1131 infectious events (including 551 hospitalizations for sepsis) occurred in 112, 085 patient-months. The hazards for both complication types declined over time in all access types: They were 5–10 times greater in the first 3–6 months than in later periods after access placement or a remedial accessrelated procedure. The hazards declined more quickly with fistulas than with grafts and catheters ($P < 0.\ 001$; Weibull regression). These data indicate that risks for noninfectious and infectious complications of the hemodialysis access decline over time with all access types and suggest that prevention strategies should target the first 6 months after access placement or a remedial access-related procedure.

▶ With the increasing life expectancy in the United States, there is a corresponding increase in the number of older persons needing hemodialysis. Unfortunately, there may not be a suitable vein for creation of an autogenous fistula, and prosthetic material implantation becomes a necessary. The morbidity and mortality associated with grafts and temporary or tunneled catheters are well known mainly because of infectious complications. This study is a large database analysis of infectious and noninfectious complications over time in an international cohort of dialysis patients. The risk of any complication is much higher in the first 3 to 6 months after access placement. The risks are obviously higher in those with a catheter or graft, but, even so, risk of infection declines over time and, in this study, was independent of individual comorbid conditions or geographical location. Thrombosis risk also declined over time with all forms of access. The main recommendation to be gleaned from this interesting study is that special and close attention should be given to newly formed accesses of all types. Preventative measures, such as early interventions in fistulae failing to mature or aggressive wound care and meticulous technique in those with grafts and catheters, should be instituted.

R. L. Bush, MD, JD, MPH

Fistula First Is Not Always the Best Strategy for the Elderly

DeSilva RN, Patibandla BK, Vin Y, et al (Harvard Med School, Boston, MA)

J Am Soc Nephrol 24:1297-1304, 2013

Whether placing a fistula first is the superior predialysis approach among octogenarians is unknown. We analyzed data from a cohort of 115,425 incident hemodialysis patients ≥67 years old derived from the US Renal Data System with linked Medicare claims, which allowed us to identify the first predialysis vascular access placed rather than the first access used. We used proportional hazard models to evaluate all-cause mortality outcomes based on first vascular access placed, considering the fistula group as the reference. In the study population, 21,436 patients had fistulas as the first predialysis access placed, 3472 had grafts, and 90,517 had catheters. Those patients with a catheter as the first predialysis access placed had significantly inferior survival compared with those patients with a fistula (HR = 1.77; 95% CI = 1.73 to 1.81; $P < 0.001$). However, we did not detect a significant mortality difference between those patients with a graft as the first access placed and those patients with a fistula (HR = 1.05; 95% CI = 1.00 to 1.11; $P = 0.06$). Analyzing mortality stratified by age groups, grafts as the first predialysis access placed had inferior mortality outcomes compared with fistulas for the 67 to ≤79-years age group (HR = 1.10; 95% CI = 1.02 to 1.17; $P = 0.007$), but differences between these groups were not statistically significant for the 80 to ≤89- and the >90-years age groups.

In conclusion, fistula first does not seem to be clearly superior to graft placement first in the elderly, because each strategy associates with similar mortality outcomes in octogenarians and nonagenarians.

▶ Since implementation of the National Kidney Foundation's Disease Outcomes Quality Initiative Vascular Access Guidelines in 1997, the Fistula First Breakthrough Initiative (FFBI) has been both encouraged to and implemented by providers and third-party payers alike. Although most vascular surgeons who perform dialysis access procedures agree that an autogenous fistula is a superior recommendation with definitely better outcomes and an improved complication profile over other forms of access, every patient needs to be regarded as an individual. Dialysis is being offered to older patients who may have more comorbidities than the younger cohorts. It is well known that fistula failure rates are higher in this group, and the patient may even die before ever needing to be placed on dialysis. Thus, 2 questions are raised: (1) Should dialysis be initiated? (2) Should these older, sicklier patients undergo prophylactic dialysis access placement? These are difficult questions to answer and involve patient views, family input, and physician opinion, and often ethical decisions complicate matters further. This article attempts to answer the latter question in that in the patients who were in cohorts older than 80 years, there was no difference in mortality outcomes for fistulas or grafts. A major conclusion and concern is that in the cases of fistula failure or lack of maturation, many patients had to have initiation of hemodialysis with a catheter. This likelihood was 77% greater if a fistula was placed first rather than a graft. This study certainly adds food for thought to those of us performing many dialysis procedures.

R. L. Bush, MD, JD, MPH

The Initial Impact of Medicare's New Prospective Payment System for Kidney Dialysis

Hirth RA, Turenne MN, Wheeler JRC, et al (Univ of Michigan, Ann Arbor; et al)
Am J Kidney Dis 62:662-669, 2013

Background.—Medicare implemented a new prospective payment system (PPS) on January 1, 2011. This PPS covers an expanded bundle of services, including services previously paid on a fee-for-service basis. The objectives of the new PPS include more efficient decisions about treatment service combinations and modality choice.

Methods.—Primary data for this study are Medicare claims files for all dialysis patients for whom Medicare is the primary payer. We compare use of key injectable medications under the bundled PPS to use when those drugs were separately billable and examine variability across providers. We also compare each patient's dialysis modality before and after the PPS.

Results.—Use of relatively expensive drugs, including erythropoiesis-stimulating agents, declined substantially after institution of the new PPS, whereas use of iron products, often therapeutic substitutes for erythropoiesis-stimulating agents, increased. Less expensive vitamin D products were substituted for more expensive types. Drug spending overall decreased by ~$25 per session, or about 5 times the mandated reduction in the base payment rate of ~$5. Use of peritoneal dialysis increased in 2011 after being nearly flat in the years prior to the PPS, with the increase concentrated in patients in their first or second year of dialysis. Home hemodialysis continued to increase as a percentage of total dialysis services, but at a rate similar to the pre-PPS trend.

Conclusion.—The expanded bundle dialysis PPS provided incentives for the use of lower cost therapies. These incentives seem to have motivated dialysis providers to move toward lower cost methods of care in both their use of drugs and choice of modalities.

▶ Vascular surgeons are all too familiar with bundling of services—those that were previously paid on a fee-for-service schedule. This is also affecting many of the specialty services that we work closely with on a daily basis. Understanding their external payment forces will enable vascular surgeons to work more collaboratively. The new dialysis prospective payment system (PPS) introduced by Medicare in 2010 changed the payment to dialysis centers for those under their care. The bundling and reduction in payments for those needing dialysis services had a positive effect. This effect was beneficial for the dialysis centers, for Medicare, and for the patients. The reduction in payment was a financial incentive for the providers of dialysis care to use lower cost pharmacologic agents, in fact, the reduction in spending was approximately $25 per patient per dialysis session. It appears the providers actually took the initiative to use less-expensive, albeit equally effective, medications. Interestingly, peritoneal dialysis increased after the initiation of the PPS. Home dialysis is much less expensive, essentially cost neutral for the dialysis centers, and completely reimbursable to the patient. This trend will undoubtedly persist and be extended to other specialties as well. In terms of vascular surgeons, counseling patients on the possibility of peritoneal dialysis, especially those in their first year or 2 of dialysis, will require outcomes tracking, complications, and other key quality measures. Although this article discussed dialysis centers, it is interesting to see how the centers adapted to bundling increases, cost reduction strategies, and, ultimately, an increase in revenue streams.

R. L. Bush, MD, JD, MPH

Trends in Relative Mortality Between Hispanic and Non-Hispanic Whites Initiating Dialysis: A Retrospective Study of the US Renal Data System

Arce CM, Goldstein BA, Mitani AA, et al (Stanford Univ School of Medicine, Palo Alto, CA)

Am J Kidney Dis 62:312-321, 2013

Background.—Hispanic patients undergoing long-term dialysis experience better survival compared with non-Hispanic whites. It is unknown whether this association differs by age, has changed over time, or is due to differential access to kidney transplantation.

Study Design.—National retrospective cohort study.

Setting & Participants.—Using the US Renal Data System, we identified 615,618 white patients 18 years or older who initiated dialysis therapy between January 1, 1995, and December 31, 2007.

Predictors.—Hispanic ethnicity (vs non-Hispanic whites), year of end-stage renal disease incidence, age (as potential effect modifier).

Outcomes.—All-cause and cause-specific mortality.

Results.—We found that Hispanics initiating dialysis therapy experienced lower mortality, but age modified this association ($P < 0.001$). Compared with non-Hispanic whites, mortality in Hispanics was 33% lower at ages 18-39 years (adjusted cause-specific HR [HR_{cs}], 0.67; 95% CI, 0.64-0.71) and 40-59 years (HR_{cs}, 0.67; 95% CI, 0.66-0.68), 19% lower at ages 60-79 years (HR_{cs}, 0.81; 95% CI, 0.80-0.82), and 6% lower at 80 years or older (HR_{cs}, 0.94; 95% CI, 0.91-0.97). Accounting for the differential rates of kidney transplantation, the associations were attenuated markedly in the younger age strata; the survival benefit for Hispanics was reduced from 33% to 10% at ages 18-39 years (adjusted subdistribution-specific HR [HR_{sd}], 0.90; 95% CI, 0.85-0.94) and from 33% to 19% among those aged 40-59 years (HR_{sd}, 0.81; 95% CI, 0.80-0.83).

Limitations.—Inability to analyze Hispanic subgroups that may experience heterogeneous mortality outcomes.

Conclusions.—Overall, Hispanics experienced lower mortality, but differential access to kidney transplantation was responsible for much of the apparent survival benefit noted in younger Hispanics.

▶ With the ever-increasing diversity of the US population, an understanding of the ethnic differences in outcomes to various disease processes is crucial. This article examines the mortality differences between Hispanic and non-Hispanic white population undergoing long-term hemodialysis. Although many of us would consider Hispanics to have a higher mortality rate given the increased prevalence of diabetes mellitus, uncontrolled hypertension, and obesity in this group, this is not the case because of a lower cardiovascular disease burden. Hispanics have also been found to have increased barriers to health care, later referrals to nephrologists given chronic kidney disease, and less predialysis care. Hispanics also have a lower rate of kidney transplantation; however, this trend is not seen with the younger population. Older Hispanics remain on dialysis longer because of the transition of non-Hispanic whites to transplantation. This fact results in more catheter usage, worse anemia, and thus, worse mortality. We, as a society and medical profession, need to address these racial differences in health care. The approach is going to have to be multipronged, looking at access to care, disease prevalence differences, familial and cultural ideologies and traditions, and other social issues. This type of health care disparity can be seen in other populations as well. It will be vital as health care reform initiatives get underway, to focus efforts on improving access, communication, education, and ultimately outreach to vulnerable populations.

R. L. Bush, MD, JD, MPH

A "Christmas Tree" Band for the Treatment of Arteriovenous Dialysis Access–Related Steal Syndrome

Smith GE, Barnes R, Green L, et al (Hull and York Med School, UK; et al)
Ann Vasc Surg 27:239.e9-239.e12, 2013

Background.—Dialysis access steal syndrome (DASS) is an uncommon but often debilitating complication of dialysis access formation. We present a technical description of a novel arteriovenous fistula (AVF) banding technique for the treatment of DASS and the results of a short case series.

Methods.—A polyethylene terephthalate carotid patch is shaped with a slit at 1 end and saw tooth edges (resulting in a "Christmas tree" shape) so as to provide a ratchet mechanism to progressively constrict the draining vein of the AVF. This is performed with finger perfusion pressure measures to allow optimal compromise between distal extremity and AVF perfusion. Data on 6 patients with brachiocephalic AVF treated with this technique are included in a case series.

Results.—During the follow-up of mean of 14 months (range, 2–36 months), all AVFs remained patent and in active use for dialysis. No alternative access was required in the immediate post- or perioperative period. All patients had relief of rest pain or evidence of healing at the last follow-up.

Conclusions.—Christmas tree banding with finger pressure measurements can offer successful treatment for DASS.

▶ Dialysis access procedures are very imperfect operations with many secondary complications that can occur, including failure of maturation, thrombosis, infection, outflow and central venous stenoses, and steal syndrome. This article describes a novel method for treating steal syndrome that is simple and does not require a major revascularization procedure. Fortunately, patients with end-stage renal disease now enjoy longer life expectancies because of tremendous advances in medical management. However, this translates into a need for maintenance of, or creation of new, permanent access sites for many years. The ongoing development of this field of surgery is imperative for the care of this ever-increasing cohort of patients.

These authors have studied dialysis steal syndrome, which can result in severe hand pain, muscle atrophy, and possible tissue loss in up to 8% of dialysis access patients. Banding, which they have studied, has been tried with little success in the past. Quantification of the needed amount of flow will vary per patient and with blood pressure and dialysis flow rates. The technique that these Scottish physicians developed involves a controlled method of banding for the treatment of steal syndrome and their short-term results. The device that they modify functions like a belt that they call a "Christmas tree" band because of its configuration. The authors are able to fine tune the tie while concomitantly measuring the flow. By balancing flow rate monitoring with the banding, the authors are able to accurately measure the best flow rates, using a digital perfusion pressure of 80 mm Hg. Salvage of a functioning arteriovenous access is crucial to the survival of the patient, as the number of access sites are not infinite.

R. L. Bush, MD, JD, MPH

A systematic review of preoperative duplex ultrasonography and arteriovenous fistula formation

Wong CS, McNicholas N, Healy D, et al (Univ Hosp Limerick, Ireland; et al)
J Vasc Surg 57:1129-1133, 2013

Background.—Arteriovenous fistula (AVF) formation for dialysis access is a common procedure. Fistula maturation is unpredictable. Preoperative duplex mapping may increase procedural success. We undertook a systematic review to assess the effect of preoperative duplex mapping on subsequent AVF patency.

Methods.—The published literature was searched on PubMed and the Cochrane Library using the following keywords: 'arteriovenous fistula,' 'venous mapping,' 'ultrasound,' 'hemodialysis,' 'vascular access,' and 'perioperative vessel mapping.' Conference proceedings were hand searched for otherwise unpublished trials. Only randomized controlled trials in which preoperative duplex mapping was compared with clinical evaluation were eligible.

Results.—Three trials (402 patients) were identified. More patients who underwent ultrasound successfully started using their fistula for dialysis access, although the difference did not reach statistical significance (174/214 vs 130/188; pooled odds ratio, 1.96; $P=.11$).

Conclusions.—Preoperative duplex mapping may improve fistula maturation rates. However, the results do not reach statistical significance and there are no cost-effectiveness data. Further work is required.

▶ The ability to predict arteriovenous fistula (AVF) maturation rates has remained elusive at best. Although guidelines emphasize the superiority of autogenous access, the aging population with multiple medical comorbidities makes this even more challenging. The easiest and most cost-efficient pre-procedural planning tool, besides a good physical examination, is that of duplex ultrasonography. Those of us who routinely perform access procedures usually choose to do our own ultrasound scans as we are evaluating patients for an operation. This article is a systematic review looking at whether preoperative duplex ultrasonography actually improves maturation rates. The article inclusion criteria were strict, so of 2079 articles initially identified, only 3 randomized, controlled trials were included for study. The total cohort was only 402 patients with no statistical significance found in the subgroups that had ultrasound scan and those who did not. Although I agree with many of the comments in the discussion about the advantages of a successful AVF, I disagree with the comments about overburdening a radiology department. Sending patients out for dialysis access vein mapping delays procedures, does not provide real-time data for the surgeon, and may overly burden a patient who has to travel a distance multiple times for evaluation, testing, and then the procedure. As for cost effectiveness, sending the patients out for an ultrasound scan is clearly more expensive than a quick study performed in the clinic. Today's vascular fellows and residents are appropriately trained in ultrasound techniques and should be performing this quick and simple imaging study themselves at the time of consultation.

R. L. Bush, MD, JD, MPH

The optimal initial choice for permanent arteriovenous hemodialysis access

Sgroi MD, Patel MS, Wilson SE, et al (Univ of California, Orange; et al)
J Vasc Surg 58:539-548, 2013

The role of prosthetic AV hemodialysis accesses (AV grafts) in the current era of the Kidney Disease Outcome Quality Initiative and the Fistula First Breakthrough Initiative remains unresolved. As a direct result of these initiatives, a tremendous amount of pressure has been placed on access surgeons to create autogenous AV accesses (AV fistulas), with a national target rate of 66% (prevalence). Indeed, the prevalence of AV fistulas and, perhaps more importantly, the prevalence of central venous dialysis catheters, have become markers for qualitydor lack thereof in the cases of the cathetersdamong dialysis units. It is unclear whether this AV fistula target is realistic or appropriate, and the anecdotal impression has been that the increased emphasis on AV fistulas has inadvertently resulted in an increased failure-to-mature rate and a prolonged dependence on dialysis catheters. These concerns are underscored by the 61% AV fistula failure-to-mature rate reported by the Dialysis Access Consortium from their National Institution of Health, randomized, controlled trial examining the role of clopidogrel.1 The data largely support the superiority of AV fistulas over AV grafts in terms of almost every outcome measure, including patency, morbidity, mortality, and cost. However, the choice of permanent access configurations may not be quite as clearcut or black-and-white as the initiatives suggest. As Dr Wilson and colleagues point out, appropriate comparison of the patency rates mandates inclusion of all accesses that fail to mature, not just those that are successfully cannulated. Accurate patency assessment also mandates comparing comparable patient cohorts, including those deemed high risk for failure after both AV fistula and graft creation, including elderly patients, diabetic patients, women, and amputees. Similarly, the appropriate comparison of the infectious complication rates likely mandates including the catheter-related infections incurred during the fistula maturation period that frequently extends up to 6 months, again potentially diluting or reducing the perceived benefit of AV fistulas. Lastly, AV grafts have several relative advantages over AV fistulas, including an essentially unlimited supply, a shorter maturation period, increased surface area for cannulation, and greater ease of cannulation. The debate about the role of AV grafts relative to AV fistulas may be somewhat artificial or moot, as suggested by both Drs Jennings and Wilson. AV fistulas and grafts should be viewed as alternative options for providing effective, long-term hemodialysis. A mature AV fistula is the ideal choice for most patients and, fortunately, an AV fistula can usually be created or successfully achieved in most patients, as emphasized in the debate. However, AV grafts are a very acceptable alternative that may be more appropriate for certain subsets of patients. The current challenge is to select the most appropriate access type or configuration for a specific patient to ensure a functional access while minimizing morbidity. It is the hope that the results of the Hemodialysis Fistula Maturation study, a prospective National Institutes of Health-funded observation study of fistula maturation, will help refine the clinical decision making for dialysis access, complementing the adverse findings from its predecessor, the Dialysis Access Consortium. However, it is important to emphasize that maintaining permanent hemodialysis access is a difficult problem that requires committed providers and a lifelong plan.

▶ The need for permanent vascular access for hemodialysis has increased dramatically in our society. As such, surgeons are seeing more and more new consults and then the need for secondary procedures, a secondary access, or a revision of the initial access. The determination of the best site and type of access must be individualized; however, the national guidelines through the Kidney Disease Outcome Quality Initiative (KDOQI) and others enthusiastically recommend an arteriovenous fistula as the optimal access because of improved patency rates and a lower complication profile than prosthetic access, including catheters. Unfortunately, not all patients are created equal, and the life expectancy of patients with end-stage renal disease has increased over the last few decades. As most surgeons who perform access procedures well know, arteriovenous fistulas (AVFs) do not always mature and if they do, have a limited life and usage expectancy, and, even more often, suitable venous conduits are not always available. This article is a fabulous review about the current challenges of AVFs and when an arteriovenous graft (AVG) may be more appropriate. This statement in and of itself seems a contradiction to the KDOQI guidelines, albeit a realistic one. The authors also discuss the 2008 Guidelines published by Sidawy et al, which recommend a prosthetic graft when an adequate vein is unsuitable. An AVG also leads to faster cannulation times and faster catheter removal times; both are desirable outcomes in a perfect world. I believe that this article is a "must read," as it discusses the current guidelines and need for autogenous access but real world surgical experience. The guidelines must be used as a goal but not as a penalty.

R. L. Bush, MD, JD, MPH

Using distal revascularization with interval ligation as the primary treatment of hand ischemia after dialysis access creation

Aimaq R, Katz SG (Huntington Hosp, Pasadena, CA; Univ of Southern California, Los Angeles, CA)

J Vasc Surg 57:1073-1078, 2013

Background.—Arterial steal syndrome after angioaccess surgery can lead to potentially devastating complications. Past treatments either ensured loss of the newly created access through ligation or attempted salvage by increasing resistance within the fistula. None of these proved to be entirely satisfactory. In 1994, we began to employ distal revascularization with interval ligation (DRIL) as our primary method of relieving hand ischemia after dialysis access creation. Described here is our experience with this procedure.

Methods.—After institutional review board approval, the charts of patients undergoing the DRIL procedure for relief of hand ischemia after dialysis access surgery were reviewed. Patient demographics, risk factors, types of fistulas, and indications for operation were recorded. The clinical results of DRIL surgery, as well as fistula and bypass graft patency, were noted.

Results.—Between May 1994 and August 2011, 81 DRIL procedures were performed on 77 patients ranging from 37 to 94 (mean, 65) years of age. Forty-four were female and 33 were male, with diabetes present in 83.3%. DRIL procedures were performed for ischemic symptoms after 37 autogenous brachiocephalic, 30 prosthetic bridge, and 14 autogenous brachiobasilic fistulas. Thirty-eight DRIL procedures were performed for ischemic rest pain (46.9%), 21 for digital ulceration (25.9%), 16 for neurological deficits (19.7%), and six for digital gangrene (7.4%). Complete symptom resolution was seen in 31 patients with ischemic rest pain (81.6%), 19 patients with digital ulcerations (90.5%), nine patients with neurological deficits (56.3%), and five patients with digital gangrene (83.3%). Fistula and brachial-brachial bypass survival 60 months after the DRIL procedure was 56% and 96.9%, respectively. The overall complication rate was 17.2%, and no patients died within 30 days of operation.

Conclusions.—The DRIL procedure is a very effective treatment for symptomatic steal syndrome and is associated with low morbidity and mortality. It is extremely effective in the treatment of ischemic hand pain and tissue loss, but less so for neurological sequelae. It can allow for prolonged fistula utilization.

▶ Over the last 2 decades, tremendous improvements have been made in patient management for patients with end-stage renal disease. These medical improvements have resulted in longer lives that are of better quality. The downside is that patients dependent on hemodialysis rely on a functioning vascular access. Any type of access has a definite life expectancy, although we have improved interventions to preserve and maintain an access site. One of the more serious complications is described in this report as well as the authors' single center experience with treatment. Hand ischemia, neurological issues, ulcers, and eventually gangrene can occur. All of these complications of steal can be devastating, leading to decreased quality of life, pain, and even loss of digits or the extremity. Fortunately, only a small portion of patients will get upper extremity vascular steal syndrome after either autogenous or prosthetic access creation. The extensive experience described herein emphasizes what many of us know to be true. Fistula ligation is no longer acceptable as a primary option because of the need to preserve access sites in this population. Banding and plication procedures often are short-lived or result in thrombosis. It is also very difficult to ascertain how tight to band or plicate the arterial anastomosis to relieve the reversal of flow. The distal revascularization with interval ligation procedure, well described in textbooks and in this article, is fairly easy to perform and only requires a small segment bypass, thus, just a short segment of vein needs to be harvested. The complication profile is basically related to the vein harvest site, with hematomas, seromas, and wound infection most commonly occurring. Because these complications are usually associated with only minor morbidity and can be treated conservatively, they are a small price to pay for relief of the patient's symptoms and preservation of a patent fistula.

R. L. Bush, MD, JD, MPH

11 Carotid and Cerebrovascular Disease

Contralateral carotid artery occlusion is not a contraindication to carotid endarterectomy even if shunts are not routinely used

Samson RH, Cline JL, Showalter DP, et al (Florida State Univ Med School, Sarasota)

J Vasc Surg 58:935-940, 2013

Objective.—Although controversial, carotid artery stenting (CAS) has been proposed as being safer than carotid endarterectomy (CEA) for patients with a contralateral internal carotid occlusion (CCO). Arguably, with a CCO, CAS should be even safer than CEA if a shunt is not used. Accordingly, we reviewed our experience with 2183 CEAs performed routinely without a shunt to evaluate the risk of CEA performed in a subset of 147 patients with a CCO.

Methods.—Between 1988 and 2011, 147 CEAs (111 men [75%], 36 women [25%]) were routinely performed without a shunt despite CCO. Of these patients, 76% were asymptomatic. CEAs were performed by seven surgeons using standard techniques (not eversion), with patients under general anesthesia and blood pressure maintained at >130 mm Hg. All patients received heparin (7500 U), and protamine reversal was routine. Median cross-clamp time was 20 minutes (range, 14-40 minutes).

Results.—Three neurologic events occurred ≤30 days (2.0%). One transient ischemic attack (TIA) occurred immediately, and one occurred on the first postoperative day due to occlusion of the endarterectomy site. One patient sustained an immediate stroke and died of a large computed tomography-documented atheroembolic shower.

Conclusions.—Our data demonstrate the safety of CEA in the presence of a CCO, even when performed without a shunt. It is unlikely that the stroke or delayed TIA could be attributed to nonshunting or CCO. Even if so, the stroke and death rates would be lower than those previously reported for patients undergoing CEA in the presence of a CCO. This may be due to short cross-clamp times, careful technique, general anesthesia, and blood pressure support. Given these low adverse event rates, our experience refutes the assumption that patients with a CCO are at such a high risk for CEA that the only alternative is CAS.

▶ Some have suggested that contralateral carotid occlusion (CCO) puts patients at high risk for stroke during carotid endarterectomy (CEA) and argue that carotid artery stenting (CAS) is a better alternative in this setting. This article clearly demonstrates that patients with CCO can safely undergo CEA without shunting under general anesthesia.

Over a 23-year period, 147 patients with CCO underwent CEA without shunting. All procedures were performed under general anesthesia, taking care to maintain a systolic blood pressure greater than 130 mm Hg. In this group of patients, there were only 3 neurologic adverse events (2.0%), a much lower incidence than that reported by groups arguing for CAS—some report stroke rates as high as 10%. Furthermore, only 1 of the 3 events in this series could possibly be attributed to watershed hypoperfusion.

How could this possibly be true? The answer lies in the etiology of stroke in the setting of carotid artery disease. It's a thromboembolic event, *not* malperfusion from a critical stenosis. Unfortunately, many nonvascular surgeons treating this disease do not understand the etiology of cerebral vascular accident in the setting of carotid artery disease and make treatment decisions based on algorithms for treatment of vascular lesions found in other locations.

The results presented in this must-read article clearly demonstrate that CEA can be performed safely in patients with CCO and that CCO should not be included on the list of "high-risk" criteria when contemplating carotid artery interventions.

B. Peterson, MD

Contralateral carotid artery occlusion is not a contraindication to carotid endarterectomy even if shunts are not routinely used

Samson RH, Cline JL, Showalter DP, et al (Florida State Univ Med School, Sarasota)

J Vasc Surg 58:935-940, 2013

Objective.—Although controversial, carotid artery stenting (CAS) has been proposed as being safer than carotid endarterectomy (CEA) for patients with a contralateral internal carotid occlusion (CCO). Arguably, with a CCO, CAS should be even safer than CEA if a shunt is not used. Accordingly, we reviewed our experience with 2183 CEAs performed routinely without a shunt to evaluate the risk of CEA performed in a subset of 147 patients with a CCO.

Methods.—Between 1988 and 2011, 147 CEAs (111 men [75%], 36 women [25%]) were routinely performed without a shunt despite CCO. Of these patients, 76% were asymptomatic. CEAs were performed by seven surgeons using standard techniques (not eversion), with patients under general anesthesia and blood pressure maintained at > 130 mm Hg. All patients received heparin (7500 U), and protamine reversal was routine. Median cross-clamp time was 20 minutes (range, 14-40 minutes).

Results.—Three neurologic events occurred ≤30 days (2.0%). One transient ischemic attack (TIA) occurred immediately, and one occurred on the first postoperative day due to occlusion of the endarterectomy site. One patient sustained an immediate stroke and died of a large computed tomography-documented atheroembolic shower.

Conclusions.—Our data demonstrate the safety of CEA in the presence of a CCO, even when performed without a shunt. It is unlikely that the stroke or delayed TIA could be attributed to nonshunting or CCO. Even if so, the stroke and death rates would be lower than those previously reported for patients undergoing CEA in the presence of a CCO. This may be due to short cross-clamp times, careful technique, general anesthesia, and blood pressure support. Given these low adverse event rates, our experience refutes the assumption that patients with a CCO are at such a high risk for CEA that the only alternative is CAS.

▶ The authors' practice of never shunting patients during a carotid endarterectomy (CEA) is certainly controversial, but their remarkable 2% stroke rate in the presence of a contralateral carotid occlusion is impressive. They certainly show that CEA is no more risky than carotid artery stenting (CAS) with a contralateral occlusion, their stated chief objective. I think 2 other points can be made. First, performing CEA the same way, every single time, is key to good results. Second, attention to detail by the surgeon and the anesthesia team are essential. Although I have no intentions of changing my use of shunts, I found that the outspoken opinions of the authors regarding their practice challenged me to thoughtfully reexamine my own practice.

P. White, MD, FACS

Contralateral carotid artery occlusion is not a contraindication to carotid endarterectomy even if shunts are not routinely used

Samson RH, Cline JL, Showalter DP, et al (Florida State Univ Med School, Sarasota)

J Vasc Surg 58:935-940, 2013

Objective.—Although controversial, carotid artery stenting (CAS) has been proposed as being safer than carotid endarterectomy (CEA) for patients with a contralateral internal carotid occlusion (CCO). Arguably, with a CCO, CAS should be even safer than CEA if a shunt is not used. Accordingly, we reviewed our experience with 2183 CEAs performed routinely without a shunt to evaluate the risk of CEA performed in a subset of 147 patients with a CCO.

Methods.—Between 1988 and 2011, 147 CEAs (111 men [75%], 36 women [25%]) were routinely performed without a shunt despite CCO. Of these patients, 76% were asymptomatic. CEAs were performed by seven surgeons using standard techniques (not eversion), with patients under general anesthesia and blood pressure maintained at >130 mm Hg.

All patients received heparin (7500 U), and protamine reversal was routine. Median cross-clamp time was 20 minutes (range, 14-40 minutes).

Results.—Three neurologic events occurred ≤30 days (2.0%). One transient ischemic attack (TIA) occurred immediately, and one occurred on the first postoperative day due to occlusion of the endarterectomy site. One patient sustained an immediate stroke and died of a large computed tomography-documented atheroembolic shower.

Conclusions.—Our data demonstrate the safety of CEA in the presence of a CCO, even when performed without a shunt. It is unlikely that the stroke or delayed TIA could be attributed to nonshunting or CCO. Even if so, the stroke and death rates would be lower than those previously reported for patients undergoing CEA in the presence of a CCO. This may be due to short cross-clamp times, careful technique, general anesthesia, and blood pressure support. Given these low adverse event rates, our experience refutes the assumption that patients with a CCO are at such a high risk for CEA that the only alternative is CAS.

▶ In this day and age of carotid stent (CAS) placement for carotid stenosis being a revascularization alternative to endarterectomy (CEA), several anatomic criteria have emerged as contraindications to CEA. One such high-risk anatomic condition is that of contralateral carotid occlusion (CO). The safety of CEA in the presence of a CO has been used as an argument for the performance of CAS in these patients. Samson et al refute this argument with their well-presented data on 147 consecutive CEAs in patients with COs. They routinely do not shunt their patients, use general anesthesia, make a longitudinal arteriotomy, and use a patch to close the artery. This vascular group comprised of 7 surgeons also performed 2036 CEAs during the same 23-year timeframe in patients who had a patent contralateral carotid artery. The cohort with a CO had 3 neurologic events occurring during the perioperative (< 30 days) period. This represents a 2% event rate. Regardless of the etiology of the neurologic event, use of shunt, and/or presence of CO, this is a much lower event rate than other reports have suggested in the presence of a CO. Our cardiology colleagues endorse CAS as the only safe procedure for patients with CO or excluding patient with CO. However, the data have not supported this with many of the CAS trials not reporting event rates in the subsets of patients with CO or excluding patient with CO. Furthermore, the patients with CO also had other risk factors that would place them at higher risk for adverse neurologic events, regardless of type of revascularization.

R. L. Bush, MD, JD, MPH

A Direct Comparison of Early and Late Outcomes With Three Approaches to Carotid Revascularization and Open Heart Surgery

Shishehbor MH, Venkatachalam S, Sun Z, et al (Cleveland Clinic, OH; et al)

J Am Coll Cardiol 62:1948-1956, 2013

Objectives.—The aim of this study was a comparison of risk-adjusted outcomes of 3 approaches to carotid revascularization in the open heart surgery (OHS) population.

Background.—Without randomized clinical trials, the best approach to managing coexisting severe carotid and coronary disease remains uncertain. Staged carotid endarterectomy (CEA) followed by OHS or combined CEA and OHS are commonly used. A recent alternative is carotid artery stenting (CAS).

Methods.—From 1997 to 2009, 350 patients underwent carotid revascularization within 90 days before OHS at a tertiary center: 45 staged CEA-OHS, 195 combined CEA-OHS, and 110 staged CAS-OHS. The primary composite endpoint was all-cause death, stroke, and myocardial infarction (MI). Staged CAS-OHS patients had higher prevalence of previous stroke ($p = 0.03$) and underwent more complex OHS. Therefore, the propensity score adjusted multiphase hazard function models with modulated renewal to account for staging, and competing risks were used.

Results.—Using propensity analysis, staged CAS-OHS and combined CEA-OHS had similar early hazard phase composite outcomes, whereas staged CEA-OHS incurred the highest risk driven by interstage MI. Subsequently, staged CAS-OHS patients experienced significantly fewer late hazard phase events compared with both staged CEA-OHS (adjusted hazard ratio: 0.33; 95% confidence interval: 0.15 to 0.77; $p = 0.01$) and combined CEA-OHS (adjusted hazard ratio: 0.35; 95% confidence interval: 0.18 to 0.70; $p = 0.003$).

Conclusions.—Staged CAS-OHS and combined CEA-OHS are associated with a similar risk of death, stroke, or MI in the short term, with both being better than staged CEA-OHS. However, the outcomes significantly favor staged CAS-OHS after the first year.

▶ In this single-center, retrospective study, the authors attempt to demonstrate the best approach to the treatment of patients with combined severe carotid and coronary artery disease. To do so, 3 treatment groups were compared: staged carotid endarterectomy before open-heart surgery (staged CEA-OHS), staged carotid artery stenting before open-heart surgery (staged CAS-OHS), and combined carotid endarterectomy and open-heart surgery (combined CEA-OHS). Results demonstrate that staged CEA-OHS was associated with a significantly higher incidence of combined stroke, death, and myocardial infarction compared with the other 2 groups. This difference in groups could largely be attributed to a higher incidence of interstage myocardial infarction experienced by the staged CEA-OHS group. Additionally, after 1 year, the staged CAS-OHS group had significantly fewer patients reach the composite end point of death, stroke, and myocardial infarction (largely because of significantly fewer deaths seen in this group). Therefore, the authors suggest that a staged approach using carotid artery stenting before open-heart surgery should be considered a first-line strategy in treating patients with severe, concomitant carotid and coronary artery disease if a 3- to 4-week delay in open-heart surgery following carotid artery stenting is possible to allow for antiplatelet therapy.

Based on the evidence presented, this may be an appropriate approach; however, a fourth group has to be added into this comparison: a group that does not undergo any carotid intervention. Perhaps the reason why the staged CAS-OHS group experienced fewer myocardial infarctions than the staged CEA-OHS group lies in the fact that the CAS patients were treated with dual antiplatelet therapy, and medical management is the optimal approach to these patients. Additionally, this study largely ignores clinical decision making based on the presence or absence of symptoms. Nevertheless, this study does serve as a starting point in determining how best to treat patients with concomitant, asymptomatic carotid and coronary artery disease.

B. Peterson, MD

Delay to Carotid Endarterectomy in Patients with Symptomatic Carotid Artery Stenosis

den Hartog AG, Moll FL, van der Worp HB, et al (Univ Med Ctr Utrecht, The Netherlands)

Eur J Vasc Endovasc Surg 47:233-239, 2014

Objective.—In patients with recently symptomatic carotid artery stenosis, guidelines recommend carotid revascularization within 2 weeks of the index event. The "index event" may be defined as either the first or the most recent event. The delay between the index event and carotid endarterectomy (CEA) over a period of 6 years in a single centre was evaluated and the effect of defining the index event as either the first or the most recent event was assessed.

Design.—Observational Study.

Methods.—555 consecutive patients with symptomatic carotid stenosis ≥50% treated with CEA between 2007 and 2012 were assessed. In 2010, changes to the in-hospital process of care to reduce delays in referral and CEA were introduced. These changes included, for example, improving access to physicians, imaging, and operating rooms. The delay from symptoms to surgery was expressed in days.

Results.—The median time between the first event and surgery was reduced from 53 days (interquartile range [IQR] 30–78) in 2007 to 21 days (IQR 12–45) in 2012, and between the most recent event and CEA from 45 days (IQR 28–67) to 17 days (IQR 9–28). Patients referred directly by their general practitioner more often underwent CEA within 2 weeks than patients referred by specialists from other hospitals. Compared to patients with transient ischaemic attack or ocular symptoms, patients with ischaemic stroke more often underwent CEA within 2 weeks.

Conclusions.—A small change in the process of care significantly reduced the delay from the index event to CEA, but in 2012 it still exceeded 14 days in the majority of patients. The definition of the "index event" has a large impact on the total duration of delay, and should therefore be uniform across studies.

▶ There are guidelines suggesting that carotid endarterectomy should be performed within 2 weeks of an index event. This study attempts to identify what factors led to delay in carotid endarterectomy (CEA). This observational study evaluated a large patient population at a tertiary vascular referral hospital in which a structured system was developed to evaluate symptomatic patients promptly. To facilitate evaluation of these patients, specific time slots for CEA evaluation were set up by a neurologist, a vascular surgeon, and an anesthesiologist. Indirect referrals from regional hospitals were made by fax or letter to the tertiary referral center. Risk factors in greater than 2-week delay in carotid endarterectomy from an index event included all of these indirect referrals. Most directly referred patients underwent CEA within 2 weeks of the first event. Patients who were referred for stroke were most likely to undergo CEA within 2 weeks when compared with patients who experienced a transient ischemic attack. Eleven of 15 patients who died after carotid endarterectomy had recurrent symptoms during their waiting time. Among these 15 patients who died within 30 days of carotid endarterectomy, the overall delay between the symptom and CEA was 43 days. Despite these findings, a statistically significant relationship could not be established between poor clinical outcome and delay in referral time. Over the duration of the study, the time from the index event to CEA did decrease; however, the definition of an index event seemed to be controversial. In some instances, the index event was defined as the event that led the patient to seek medical attention, and in others it was the time when the diagnosis of carotid stenosis was established. This study provides interesting perspective on the difficulties encountered in attempting to streamline care and may have medicolegal consequences in litigious societies.

M. T. Watkins, MD

Patching plus extended exposure and tacking of the common carotid cuff may reduce the late incidence of recurrent stenosis after carotid endarterectomy

Hertzer NR, Bena JF (Cleveland Clinic, OH)
J Vasc Surg 58:926-934.e2, 2013

Objective.—The safety and durability of carotid endarterectomy (CEA) require attention to certain technical details that may evolve over time. The objective of this study was to determine whether routine patch angioplasty and precautions related to the common carotid cuff could reduce the risks for perioperative stroke, internal carotid artery (ICA) thrombosis, or recurrent carotid stenosis.

Methods.—The senior author (N.H.) performed 1959 consecutive isolated CEAs at the Cleveland Clinic from 1976 to 2004. This series can be divided into three distinct eras with respect to patching and management of the proximal common carotid cuff: (1) primary arteriotomy closure with selective patching in only 38 of 653 CEAs (5.8%) from 1976 to 1983 (group 1); (2) routine patching without any special precautions related to the common carotid cuff in 568 CEAs from 1983 to 1990 (group 2); and (3) routine patching with extended exposure and tacking sutures to secure the carotid cuff in 738 CEAs from 1990 to 2004 (group 3).

Results.—Although vein patching alone seemed to have less risk for perioperative stroke (1.2% vs 2.4%) or ICA thrombosis (0.6% vs 1.8%) than primary closure, these differences did not attain statistical significance. There also were no significant differences in the perioperative stroke and ICA thrombosis rates among the three eras in which changes occurred in patch use and in the management of the carotid cuff. After adjusting for the various lengths of follow-up in the study groups, however, group 3 had a significantly lower risk for recurrent 60% to 99% stenosis or ICA occlusion at > 5 years after CEA (odds ratio [OR], 0.09; 95% confidence interval [CI], 0.04-0.22; $P < .001$). On multivariable analysis, group 3 (OR, 0.23; 95% CI, 0.09-0.60; $P = .003$) and advancing age (OR, 0.89 per year; 95% CI, 0.85-0.92 per year; $P < .001$) had less risk for late recurrent stenosis, whereas this risk was higher in women (OR, 2.23; 95% CI, 1.23-4.06; $P = .009$) and in patients who had undergone previous ipsilateral CEA (OR, 6.02; 95% CI, 1.63-22.2; $P = .007$).

Conclusions.—Routine patching plus extended exposure and tacking of the common carotid cuff appear to significantly reduce the long-term incidence of recurrent 60% to 99% stenosis or ICA occlusion after CEA.

▶ The objective of this study was to determine whether routine patch angioplasty and precautions related to the common carotid cuff could reduce the risks for perioperative stroke, internal carotid artery (ICA) thrombosis, or recurrent carotid stenosis. The concept of specific attention to the management of the proximal carotid cuff during carotid endarterectomy (CEA) was originally published by Archie in the 1990s. In this report, the personal experience of the senior author in the management of 2262 bifurcation CEAs at the Cleveland Clinic from 1976 to 2004, including 303 procedures in conjunction with simultaneous coronary bypass surgery, is provided with specific attention 3 three groups:

1 Before routine patching (group 1): Primary arteriotomy closure was customarily performed from 1976 to 1983, with selective patching in only 38 (5.8%) of these 653 CEAs (559 patients).

2 Patching without carotid cuff precautions (group 2): Routine patch angioplasty was done without any special precautions with respect to the common carotid cuff during 568 CEAs (481 patients) from 1983 to 1990.

3 Patching with extended carotid cuff exposure and tacking (group 3). In 738 CEAs (648 patients) from 1990 to 2004, the carotid cuff was divided far enough above the lower end of the arteriotomy to incorporate it beneath

the full diameter of a patch. The cuff also was secured with several 7-0 sutures to prevent mobility.

This report concludes that extended exposure and patching of a common carotid cuff secured by tacking sutures may give better protection against late recurrent stenosis than routine patching alone. This study failed to demonstrate a statistically significant reduction in the incidence of perioperative stroke or ICA thrombosis after the transition from selective patching to routine patching. Of great importance when considering this patient population are the mortality, severe restenosis, and reintervention data. The complete 10-year Kaplan-Meier estimates for mortality, severe recurrent stenosis (> 60%), and reintervention can be found in the Supplementary Table (online only). The 10-year mortality, severe recurrence, and reintervention rates were 56% ± 2.2%, 27% ± 4.0%, and 14% ± 2.7% in group 1; 56% ± 2.4%, 18% ± 3.3%, and 13% ± 2.5% in group 2; and 62% ± 3.2%, 13% ± 3.6%, and 5.8% ± 2.4% in group 3. Given the large numbers of patients in this report, in addition to the results from the earlier report from Archie, more attention to management of the proximal carotid cuff is warranted.

M. T. Watkins, MD

Neurocognitive Changes After Eversion Carotid Endarterectomy Under Local Anesthesia

Migliara B, Trentin M, Idone D, et al (Casa di Cura, "Dott. Pederzoli," Peschiera del Garda, Verona, Italy)
Ann Vasc Surg 27:727-735, 2013

Background.—The effects of carotid endarterectomy (CEA) on cognitive function have yet to be fully elucidated. The aim of our study was to administer a battery of cognitive tests to identify any cognitive changes occurring in a consecutive series of patients who underwent CEA using the eversion technique under local anesthesia.

Methods.—This prospective study was designed to analyze a consecutive series of patients undergoing eversion CEA under local anesthesia for significant carotid stenosis at our vascular surgery unit over a period of 6 months. Patients underwent tests to rule-out those who already had cognitive impairments or states of depression/anxiety capable of interfering with cognitive testing outcomes. Patients then completed a battery of 10 neurocognitive tests preoperatively and again 30 days and 4 months after surgery to assess the functions of both cerebral hemispheres as thoroughly as possible.

Results.—Of the 48 patients initially considered for our study, 39 completed the follow-up. They were 71.4 ± 8.2 (mean ± SD) years of age; 30 were men and 9 were women. Six were symptomatic for carotid stenosis and 33 were asymptomatic. All patients were examined by a neurologist and underwent pre- and postoperative nuclear MRI or CT scan of the brain to identify any cerebral ischemia potentially correlated with the surgical procedure. In all cases, the cognitive test findings tended to improve postoperatively; this improvement was statistically significant in 7 tests. Post-hoc analysis confirmed an improvement between the pre- and postoperative test results. Among the different variables considered, only age <75 years seems to have influenced cognitive improvement.

Conclusions.—The effects on cognitive function of carotid stenosis, particularly CEA, is still a much debated issue. The data reported in the literature vary considerably, preventing any final conclusions from being drawn. The mechanisms capable of inducing changes in cognitive status after CEA have yet to be precisely clarified. In our study, a suitable battery of tests were used to analyze the trend of cognitive function correlating with eversion CEA under local anesthesia. Our results demonstrate substantially improved cognitive function after CEA, which was statistically significant in 7 of 10 tests. We surmise that the CEA procedure, per se, can help to protect patients against cognitive deterioration, especially in those <75 years of age.

▶ It has been shown that cognitive changes do happen after carotid endarterectomy (CEA), and such changes may be imperceptible unless specifically targeted by physical examination or testing protocols. This labor-intensive study used 10 cognitive tests after CEA performed under local anesthesia. Interestingly, the cohort is small (39 patients completed the study), and 33 (84.6%) were asymptomatic from the standpoint of their carotid lesion. The patients improved their cognitive function in 7 of the tests when compared with baseline or preoperatively. So is it fair with this small study to say that prophylactic CEA should be done to prevent cognitive deterioration or be done to prevent the small incidence of stroke associated with an asymptomatic lesion? Additionally, there are several confounding variables that may limit the interpretation of these results, including the use of local anesthesia. I would recommend repeating this study with a control group, one undergoing CEA under general anesthesia. I would also recommend perhaps making comparisons with carotid stenting. Of course, delaying or decreasing the deterioration of cognition is a laudable goal, but can this delay or decrease be quantified? These patients need to be studied over time. Moreover, the risk of stroke inherent with a CEA performed in an asymptomatic patient needs to be weighed against any perceived improvements in cognition.

R. L. Bush, MD, JD, MPH

Management of common carotid artery dissection due to extension from acute type A (DeBakey I) aortic dissection

Charlton-Ouw KM, Azizzadeh A, Sandhu HK, et al (Univ of Texas Med School at Houston)

J Vasc Surg 58:910-916, 2013

Background.—Acute type A aortic dissection can extend into arch vessels, including the common carotid arteries. Although several reports describe concomitant endovascular repair of common carotid artery dissection (CCAD) during open ascending aortic repair, the criteria for repair, natural history, and risk of stroke are unclear. We examine the literature and our experience with nonoperative management of CCAD after acute aortic dissection repair to determine the risk of stroke and the need for carotid revascularization.

Methods.—We queried our cases of type A aortic dissection over a 10-year period from January 2002 to December 2011. Imaging was reviewed to determine the presence of CCAD and degree of true-lumen stenosis. Analysis was performed to determine risk of stroke and survival on initial presentation and during follow-up. Survival functions between excluded groups and those with and without CCAD were compared using log-rank statistics.

Results.—We repaired 288 cases of acute type A aortic dissection during the study period. Adequate carotid imaging was available in 179 patients and comprised the study group. We identified 43 cases with CCAD (group A, 24.0%) and 136 cases without it (group B, 76.0%). History of previous stroke was not a risk factor for new stroke in either group ($P = .517$). Bilateral CCAD occurred in 16 cases (37.2%). Stroke on initial presentation was more common in group A (18.6%) than in group B (8.1%; odds ratio, 2.6; 95% confidence interval, 0.97-6.95; $P = .051$). Degree of stenosis or false-lumen thrombosis did not affect rate of stroke on presentation. The degree of postoperative true-lumen stenosis ranged from 0% (resolution) to 90%. No patient with CCAD had stroke or required carotid revascularization after discharge on follow-up. The 5-year, stroke-free survival rates in groups A and B were 69.7% and 73.6% ($P = .820$), respectively.

Conclusions.—CCAD, due to extension from aortic arch dissection, has a low risk of subsequent stroke after the initial event. Based on current data, there is little evidence to suggest that aortic origin CCAD requires repair in the absence of recurrent symptoms, regardless of the degree of stenosis or false-lumen patency. Recommended optimal medical therapy includes either aspirin or anticoagulation for 6 months after initial presentation. Additional longitudinal studies are needed.

▶ Acute aortic dissection is a terrifying disease process that can often be unpredictable in terms of extension of the dissection and presence of symptoms. This retrospective analysis comes from a high-volume center that has considerable expertise in the medical and surgical management of acute aortic dissection. In their cohort, 24% of patients had extension of the dissection into the common carotid artery (CCAD), with more than one-third of patients having bilateral CCAD. Their data show that after the initial event, there is no evidence supporting ongoing risk of stroke regardless of residual luminal diameter or thrombosis. After management of the initial presentation of a type A dissection, surgical repair is recommended of the carotid origin in addition to the proximal aortic repair only if the patient has symptoms of cerebral ischemia. For all patients, maximal medical management with antihypertensive drugs and anticoagulant or antiplatelet therapy should be undertaken. These cases are challenging, and it is clear that this group represents a center of excellence with available resources to ensure optimal patient outcomes. Unfortunately, in acute situations, referral and transfer to such regional centers is not always feasible. However, these centers need to be identified for consultation and safe transfer when the patient is stable.

R. L. Bush, MD, JD, MPH

Safety and Efficacy of Carotid Endarterectomy in Octogenarians

Pol RA, Reijnen MMPJ, Lont M, et al (Univ of Groningen, The Netherlands; Rijnstate Hosp, Arnhem, The Netherlands)

Ann Vasc Surg 27:736-742, 2013

Background.—To evaluate the outcome of carotid endarterectomy (CEA) in octogenarians.

Method.—Between January 2005 and July 2010, all CEA patients were prospectively recorded. Patients were categorized into those <80 and ≥80 years of age. Primary outcome measures were hospital duration of stay (HDOS), mortality, any stroke, and postprocedural complications.

Results.—In total, 477 patients with carotid artery stenosis were treated with CEA. Seventy-one patients (13%) were ≥80 years of age and 477 (87%) patients were <80 years of age. Median HDOS was 3.0 days (interquartile range [IQR], 2–5) for the entire cohort with a median of 3 days (IQR, 2–4) for patients <80 years of age and 4 days (IQR, 2–7) for patients ≥80 years of age ($P = 0.0001$). Fifteen patients (3%) had an early adverse neurologic event, with 7 patients (1.3%) developing a transient ischemic attack, 2 patients (0.3%) a minor stroke with full neurologic recovery, and 6 patients (1.1%) had a major stroke. Forty patients (6.8%) had a postoperative nerve injury. No statistical differences were observed between the younger (<80 years of age) and older (≥80 years of age) group despite a significant difference in postoperative delirium ($P < 0.0001$). During follow-up, more fatal cardiac events occurred in the octogenarians group (4.2% vs. 0.4%; $P = 0.02$). Kaplan–Meier analysis revealed a significantly better survival for the younger patients (log rank test; $P = 0.04$).

Conclusions.—Octogenarians who suffer from carotid artery stenosis can be safely treated by CEA. The increased incidence of postoperative delirium is an important finding and requires extra attention in this vulnerable group.

▶ Carotid revascularization in the elderly is controversial at best. Recently published trials have shown carotid endarterectomy (CEA) to be the preferred treatment over carotid stenting in those who are of older age. This study examines the outcomes of CEA in octogenarians, although the authors reconcile that many studies define an elderly cohort as ≥70 years of age. The older segments of the population are increasing with more people living longer; thus, surgeons will be consulted on these patients and need to be able to give evidence-based recommendations on the safety and efficacy of carotid interventions. In this cohort, 13% of all patients undergoing CEA were ≥80 years of age (elderly group). The elderly group had a statistically significantly longer length of hospital stay than younger patients. However, there were no differences seen in postoperative complications, including the rate of adverse neurologic events. Interestingly, the elderly group had a higher rate of postoperative delirium ($P < .0001$) and an increased rate of fatal cardiac event ($P = .02$), whereas younger patients had a significantly better survival. These are not surprising results given the average age difference between the groups of 15 years. The bottom line is that CEA can be performed with acceptable results. The major question that I believe should be considered in an older person is not which procedure to perform but whether to perform any at all, especially if the patient has an asymptomatic stenosis.

R. L. Bush, MD, JD, MPH

Management of Carotid Stenosis in Women

Kuy S, Seabrook GR, Rossi PJ, et al (Med College of Wisconsin, Milwaukee)
JAMA Surg 148:788-790, 2013

The management of carotid stenosis in women remains a topic of controversy. In this review article, we aimed to define carotid disease burden in women, review outcomes of carotid endarterectomy and carotid artery stenting in women, discuss differences in practice patterns based on sex, and provide guidelines for management of women with carotid stenosis. Symptomatic women with high-grade stenosis derive benefit from carotid endarterectomy, although they have different risk profiles than men and are often not taking appropriate medical therapy. Women with asymptomatic carotid artery stenosis have less stroke risk reduction with CEA than their male counterparts; therefore, they should be screened for other treatable risk factors for stroke, with the institution of lifestyle changes and the appropriate medical therapy. After medical optimization, the decision to proceed with CEA in asymptomatic women must be made by carefully assessing that the benefits of stroke risk reduction outweigh perioperative risks.

▶ This article represents an excellent review of what is currently known and recommended for the management of carotid artery occlusive disease in women. Many of the early studies assessing the treatment, whether medical or surgical, of carotid stenosis had a paucity of women enrolled. Thus, extrapolations have been made from male cohorts, but the topic remains controversial despite screenings showing a higher prevalence of disease in women. Other studies have been published with conflicting results concerning the efficacy of carotid interventions as well as complication rates in women. There are no firm conclusions to be made from this article, just an overview of what is known to date and a plea for further research to be done. Health disparities for women do exist, some placed by the providers and some placed by the patients themselves. Women tend to put off their own personal care to care for their children, spouse, and/or parents. Additionally, combined with the fact that women tend to have smaller-caliber blood vessels, the decision to intervene on an asymptomatic lesion is highly debatable. Until further evidence is forthcoming, vascular surgeons should appropriately counsel female patients and inform them of the lack of evidence for revascularization in women.

R. L. Bush, MD, JD, MPH

The role of completion imaging following carotid artery endarterectomy

Ricco J-B, Schneider F, Illuminati G, et al (Univ of Poitiers, France; Univ Hosp la Sapienza, Rome, Italy; et al)

J Vasc Surg 57:1432-1439, 2013

A variety of completion imaging methods can be used during carotid endarterectomy to recognize technical errors or intrinsic abnormalities such as mural thrombus or platelet aggregation, but none of these methods has achieved wide acceptance, and their ability to improve the outcome of the operation remains a matter of controversy.

It is unclear if completion imaging is routinely necessary and which abnormalities require re-exploration. Proponents of routine completion imaging argue that identification of these abnormalities will allow their immediate correction and avoid a perioperative stroke. However, much of the evidence in favor of this argument is incidental, and many experienced vascular surgeons who perform carotid endarterectomy do not use any completion imaging technique and report equally good outcomes using a careful surgical protocol. Furthermore, certain postoperative strokes, including intracerebral hemorrhage and hyperperfusion syndrome, are unrelated to the surgical technique and cannot be prevented by completion imaging. This controversial subject is now open to discussion, and our debaters have been given the task to clarify the evidence to justify their preferred option for completion imaging during carotid endarterectomy.

▶ As a vascular surgeon who has ALWAYS done completion ultrasound imaging after a carotid endarterectomy, I read this article with interest and then with perplexity. The authors make very good points arguing for and against imaging, either with angiography or with ultrasound scan. The argument for imaging is mainly what I was trained to do, then any technical abnormality can be immediately repaired, thus, perhaps preventing a postoperative complication and need for return to the operating room. However, these authors raise a few questions in their argument against completion imaging: What good is it really? There have been no studies or any data that have suggested improved outcomes and lower complication profiles with completion imaging. Furthermore, they make a point of stating that some of the complications, hyperperfusion syndrome and intracerebral hemorrhage, are not related to the surgical technique and thus would not be found on imaging studies. I am left to ponder the decision of the utility of completion imaging. Because ultrasound scan is cheap and easy to perform, I do the study myself. It takes only a few minutes, and I have peace of mind about the integrity of the repair. I will continue to use this completion imaging modality and teach my trainees to do so as well.

R. L. Bush, MD, JD, MPH

Usefulness of Contrast-Enhanced Ultrasound for Detection of Carotid Plaque Ulceration in Patients With Symptomatic Carotid Atherosclerosis

ten Kate GL, van Dijk AC, van den Oord SCH, et al (Erasmus Med Ctr, Rotterdam, The Netherlands)

Am J Cardiol 112:292-298, 2013

Previous data have indicated that carotid plaque ulceration is a strong predictor of cerebrovascular events. Standard ultrasound and color Doppler ultrasound (CDUS) scans have poor diagnostic accuracy for the detection of carotid plaque ulceration. The aim of the present prospective study was to assess the value of contrast-enhanced ultrasound (CEUS) scans for the detection of carotid plaque ulceration. The Institutional Ethics Committee approved the study protocol, and all patients provided informed consent. The patients had symptomatic stenosis of the internal carotid artery and underwent carotid computed tomographic angiography as part of their clinical evaluation. All patients underwent a CDUS examination in conjunction with CEUS. Carotid plaque ulceration was defined as the presence of ≥1 disruptions in the plaque–lumen border ≥1 × 1 mm. Carotid computed tomographic angiography was used as reference technique. The study population consisted of 20 patients (mean age 64 ± 9 years, 80% men), and 39 carotid arteries were included in the present analysis. Computed tomographic angiography demonstrated that the plaque surface was smooth in 15 (38%), irregular in 7 (18%) and ulcerated in 17 (44%) carotid arteries. The sensitivity, specificity, accuracy, positive predictive value, and negative predictive value of CDUS for the detection of ulceration was 29%, 73%, 54%, 46%, and 57%, respectively. The sensitivity, specificity, accuracy, positive predictive value, and negative predictive value of CEUS for the detection of ulceration was 88%, 59%, 72%, 63%, and 87%, respectively. CEUS had superior sensitivity and diagnostic accuracy for the assessment of carotid plaque ulceration compared with CDUS. CEUS improved the intra-reader and inter-reader variability for the assessment of carotid plaque ulceration compared with CDUS. In conclusion, CEUS could be an additional method for the detection of carotid plaque ulceration. The role of CDUS for the assessment of carotid plaque ulceration seems limited.

► This article is one of many that tries to enhance the decision-making process for carotid interventions by utilizing duplex ultrasound findings. This study compares contrast-enhanced ultrasound with standard carotid computed tomographic angiography (CTA) in the ability to detect carotid plaque ulceration. Many studies have documented that the presence of carotid plaque ulceration represents a more vulnerable lesion and is a strong predictor of a future cerebrovascular event. Contrast enhancement of ultrasonography has been assessed in both cardiac examinations (echocardiography) as well as endoleak detection after endovascular repair of abdominal aortic aneurysms. This study found that contrast could be used reliably in the detection of plaque ulceration and, thus, increases the sensitivity of regular duplex. However, there are caveats to performing contrast-enhanced ultrasound scan, and perhaps many of these limitations are reasons that the use of contrast is not widespread. First and foremost, contrast is not approved for this type of use. This would be considered off-label use and, thus, potentially experimental. The injection requires an intravenous catheter to be inserted, which is a skill usually not performed by an ultrasound technician. A consent document for the procedure would be necessary as well. Both of these requirements would necessitate additional personnel and time, with no potential for increased reimbursement. These facts would prohibit most from pursuing the use of contrast in ultrasound scan. However, clearly, we need better means of identifying those persons who have asymptomatic carotid lesions who are at high risk for associated cerebrovascular events. I applaud these authors for their compelling and interesting data and do hope that they continue to study this technique.

R. L. Bush, MD, JD, MPH

Race as a predictor of morbidity, mortality, and neurologic events after carotid endarterectomy

Brown HA, Sullivan MC, Gusberg RG, et al (Yale Univ School of Medicine, New Haven, CT)

J Vasc Surg 57:1325-1330, 2013

Objective.—Racial disparities in the outcomes of patients undergoing carotid endarterectomy (CEA) have been reported. We sought to examine the contemporary relationship between race and outcomes and to report postdischarge events after CEA.

Methods.—The American College of Surgeons National Surgical Quality Improvement Program Participant Use Data Files were reviewed to identify all CEAs performed from 2005 to 2010 by vascular surgeons. The influence of race on outcomes was examined. Multivariate analysis was performed using variables found to be significant on bivariate analysis. The primary outcomes were stroke and mortality. Secondary outcomes were other 30-day complications, including postdischarge events.

Results.—CEA was performed on 29,114 white patients (95.7%) and on 1316 black patients (4.3%); the overall stroke and mortality rates were 1.65% and 0.7%, respectively. The stroke rate was 1.6% for whites and 2.5% blacks ($P = .009$). The 30-day mortality rate was 0.7% for whites and 1.4% for blacks ($P = .002$). There was a longer operating time ($P < .001$) and total length of stay ($P < .001$), more postoperative pneumonias ($P = .049$), unplanned intubations ($P < .001$), ventilator dependence ($P < .001$), cardiac arrests ($P < .001$), bleeding requiring transfusions ($P = .024$), and reoperations within 30 days ($P = .021$) among black patients. Multivariate logistic regression modeling identified black race as an independent risk factor for 30-day mortality (odds ratio, 1.9; $P = .007$). Black patients also had a greater proportion of in-hospital deaths than white patients (73.7% vs 43.1%; $P = .01$). There was no between-group difference in the rate of postdischarge strokes. Thirty-six percent of all strokes occurred after discharge at a mean of 8.3 days, and 54.3% of deaths occurred after discharge at a mean of 11 days.

Conclusions.—Black race is an independent risk factor for 30-day mortality after CEA. A significant proportion of strokes and deaths occur after discharge in both racial groups evaluated.

▶ Literature concerning racial disparities in health care availability, evaluation, treatment, and outcomes is not unusual or new. The concept about inequality in access has been well discussed and proven; however, this study takes racial differences one step further. These authors show that black race is an independent risk factor for ongoing events following hospital discharge after carotid endarterectomy (CEA). A large, robust, validated database, the American College of Surgeons National Surgical Quality Improvement Project, was used to identify a cohort of more than 29 000 patients who had undergone CEA. Even though this data set has the limitations inherent with administrative data and subsequent retrospective analysis, it is comprehensive in the number of perioperative variables recorded, including 30-day mortality. One major shortcoming is the fact that smaller hospitals may not be part of this data set; thus, many possible treatment facilities for some minorities may be missed. And the data set thus represents a selected group of physicians and their patients. An important take-home message from this study's conclusions is that morbidity and mortality after CEA continue long after the operation is complete. Stroke and death risks clearly do not end with hospital discharge. Strategies for 30-day surveillance should be in place for ensuring follow-up and identification of signs of difficulty.

R. L. Bush, MD, JD, MPH

Simulator training on pulsatile vascular models significantly improves surgical skills and the quality of carotid patch plasty

Duschek N, Assadian A, Lamont PM, et al (Dept of Vascular and Endovascular Surgery, Wilhelminenspital, Vienna, Austria; Bristol Royal Infirmary, Bristol, UK; et al)

J Vasc Surg 57:1148-1154, 2013

Objective.—Vascular surgeons perform numerous highly sophisticated and delicate procedures. Due to restrictions in training time and the advent of endovascular techniques, new concepts including alternative environments for training and assessment of surgical skills are required. Over the past decade, training on simulators and synthetic models has become more sophisticated and lifelike. This study was designed to evaluate the impact of a 3-day intense training course in open vascular surgery on both specific and global vascular surgical skills.

Methods.—Prospective observational cohort analysis with various parameter measurements of both surgical skills and the technical quality of the finished product, performed before and after 3 days of simulator training of 10 participants (seven male and three female) in a vascular surgery training course. The simulator model used was a conventional carotid endarterectomy with a Dacron patch plasty on a lifelike carotid bench model under pulsatile pressure. The primary end points were assessment of any changes in the participants' surgical skills and in the technical quality of their completed carotid patches documented by procedure-based assessment forms. Scores ranging from 1 (inadequate) to 5 (excellent) were compared by a related-sample Wilcoxon signed test. Interobserver reliability was estimated by Cronbach's alpha (CA).

Results.—A significant improvement in surgical skills tasks was observed ($P < .001$). The mean score increased significantly by 21.5% from fair (3.43 ± 0.93) to satisfactory (4.17 ± 0.69; $P < .001$). The mean score for the quality of the carotid patch increased significantly by 0.96 (27%) from fair (3.55 ± 0.87) to satisfactory (4.51 ± 0.76; $P < .01$). The median interassessor reliability for the quality of the carotid patch was acceptable (CA = 0.713) and for surgical skills was low (CA = 0.424).

Conclusions.—This study shows that lifelike simulation featuring pulsatile flow can increase surgical skills and technical quality in a highly sophisticated multistep vascular intervention. This training provides comparatively inexpensive and lifelike training possibilities for the adoption and assessment of surgical skills required to perform delicate vascular surgical procedures.

▶ The importance and utility of medical simulation training is clearly established both for individual as well as team-based skills. Given the limitations on resident duty hours by the Accreditation Council for Graduate Medical Education, simulation training and the need for high-level complex simulators in a virtual reality system are paramount to ensure training and improvement in skills needed for the operating room. Vascular simulators have mainly focused on endovascular training with the recent addition of open surgical simulators for conventional surgical training. This study addresses the outcomes of simulator training using a realistic pulsatile model of carotid endarterectomy and patch angioplasty. The authors evaluated a 3-day intense training program looking at the skill improvement and technical quality of more junior trainees. The results are excellent with trainees improving their skill set. However, as the authors state, one of the keys of simulator training is continued practice of the newly acquired skills to ensure reinforcement and expertise. It will be prudent for US training programs to adopt regular simulator training and practice within their curricula for time and cost considerations.

R. L. Bush, MD, JD, MPH

Urgent Best Medical Therapy May Obviate the Need for Urgent Surgery in Patients With Symptomatic Carotid Stenosis

Shahidi S, Owen-Falkenberg A, Hjerpsted U, et al (Univ Hosp Roskilde, Region Zealand, Denmark)

Stroke 44:2220-2225, 2013

Background and Purpose.—The purpose of this study was to analyze the 30-day outcome after introduction of a rapid carotid endarterectomy (CEA) program. Reasons for delay in CEA and the incidence of early recurrence neurological symptoms were recorded.

Methods.—This is a prospective population-based study of delays to CEA and 30-day outcome in patients with symptomatic carotid stenosis. Neurological recurrence (NR) rate was determined after initiation of urgent best medical treatment (loading dose aspirin/clopidogrel and duel therapy with aspirin plus clopidogrel with a statin) until CEA and compared with NR ≤90 days prior index event.

Results.—Of a total of 4905 (transient ischemic attack/ischemic stroke, and ocular events) patients, 115 symptomatic patients underwent CEA, 42% within 14 days of the index event and 99% within 14 days of surgical referral. The overall NR from index event to CEA in symptomatic carotid stenosis patients was significantly lower (2.5% [95% confidence interval, 1%–6%]) after best medical treatment when compared with NR ≤90 days in those before referral to a stroke clinic (29% [95% confidence interval, 22%–37%]; $P < 0.00001$). There were no significant differences in outcomes among 48 early (<14 days), 46 intermediate (14–30 days), and 21 delayed (>30 days) CEAs.

Conclusions.—CEA can be performed in the subacute period without significantly increasing the operative risk. The urgent best medical treatment was associated with significant reduction in the risk of early NR in CEA patients. It seems that urgent aggressive best medical treatment may obviate the need for urgent CEA.

▶ This is an interesting study that both contradicts and supports literature concerning the timing of surgical intervention for patients with symptomatic carotid artery stenosis. Currently, the controversy surrounds the risk of recurrent neurologic events, with many providers supporting early intervention and others holding fast to a 4- to 6-week waiting period for performing an endarterectomy. This study looked at a population of patients in Denmark who are treated within a closed health care system. They found that early intervention, defined as within 14 days, did not result in an increased risk to the patient. This study also analyzed why some patients were delayed, because of a lack of patient knowledge, provider recognition, and even the waiting period necessary to get a noninvasive carotid ultrasound.

Regardless of the limitations of this study and the differences in the Danish health care system described herein and other systems, the aspect of the article that fascinated me was the aggressive early institution of best medical therapy. This was defined in this study as dual antiplatelet therapy with a statin, both being started when the patient initially presented and was determined to have had an embolic event. Despite some of the data concerning dual antiplatelet therapy that is less than supportive, the data presented are compelling. The therapy, according to these investigators, is safe from hemorrhagic risk in the short term, which may obviate the need for urgent carotid endarterectomy (CEA). In a situation with a lack of qualified surgeons and a need for transport to another facility, as well as a possible reduction in resources, this article supports that aggressive medical therapy is safe and perhaps has a protective effect for neurologic event recurrence before CEA.

R. L. Bush, MD, JD, MPH

Clinical characteristics and strategy for treatment of functional carotid body tumours

Zeng G, Feng H, Zhao J, et al (Sichuan Univ, Chengdu, PR China; Hosp of China Natl Nuclear Corporation, Chengdu, Sichuan Province, PR China)
Int J Oral Maxillofac Surg 42:436-439, 2013

Functional carotid body tumours are rare, but linked to malignant hypertension, postoperative persistent hypotension, cranial nerve injury and stroke. The aim of this study is to analyze the treatment options for functional carotid body tumours. Six patients with functional carotid body tumours who underwent surgical procedures were studied retrospectively. They all had abnormal levels of preoperative catecholamine (norepinephrine, 721 ± 452.2 ng/l). One patient presented preoperative hypertension. Preoperative alpha- and beta-adrenergic blockade was carried out. Surgical methods included complete resection (6), saphenous vein interposition (3) and carotid shunt (1). With thorough supervision and treatment, the 6 patients underwent tumour resection. They all experienced intraoperative hypertension while the tumours were being resected. Postoperative problems included endurance hypotension (3/6, 50%), coughing when drinking (3/6, 50%) and deviation of the tongue on protrusion (3/6, 50%). The clinical highlights of functional carotid body tumour include preoperative abnormal catecholamine, peroperative fluctuations of blood pressure level, and regime issues. Operative resection could be the best option for functional carotid body tumours. Careful preoperative evaluation, measurement of serum catecholamine, treatment for alpha- and beta-adrenergic blockade, and gentle intraoperative manipulation are essential to avoid life-threatening complications.

▶ Vascular surgeons often are the surgeons for carotid body tumors, albeit an infrequent diagnosis and operation. This article would likely be missed by vascular surgeons because of its publication in the *International Journal of Oral and Maxillofacial Surgery*. It is a very interesting article about the treatment of functional carotid body tumors, an entity of which I was unaware, as most carotid body tumors are nonfunctional. This represents a special group of patients who must have special preoperative evaluation and postoperative care because of the consequences of catecholamine release. Patients with functional tumors also will require aggressive care by the anesthesia team for intraoperative blood pressure fluctuations, which may increase the risk of cranial nerve injury and stroke. Similar to other paragangliomas, preoperative α- and β-blockade may be started to help avoid malignant hypertensive episodes during resection. The type of resection with possible need for carotid artery reconstruction is similar to that of nonfunctional carotid body tumors, which varies according to Shamblin classification. I recommend this article, as it describes the diagnosis, evaluation, and care of a rare entity.

This group describes their experience with 6 patients having this rare but functional paraganglioma. Symptomatology may be variable or absent at time of diagnosis, but a high degree of suspicion should warrant measurement of plasma catecholamines.

R. L. Bush, MD, JD, MPH

In-hospital versus postdischarge adverse events following carotid endarterectomy

Fokkema M, Bensley RP, Lo RC, et al (Beth Israel Deaconess Med Ctr, Boston, MA; et al)

J Vasc Surg 57:1568-1575.e3, 2013

Objective.—Most studies based on state and nationwide registries evaluating perioperative outcome after carotid endarterectomy (CEA) rely on hospital discharge data only. Therefore, the true 30-day complication risk after carotid revascularization may be underestimated.

Methods.—We used the National Surgical Quality Improvement Program database 2005-2010 to assess the in-hospital and postdischarge rate of any stroke, death, cardiac event (new Q-wave myocardial infarction or cardiac arrest), and combined stroke/death and combined adverse outcome (S/D/CE) at 30 days following CEA. Multivariable analyses were used to identify predictors for in-hospital and postdischarge events separately, and in particular, those that predict postdischarge events distinctly.

Results.—A total of 35,916 patients who underwent CEA during 2005-2010 were identified in the National Surgical Quality Improvement Program database; 59% were male, median age was 72 years, and 44% had a previous neurologic event. Thirty-day stroke rate was 1.6% (n = 591), death rate was 0.8% (n = 272), cardiac event rate was 1.0% (n = 350), stroke or death rate was 2.2% (n = 794), and combined S/D/CE rate was 2.9% (n = 1043); 33% of strokes, 53% of deaths, 32% of cardiac events, 40% of combined stroke/death, and 38% of combined S/D/CE took place after hospital discharge. Patients with a prior stroke or transient ischemic attack had similar proportions of postdischarge events compared with patients without prior symptoms. Independent predictors for postdischarge events, but not for in-hospital events were female sex (stroke [odds ratio (OR), 1.6; 95% confidence interval (CI), 1.2-2.1] and stroke/death [OR, 1.4; 95% CI, 1.1-1.7]), renal failure (stroke [OR,

3.0; 95% CI, 1.4-6.2]) and chronic obstructive pulmonary disease (death [OR, 2.5; 95% CI, 1.6-3.7], stroke/death [OR, 1.8; 95% CI, 1.4-2.4], and S/D/CE [OR 1.8, 95% CI 1.4-2.3]).

Conclusions.—With 38% of perioperative adverse events after CEA happening posthospitalization, regardless of symptoms status, we need to be alert to the ongoing risks after discharge particularly in women, patients with renal failure, or chronic obstructive pulmonary disease. This emphasizes the need for reporting and comparing 30-day adverse event rates when evaluating outcomes for CEA, or comparing carotid stenting to CEA.

▶ Much of the medical literature is based on recommendations and conclusions from the examination and analysis of large administrative datasets. Even with their inherent flaws, these datasets offer a great deal of valuable information on patients and outcomes oftentimes reflecting real world experience outside of the confines of a controlled clinical trial. The collection and entry of the data is variable, albeit the larger size of the cohort sometimes negates this factor. The National Surgical Quality Improvement Project (NSQIP) is one such large databank but with uniformity in the collection and entry of the variables by trained nurse reviewers who undergo periodic accuracy audits. This study takes the NSQIP data on patients undergoing carotid revascularization either by stenting or endarterectomy and analyzes a smaller cohort via physician retrospective chart review. The results from the nurse entry and the physician are compared for symptom and high-risk status as well as postoperative complications. The NSQIP failed in its identification of each of these 3 very important items. These authors make the conclusion that the NSQIP should not be used to analyze these 2 operations. So why then collect the data? What other operations are falling short in data collection in this administrative set? Perhaps this study will inform those in charge of administrative data and assist in revision of data collection efforts. The NSQIP is being adjusted to capture more procedure-specific comorbidities and complications so that this limitation will be lessened.

R. L. Bush, MD, JD, MPH

Differences and Similarities Between Spontaneous Dissections of the Internal Carotid Artery and the Vertebral Artery

von Babo M, De Marchis GM, Sarikaya H, et al (Univ Hosp of Bern, Switzerland; et al)
Stroke 44:1537-1542, 2013

Background and Purpose.—To compare potential risk factors, clinical symptoms, diagnostic delay, and 3-month outcome between spontaneous internal carotid artery dissection (sICAD) and spontaneous vertebral artery dissection (sVAD).

Methods.—We compared patients with sICAD (n = 668) and sVAD (n = 302) treated in 3 university hospitals.

Results.—Patients with sICAD were older (46.3 ± 9.6 versus 42.0 ± 10.2 years; $P < 0.001$), more often men (62.7% versus 53.0%; $P = 0.004$), and presented more frequently with tinnitus (10.9% versus 3.4%; $P < 0.001$) and more severe ischemic strokes (median National Institutes of Health Stroke Scale, 10 ± 7.1 versus 5 ± 5.9; $P < 0.001$). Patients with sVAD had more often bilateral dissections (15.2% versus 7.6%; $P < 0.001$) and were more often smokers (36.0% versus 28.7%; $P = 0.007$). Thunderclap headache (9.2% versus 3.6%; $P = 0.001$) and neck pain were more common (65.8% versus 33.5%; $P < 0.001$) in sVAD. Subarachnoid hemorrhage (6.0% versus 0.6%; $P < 0.001$) and ischemic stroke (69.5% versus 52.2%; $P < 0.001$) were more frequent in sVAD. After multivariate analysis, sex difference lost its significance ($P = 0.21$), and all other variables remained significant. Time to diagnosis was similar in sICAD and sVAD and improved between 2001 and 2012 compared with the previous 10-year period (8.0 ± 10.5 days versus 10.7 ± 13.2 days; $P = 0.004$). In sVAD, favorable outcome 3 months after ischemic stroke (modified Rankin Scale, 0–2: 88.8% versus 58.4%; $P < 0.001$), recurrent transient ischemic attack (4.8% versus 1.1%; $P = 0.001$), and recurrent ischemic stroke (2.8% versus 0.7%; $P = 0.02$) within 3 months were more frequent.

Conclusions.—sICAD and sVAD patients differ in many aspects. Future studies should perform separate analyses of these 2 entities.

▶ This article published in *Stroke* emphasizes an important point that has not been followed in much of the literature on spontaneous dissections of cerebrovascular vessels. Most articles combine data on spontaneous carotid and vertebral dissections. Although the treatment strategies are similar for either vertebral or carotid dissections, the patient populations, clinical presentation, time to accurate diagnosis, associated risk factors, outcomes, and rate of recurrent ischemic events are different. Thus, to combine the 2 disease processes that occur in different arterial beds is basically combining apples and oranges for analysis. No meaningful conclusions may be made with such a heterogeneous group. This group analyzed data from large patient cohorts with spontaneous dissections: carotid, 668 patients, and vertebral, 302 patients, from only 3 hospitals. Although follow-up after 3 months was lost in 16.7%, this is still a very robust dataset. Time to diagnosis was definitely improved over the decade of reporting, probably because of improvements in imaging techniques and more aggressive imaging owing to disease recognition and a high degree of suspicion. Hopefully, all reviewers and editors will follow this group's recommendation that "future studies perform separate analyses of these entities."

R. L. Bush, MD, JD, MPH

A Model for Predicting the Risk of Carotid Artery Disease

Greco G, Egorova NN, Moskowitz AJ, et al (Mount Sinai School of Medicine, NY; et al)

Ann Surg 257:1168-1173, 2013

Objective.—To develop a model for the identification of individuals at risk for carotid stenosis (CS) that could be useful in a clinical setting when trying to decide whether screening is worthwhile.

Background.—Evidence that aggressive medical therapy and life style changes reduce the risk of stroke in individuals with CS is increasing and has led to a renewed interest in screening for CS.

Methods.—Data on demographics and risk factors were obtained from 2,885,257 individuals who had carotid Duplex scans by Life Line Screening between 2003 and 2008. Multivariable logistic regression analysis was used to identify independent risk factors for CS (>50% stenosis). A scoring system was developed where risk factors were assigned a weighted score. Predictive ability was assessed by calculating C statistics and r^2.

Results.—In the screened cohort, 71,004 patients (2.4%) had CS. Independent risk factors include advanced age, smoking, peripheral arterial disease, high blood pressure, coronary artery disease, diabetes, cholesterol, and abdominal aortic aneurysm. African Americans, Asians, and Hispanics had reduced risk than whites. Exercise and consumption of fruit, vegetables, and nuts had a modest protective effect. A predictive scoring system was created that identifies individuals with CS more efficiently (C statistic = 0.753) than previously published models.

Conclusions.—We provide a model that enables identification of individuals who have a high probability of having CS. This model can be helpful in designing targeted screening programs that are cost-effective.

▶ Stroke is not only prevalent, it is devastating. Eighty percent of strokes are embolic with carotid bifurcation disease continuing to be a major culprit. The prediction of which asymptomatic patients should undergo intervention is still an elusive concept and a controversial topic in the literature. Routine duplex ultrasound screening of so-called high risk patients is not only a hot topic; it is also not currently a reimbursed imaging test. Risk prediction models are not often used, as they are time consuming to calculate, and the question is always, whose responsibility is it to perform? These authors provide a model that includes demographic risk factors along with nutritional and exercise variables from a large cohort of more than 70 000 people who participated in a voluntary screening. Similar to other screenings, women composed two-thirds of the participants. Although the prevalence of carotid disease, defined as ≥50% luminal diameter reduction, was low (2.4%), some important data emerge. Although the risk factors for atherosclerotic disease are known, aggressive medical management is not always accomplished. Furthermore, the contribution of each risk factor to actual risk is unclear. Having a model that discriminates risk factors so that more targeted therapy and screening can be done may work toward identifying those asymptomatic patients that would benefit from intervention. I recommend reading this article to gain a better understanding of the process of prediction model development and how individualized patient care can result.

R. L. Bush, MD, JD, MPH

Cerebral monitors *versus* regional anesthesia to detect cerebral ischemia in patients undergoing carotid endarterectomy: a meta-analysis

Guay J, Kopp S (Univ of Montreal, Quebec, Canada; Mayo Clinic College of Medicine, Rochester, MN)

Can J Anesth 60:266-279, 2013

Purpose.—The aim of this meta-analysis is to compare the ability of different types of brain monitoring systems vs clinical monitoring of the brain function to detect cerebral ischemia during cross-clamping of the carotid artery under regional anesthesia.

Methods.—In May 2012, a search was conducted in PubMed, Cochrane Central Register of Controlled Trials, Cochrane Database of Systematic Reviews, and Ovid MEDLINE® for prospective trials with 20 patients or more where a cerebral monitoring system was compared with clinical brain monitoring during a carotid endarterectomy performed under regional anesthesia. The quality of the study was evaluated with the Cochrane Collaboration's tool. Data were extracted independently by the two investigators.

Results.—Data could be extracted for 4,664 measurements taken from 29 studies: transcranial Doppler (TCD) = 739; cerebral saturation = 320; stump pressure = 2,549; electroencephalography (EEG) = 742; evoked potentials = 187; jugular venous saturation = 79; and jugular venous lactate = 48. The pooled diagnostic odds ratios (DOR) and 95% confidence intervals (CI) were obtained for EEG, TCD, stump pressure, evoked potentials, and cerebral saturation: (DOR 65.3; 95% CI 20.5 to 207.7; I^2 [56.8%]); (DOR 58.1; 95% CI 23.0 to 146.3; I^2 [24.9%]); (DOR 27.8; 95% CI 13.4 to 57.9; I^2 [59.9]); (DOR 17.2; 95% CI 2.4 to 123.9; I^2 [69.1]); and (DOR 12.1; 95% CI 3.5 to 41.2; I^2 [30.8]), respectively. Sequential testing with stump pressure 25 mmHg followed by either TCD or EEG delivered the best post-test probabilities. For EEG, the DOR increases with the number of channels used ($P = 0.03$).

Conclusion.—A combination of stump pressure and either TCD or EEG appears to deliver the best results for detecting brain ischemia during carotid artery cross-clamping. Electroencephalography should be used with a high number of channels.

► The ideal method of neurologic monitoring during carotid endarterectomy (CEA) has long been debated, with many advocates for either general or regional anesthesia. Benefits and disadvantages exist for both modalities with the ultimate being cerebral monitoring, ensuring adequate cerebral perfusion during clamping, and, of course, a low complication profile. Many who perform

CEA under general anesthesia utilize neurologic monitoring, such as electroencephalography (EEG), rather than nonselectively shunt all patients. Of course, under local or regional anesthesia, the awake patient is simply monitored clinically. This meta-analysis included 29 studies that were chosen for quality based on a rigorous selection process. Prospective trials of cerebral monitoring compared with clinical monitoring were analyzed.

Interestingly, the results showed that a combination of stump pressure and either transcranial Doppler (TCD) or EEG were better at detecting cerebral ischemia during cross-clamping. Stump pressure has fallen out of favor because of its transient measurement and inability to do continuous flow monitoring. It raises the question of whether it adds any additional benefit over TCD or EEG at all. The authors did also conclude that no cerebral monitoring system is as good as clinical monitoring under regional anesthesia, my personal preference. Either way, the avoidance of shunt insertion with its inherent complications seems prudent.

R. L. Bush, MD, JD, MPH

A Risk Prediction Model for Determining Appropriateness of CEA in Patients with Asymptomatic Carotid Artery Stenosis

Conrad MF, Kang J, Mukhopadhyay S, et al (Massachusetts General Hosp, Boston)

Ann Surg 258:534-538, 2013

Objective.—The benefit of carotid endarterectomy (CEA) over medical therapy in patients with asymptomatic carotid artery stenosis is predicated upon a life expectancy of at least 5 years after the procedure. The goal of this study was to create a scoring system for prediction of 5-year survival after CEA that can be used to triage patients with ACAS.

Methods.—All patients who underwent CEA for severe asymptomatic carotid stenosis from 1989 to 2005 were identified. Long-term survival was determined by a review of hospital records and the social security death index. Because all patients had at least 5-year follow-up, a logistic regression of predictors of survival at 5 years was performed and the odds ratios associated with particular significant comorbidities were used to create a scoring system to predict survival. The scoring system was then validated within the cohort using the Hosmer-Lemeshow Test and a derivation/validation receiver operating characteristic (ROC) curve.

Results.—There were 2004 CEA performed in 1791 patients. The average follow-up was 130 ± 49 months. The clinical profile of the cohort data included 84% hypertension, 56% coronary artery disease (CAD), 24% diabetes, and 71% on statins. The 30-day stroke rate was 1.1% and the death rate was 0.7%. The actual 5-year survival was 73%. Logistic regression yielded the following predictors of mortality: age (by decade) (odds ratio [OR] = 1.8, $P < 0.0001$), CAD (OR = 1.5, $P = 0.0007$), chronic obstructive pulmonary disease (OR = 2.5; $P < 0.0001$), diabetes (OR = 1.7, $P < 0.0001$), neck radiation (OR = 2.6, $P = 0.005$), no statin (OR = 2.1, $P < 0.0001$), and creatinine more than 1.5 (OR = 2.6, $P < 0.0001$). These variables were then assigned a hierarchal point scoring system in accordance with the OR value. The 5-year survival based on the scoring system was as follows: 0 to 5 points = 92.5%, 6 to 8 points = 83.6%, 9 to 11 points = 63.7%, 12 to 14 points = 46.5%, and more than 15 points = 33.8%. The Hosmer-Lemeshow test validated the scoring system ($P = 0.26$) and there was no difference in the ROC curves (C statistic = 0.74 vs 0.73).

Conclusions.—This validated scoring system can be a useful tool for determining which patients are likely to benefit most from CEA based on the probability of long-term survival. Given that the 5-year survival of patients in the medical arm of the asymptomatic CEA trials was 60% to 70%, it is reasonable to conclude that patients who score 0 to 8 points are excellent candidates for CEA whereas most patients with ≥12 points should be managed with medical therapy alone.

▶ This is another article that attempts to give more information to guide providers in the decision-making process for patients with asymptomatic carotid stenoses. The group from Massachusetts General Hospital has been a leader in this field with this study looking at a risk prediction model for determining which patients with asymptomatic lesions may benefit from prophylactic revascularization with an endarterectomy (CEA). There are currently many proponents of modern best medical therapy for the asymptomatic patient; however, as this group points out, the benefits of CEA have been predicated on one having a life expectancy at least 5 years after the procedure. Thus, the proposed scoring system should help a provider determine the 5-year survival after a CEA to best advise a patient about whether to undergo surgery. Although based on a retrospective analysis, the data provided herein is valuable in that a scoring system is illustrated in Table 4 of the original article, which is simple, easy to calculate, can be done from a patient's medical record prior to consultation, takes just a few minutes, and can also be done by a nurse or other health assistant who is first seeing the patient in a clinic. Clearly, other information will need to be used in making an individual decision such as functional status and other clinical information. However, this scoring system does provide a good starting point and should be validated in a larger cohort.

R. L. Bush, MD, JD, MPH

The impact of Centers for Medicare and Medicaid Services high-risk criteria on outcome after carotid endarterectomy and carotid artery stenting in the SVS Vascular Registry

Schermerhorn ML, on behalf of the SVS Outcomes Committee (Beth Israel Deaconess Med Ctr, Boston, MA; et al)
J Vasc Surg 57:1318-1324, 2013

Objective.—The Centers for Medicare and Medicaid Services (CMS) require high-risk (HR) criteria for carotid artery stenting (CAS) reimbursement. The impact of these criteria on outcomes after carotid endarterectomy (CEA) and CAS remains uncertain. Additionally, if these HR criteria are associated with more adverse events after CAS, then existing comparative effectiveness analysis of CEA vs CAS may be biased. We sought to elucidate this using data from the SVS Vascular Registry.

Methods.—We analyzed 10,107 patients undergoing CEA (6370) and CAS (3737), stratified by CMS HR criteria. The primary endpoint was composite death, stroke, and myocardial infarction (MI) (major adverse cardiovascular event [MACE]) at 30 days. We compared baseline characteristics and outcomes using univariate and multivariable analyses.

Results.—CAS patients were more likely to have preoperative stroke (26% vs 21%) or transient ischemic attack (23% vs 19%) than CEA. Although age ≥80 years was similar, CAS patients were more likely to have all other HR criteria. For CEA, HR patients had higher MACEs than normal risk in both symptomatic (7.3% vs 4.6%; $P < .01$) and asymptomatic patients (5% vs 2.2%; $P < .0001$). For CAS, HR status was not associated with a significant increase in MACE for symptomatic (9.1% vs 6.2%; $P = .24$) or asymptomatic patients (5.4% vs 4.2%; $P = .61$). All CAS patients had MACE rates similar to HR CEA. After multivariable risk adjustment, CAS had higher rates than CEA for MACE (odds ratio [OR], 1.2; 95% confidence interval [CI], 1.0-1.5), death (OR, 1.5; 95% CI, 1.0-2.2), and stroke (OR, 1.3; 95% CI, 1.0-1.7), whereas there was no difference in MI (OR, 0.8; 95% CI, 0.6-1.3). Among CEA patients, age ≥80 (OR, 1.4; 95% CI, 1.02-1.8), congestive heart failure (OR, 1.7; 95% CI, 1.03-2.8), EF <30% (OR, 3.5; 95% CI, 1.6-7.7), angina (OR, 3.9; 95% CI, 1.6-9.9), contralateral occlusion (OR, 3.2; 95% CI, 2.1-4.7), and high anatomic lesion (OR, 2.7; 95% CI, 1.33-5.6) predicted MACE. Among CAS patients, recent MI (OR, 3.2; 95% CI, 1.5-7.0) was predictive, and radiation (OR, 0.6; 95% CI, 0.4-0.8) and restenosis (OR, 0.5; 95% CI, 0.3-0.96) were protective for MACE.

Conclusions.—Although CMS HR criteria can successfully discriminate a group of patients at HR for adverse events after CEA, certain CMS HR criteria are more important than others. However, CEA appears safer for the majority of patients with carotid disease. Among patients undergoing CAS, non-HR status may be limited to restenosis and radiation.

▶ This article represents another excellent study utilizing the Society for Vascular Surgery (SVS) Vascular Registry and analysis of outcomes after carotid artery revascularization procedures. Data from patients undergoing both carotid artery stenting (CAS) and carotid endarterectomy (CEA) were assessed using the Centers for Medicare and Medicaid Services (CMS) criteria for high-risk designation. Compliance with the CMS high-risk criteria are necessary for reimbursement for CAS performed in patients with symptomatic high-grade stenoses. The authors, using the SVS registry, found that the CMS high-risk criteria identified some patients who were at risk for postprocedure adverse events, but not all. Even so, the outcomes after CAS were not improved in high-risk patients compared with outcomes after CEA. Further analysis found that being at high risk for anatomic conditions, such as recurrent disease after CEA or neck radiation, is much more significant than being at high risk for medical conditions such as age, heart failure, and recent myocardial infarction to name a few. The SVS registry is important for review and policy making in that it represents real-world and real-time results across several practice situations. Hopefully, policy makers and third-party payers will read this important study and pay attention.

R. L. Bush, MD, JD, MPH

The size of juxtaluminal hypoechoic area in ultrasound images of asymptomatic carotid plaques predicts the occurrence of stroke

Kakkos SK, for the Asymptomatic Carotid Stenosis and Risk of Stroke (ACSRS) Study Group (Imperial College, London, UK; et al)

J Vasc Surg 57:609-618.e1, 2013

Objective.—To test the hypothesis that the size of a juxtaluminal black (hypoechoic) area (JBA) in ultrasound images of asymptomatic carotid artery plaques predicts future ipsilateral ischemic stroke.

Methods.—A JBA was defined as an area of pixels with a grayscale value <25 adjacent to the lumen without a visible echogenic cap after image normalization. The size of a JBA was measured in the carotid plaque images of 1121 patients with asymptomatic carotid stenosis 50% to 99% in relation to the bulb (Asymptomatic Carotid Stenosis and Risk of Stroke study); the patients were followed for up to 8 years.

Results.—The JBA had a linear association with future stroke rate. The area under the receiver-operating characteristic curve was 0.816. Using Kaplan-Meier curves, the mean annual stroke rate was 0.4% in 706 patients with a JBA <4 mm^2, 1.4% in 171 patients with a JBA 4 to 8 mm^2, 3.2% in 46 patients with a JBA 8 to 10 mm^2, and 5% in 198 patients with a JBA >10 mm^2 ($P < .001$). In a Cox model with ipsilateral ischemic events (amaurosis fugax, transient ischemic attack [TIA], or stroke) as the dependent variable, the JBA (<4 mm^2, 4-8 mm^2, >8 mm^2) was still significant after adjusting for other plaque features known to be associated with increased risk, including stenosis, grayscale median, presence of discrete white areas without acoustic shadowing indicating neovascularization, plaque area, and history of contralateral TIA or stroke. Plaque area and grayscale median were not significant. Using the significant variables (stenosis, discrete white areas without acoustic shadowing, JBA, and history of contralateral TIA or stroke), this model predicted the annual risk of stroke for each patient (range, 0.1%-10.0%). The average annual stroke risk was <1% in 734 patients, 1% to 1.9% in 94 patients, 2% to 3.9% in 134 patients, 4% to 5.9% in 125 patients, and 6% to 10% in 34 patients.

Conclusions.—The size of a JBA is linearly related to the risk of stroke and can be used in risk stratification models. These findings need to be confirmed in future prospective studies or in the medical arm of randomized controlled studies in the presence of optimal medical therapy. In the meantime, the JBA may be used to select asymptomatic patients at high stroke risk for carotid endarterectomy and spare patients at low risk from an unnecessary operation.

▶ One of the foremost controversies today in vascular surgery which is the best mode of therapy for those with significant but asymptomatic carotid artery occlusive disease. Whether to intervene with carotid artery revascularization has been widely debated by experts and key opinion leaders. On one hand, it is logical to observe those who are asymptomatic and treated with pharmacotherapy; however, the present and real, albeit small, possible risk of stroke remains. The best methodology for risk stratification of these patients has been suggested, but none has gained popularity, and none has been widely implemented. The hypothesis presented by these authors is interesting in that it uses noninvasive ultrasound capabilities to characterize carotid plaque by the size of the juxtaluminal hypoechoic (JBA- juxtaluminal black area) area. In this observational study, the size of the JBA was linearly related to the risk of stroke. Patients with high-grade stenoses who are good interventional candidates are more than likely to undergo carotid revascularization. However, in patients with a moderate but asymptomatic stenosis, the size of the JBA could be a potential factor in the treatment algorithm for the decision whether to intervene. For this technique to be useful in current practice, the recognition, measurements, and evaluation of the JBA need to be rapid, cost effective, and easily reproducible for widespread implementation. Nevertheless, a higher level of sophisticated preoperative discrimination in the stability of carotid plaques in the operative decision-making process appears to be both prudent and reasonable.

R. L. Bush, MD, JD, MPH

Progression of asymptomatic carotid stenosis despite optimal medical therapy

Conrad MF, Baloum V, Mukhopadhyay S, et al (Massachusetts General Hosp and Harvard Med School, Boston)
J Vasc Surg 58:128-135.e1, 2013

Background.—Despite level 1 evidence in support of carotid endarterectomy vs medical therapy in selected asymptomatic patients, an alternative posture is that optimal medical therapy (OMT) has not been adequately studied and that such OMT has reduced stroke risk in asymptomatic patients to levels wherein carotid endarterectomy is no longer justified. The goal of this study was to determine the natural history of patients with asymptomatic moderate (50%-69%) carotid artery stenosis (AMCAS) in a contemporary cohort as a function of their associated medical therapy.

Methods.—Patients with AMCAS determined by duplex ultrasound (DUS) from 2005-2006 were identified in our hospital database. Patients were included in the cohort if they had at least one additional DUS during the 6-year follow-up interval. Patient characteristics including medication history and lipid levels were collected. Patients were considered to have OMT if they were on aspirin and a statin with a low-density lipoprotein level that was always <100 mg/dL. Study end points included progression of carotid disease by DUS to severe stenosis (70%–100%), development of ipsilateral neurologic symptoms (INS) such as stroke or transient ischemic attack, and death.

Results.—There were 900 carotid arteries in 794 patients in the study cohort. The average age was 72.5 years, 77.2% had hypertension, 59.6% had coronary artery disease, and 87.1% were on a statin throughout the study. The low-density lipoprotein cholesterol level was always normal (<100 mg/dL) in 37.8% and accordingly, 241 (30.3%) had OMT as defined above. The 5-year actuarial survival was 81.9% ± 1.3% with no advantage seen with OMT. Multivariate analysis of survival showed statins were protective (hazard ratio [HR], 0.50; confidence interval [CI], 0.34-0.73; *P* =.0004). The 5-year freedom from plaque progression was 61.2% ± 2.1% with no benefit from OMT vs the control group. Multivariate predictors of plaque progression were chronic kidney disease (HR, 2.1; CI, 1.2-3.7; *P* =.009), aspirin use (HR, 1.9; CI, 1.2-3.0; *P* =.01), and the use of calcium channel blockers (HR, 1.4; CI, 1.1-1.8; *P* =.007). There were 90 (11.3%) patients who developed INS during follow-up (58% of these were strokes), and the 5-year freedom from INS was 88.4% ± 1.5%. Multivariate predictors of INS were diabetes (HR, 2.3; CI, 1.5-3.6; *P* =.0002) and warfarin use (HR, 1.9; CI, 1.2-2.9; *P* =.009); while statin use (HR, 0.37; CI, 0.22-0.65; *P* =.0005) was protective against symptom development.

Conclusions.—At the 5-year of follow-up, OMT failed to prevent carotid disease progression or development of ipsilateral symptoms in 45% of patients with AMCAS.

▶ I highly recommend this timely article for all to read. The treatment of moderate atherosclerotic carotid artery disease is controversial. Some surgeons still believe in intervention, whereas there is a growing popularity with so-called best medical therapy. The true definition of "optimal medical therapy" (OMT) has not been clarified and, even in this study, is limited to antiplatelet therapy and statin use. Other contributory factors remain, which are hard to elucidate from retrospective database reviews including control of hypertension, smoking cessation, tight glycemic management in diabetics, and weight control.

This study looked at the progression of atherosclerotic carotid disease in those compliant with statins and aspirin (OMT), even documenting low-density lipoprotein levels less than 100 mg/dL. The 5-year freedom from plaque progression was 61% with no difference in the cohort treated with OMT. Good information can be learned from this study; however, only 30% of patients had OMT as defined in the methods. Thus, the conclusion that OMT failed to prevent plaque progression is based on 241 patients. The overall reduction in adverse cardiovascular events is reason enough to continue medical therapy in these patients. The take-home message is that despite the best efforts of medical therapy along with the realities of patient compliance with expensive and complex management, serial carotid ultrasound scanning needs to be performed at routine intervals to monitor disease progression.

R. L. Bush, MD, JD, MPH

12 Carotid and Endovascular Disease

A Clinical Rule (Sex, Contralateral Occlusion, Age, and Restenosis) to Select Patients for Stenting Versus Carotid Endarterectomy: Systematic Review of Observational Studies With Validation in Randomized Trials

Touzé E, in Collaboration with the Carotid Stenting Trialists' Collaboration (Université Paris Descartes, France; et al)

Stroke 44:3394-3400, 2013

Background and Purpose.—Compared with carotid endarterectomy (CEA), carotid angioplasty and stenting (CAS) is associated with a higher risk of procedural stroke or death especially in patients with symptomatic stenosis. However, after the perioperative period, risk is similar with both treatments, suggesting that CAS could be an acceptable option in selected patients.

Methods.—We performed systematic reviews of observational studies of procedural risks of CEA or CAS and extracted data on 9 predefined risk factors (age, contralateral carotid occlusion, coronary artery disease, diabetes mellitus, sex, hypertension, peripheral artery disease, and type and side of stenosis). We calculated pooled relative risks of procedural stroke or death. Factors with differential effects on risk of CAS versus CEA were identified by interaction tests and used to derive a rule. The rule was tested using individual patient data from randomized trials of CAS versus CEA from the Carotid Stenting Trialists' Collaboration (CSTC).

Results.—We identified 170 studies. The effects of sex, contralateral occlusion, age, and restenosis (SCAR) on the procedural risk of stroke or death differed. Patients with contralateral occlusion or restenosis and women <75 years were at relatively low risk for CAS (SCAR negative), with all others being high risk (SCAR positive). Among the 3049 patients in the CSTC validation, 694 (23%) patients were SCAR negative. The pooled RR of procedural stroke and death with CAS versus CEA was 0.93 (0.49–1.77; $P = 0.83$) in SCAR-negative and 2.41 (1.68–3.45; $P < 0.0001$) in SCAR-positive patients (P [interaction] = 0.05).

Conclusions.—The SCAR rule is potentially useful to identify patients in whom CAS has a similar risk of perioperative stroke or death to CEA.

▶ These authors sought to develop a score to predict procedural risks between carotid artery stenting (CAS) and carotid endarterectomy (CEA). To accomplish this, they evaluated data from 170 studies (> 70 000 patients) and performed a meta-analysis. The primary outcome was procedural stroke or death during the 30-day period. In contrast to other widely quoted studies, this analysis did not consider nonfatal myocardial infarction. They analyzed 9 potential risk factors separately for studies of CAS and CEA and calculated the relative risks of a procedural event in patients versus those without the risk factor. Age was associated with the higher risks of procedural stroke or death for both CAS and CEA, but the increase in risk was greater after CAS. Contralateral occlusion and female sex were associated with a higher risk of procedural stroke or death after CEA but had little influence on the risk after CAS. Patients with restenosis after CEA had a higher risk for procedural stroke or death rate after treatment with redo CEA but a lower risk when treated by CAS. Thus the authors proposed a risk score based on sex, contralateral occlusion, age, and restenosis (SCAR rule). The limitations of the study are based on the fact that asymptomatic patients were excluded from some of the European trials. The cutoff of < 70 years may be questionable. In addition, this study precluded analysis of anatomic risk factors that might contribute to the risk of stroke in patients undergoing CEA or CAS. Despite these limitations, this scoring system as described should be more widely applied to assessing risk factors associated with either CEA or CAS.

M. T. Watkins, MD

Hispanic ethnicity is associated with increased costs after carotid endarterectomy and carotid stenting in the United States

Propper B, Black JH III, Schneider EB, et al (The Johns Hopkins Hosp, Baltimore, MD; et al)

J Surg Res 184:644-650, 2013

Objective.—We have previously demonstrated an adverse impact of black race and Hispanic ethnicity on the outcomes of carotid endarterectomy (CEA) and carotid artery stenting (CAS). The current study was undertaken to examine the influence of race and ethnicity on the cost of CEA and CAS.

Methods.—The Nationwide Inpatient Sample (2005–2009) was queried using ICD-9 codes for CEA and CAS in patients with carotid artery stenosis. The primary outcome was total hospital charges. Multivariate analysis was performed using a generalized linear model adjusting for age, sex, race, comorbidities (Charlson index), high-risk status, procedure type, symptomatic status, year, insurance type, and surgeon and hospital operative volumes and characteristics.

Results.—Hispanic and black patients were more likely to have a symptomatic presentation, and were more likely to undergo either CEA or CAS by low-volume surgeons at low-volume hospitals ($P < 0.05$, all). They were also less likely to have private insurance or Medicare ($P < 0.001$). Overall, CEA was less expensive than CAS over the 4-y study period ($29,502 ± $104 *versus* $46,713 ± $409, $P < 0.001$). Total hospital charges after CEA were increased in both blacks (\$39,562 ± \$843) and Hispanics (\$45,325 ± \$735) compared with whites on univariate analysis (\$28,403 ± \$101, $P < 0.001$). After CAS, total hospital charges were similarly increased in both blacks (\$51,770 ± \$2085) and Hispanics (\$63,637 ± \$2766) compared with whites on univariate analysis (\$45,550 ± \$412, $P < 0.001$). On multivariable analysis, however, only Hispanic ethnicity remained independently associated with increased charges after both CEA (exponentiated coefficient 1.18; 95% CI [1.15–1.20]; $P < 0.001$) and CAS (exponentiated coefficient 1.17; 95% CI [1.09–1.24]; $P < 0.001$).

Conclusion.—Hispanic ethnicity was independently associated with increased hospital charges after both CEA and CAS. The increased charges seen in black patients were explained, in part, by decreased surgeon operative volume and increased postoperative complications. Further efforts are warranted to contain costs in minorities undergoing carotid revascularization.

▶ This report is an appropriate follow-up to previous reports indicating that Hispanic ethnicity is an independent predictor of mortality following carotid endarterectomy. Hispanic ethnicity was identified as a predictor of mortality following endovascular aortic surgery and open aortic surgery. This was associated with an increase in hospital cost after aortic surgery in both Hispanic and black patients compared with white patients. These authors evaluated how ethnicity affects the cost of carotid endarterectomy (CEA) and carotid artery stenting (CAS) using the Nationwide Inpatient Sample (NIS) database. The authors hypothesized that the increased complications seen in previous studies would translate into additional costs for racial and ethnic minorities. Hispanic ethnicity proved to be an independent predictor of increased costs after both CEA and CAS. Black race was not a significant predictor of increased charges after either CEA or CAS. Interestingly, high surgeon operative volume was found to decrease costs for both CEA and CAS. The question remains as to why ethnicity should affect cost. Because this finding was independent of other variables studied, these authors conclude that their data indicate that either something genetic or other variables not found in the NIS account for this finding. I suspect the NIS database does not encompass all the relevant variables. An interesting finding is that the only variable to have a significant effect on the Hispanic ethnicity coefficient in the multivariable analysis was length of stay. When length of stay was removed from the regression analysis, there was an increase in the coefficient. Thus, length of stay was a driving factor in the cost of carotid interventions for Hispanics.

M. T. Watkins, MD

Cilostazol inhibits accumulation of triglycerides in a rat model of carotid artery ligation

Tanaka H, Zaima N, Ito H, et al (Hamamatsu Univ School of Medicine, Japan; Otsuka Pharmaceutical Co, Ltd, Tokushima, Japan)

J Vasc Surg 58:1366-1374, 2013

Objective.—Triglyceride (TG) accumulation in arterial tissue is associated with the development of cardiovascular disease; however, the underlying mechanism remains unclear. Cilostazol (CLZ), a selective inhibitor of phosphodiesterase 3, has antiplatelet and vasodilating effects and may decrease serum TG levels. We examined the effect of CLZ on TG accumulation in the arterial tissue of a rat model of carotid artery ligation.

Methods.—Rats were fed normal chow with 0.1% CLZ (CLZ group) or without CLZ (control group) for 4 weeks after unilateral carotid artery ligation near the carotid bifurcation.

Results.—At the end of this period, the control group showed 3.3-fold higher TG levels in the ligated carotid artery than in the contralateral artery; however, compared with the contralateral artery, the ligated artery in the CLZ group showed significantly lower levels of TG accumulation but similar serum levels of TG, total cholesterol, and high-density lipoprotein cholesterol. Furthermore, matrix-assisted laser desorption/ionization imaging mass spectrometry revealed that the ligated carotid artery in both groups had ubiquitous accumulation of TG in the intima, media, and adventitia, along with decreased heme B signals, which was indicative of ischemia. However, heme B signals were less reduced in the CLZ group than in the control group.

Conclusions.—Our results indicate that CLZ can inhibit the ubiquitous accumulation of TG in arterial tissues, possibly by ameliorating tissue ischemia. CLZ may be useful in improving arterial tissue hemodynamics and lipid metabolism.

▶ Elevated triglyceride levels have long been associated with an increased incidence of cardiovascular disease, and more than 30% of the US adult population has a triglyceride level ≥150 mg/dL. Hypertriglyceridemia is also important in relation to obesity and insulin resistance. Triglycerides are often found in vascular tissue, and their accumulation is often thought to promote the development of cardiovascular disease. Cilostazol (CLZ) is a selective inhibitor of phosphodiesterase-3, which is used to treat intermittent claudication due to its vasodilatory effect. Recent studies have shown that CLZ may be beneficial in preventing the progression of carotid atherosclerosis and improving the pro-atherogenic lipid profile by decreasing serum triglyceride and low-density lipoprotein cholesterol levels. The present study examined the effect of CLZ on triglyceride accumulation in the arterial tissue of a rat model of carotid artery ligation. Their results demonstrate that in a rat vascular flow—cessation model, administration of CLZ ameliorates an intra-arterial decrease in heme B and inhibits triglyceride accumulation without reducing serum triglyceride levels. This is an interesting study because this flow-cessation model mainly involves medial remodeling as a result of smooth muscle cell proliferation and hyperplasia, and this more closely recapitulates the processes involved in vascular restenosis as opposed to atherosclerosis. It has been previously demonstrated that CLZ reduces lesion development in apolipoprotein knockout mice fed a high-fat diet and also decreases the accumulation of triglycerides in the aorta and platelet aggregation in cholesterol-fed rabbits. The fact that the present study demonstrates an inhibitory effect of CLZ on arterial medial hyperplasia is extremely novel, and the potential of pharmacological therapy to prevent restenosis after angioplasty or stenting is promising.

J. Cullen, PhD

Results of carotid artery stenting with transcervical access

Sfyroeras GS, Moulakakis KG, Markatis F, et al (Attikon Univ Hosp, Athens, Greece)

J Vasc Surg 58:1402-1407, 2013

Objective.—Carotid artery stenting (CAS) is usually performed with femoral access; however, this access may be impeded by anatomic limitations. Moreover, many embolic events happen during aortic arch catheterization. To overcome these problems, transcervical access to the carotid artery can be used as an alternative approach for CAS.

Methods.—An electronic search of the literature using PubMed was performed. All studies reporting the results of CAS using the transcervical approach were retrieved and analyzed.

Results.—The analysis included 12 studies reporting the results of 739 CAS procedures performed in 722 patients (mean age, 75.5 years). Of 533 lesions reported, 235 (44%) were symptomatic, with no data regarding symptomatic status available for 206 lesions. Two techniques were used: direct CAS with transcervical access (filter protected or unprotected) in 250 patients and CAS with transcervical access under reversed flow (with arteriovenous shunt in most cases) in 489 patients. Local anesthesia was used in 464 of 739 procedures (63%), and the remaining were performed under general anesthesia or cervical block. Technical success was 96.3% for 579 procedures with available data (558 successful procedures and 21 failures: inability to cross the lesion, 10; dissection, 5; failure of predilatation, 1; stent thrombosis, 1; patient agitation, 1; and no data, 3). The incidence of conversion to open repair was 3.0% (20 of 579 procedures: 18 carotid endarterectomies and two common carotid-internal carotid bypass grafts). Stroke occurred in eight patients (two fatal) and a fatal myocardial infarction in one patient. The incidence of stroke, myocardial infarction, and death was 1.1%, 0.14%, and 0.41%, respectively. The incidence of stroke was 1.2% (3 of 250) in direct CAS with transcervical access and 1.02% (5 of 489) in CAS under reversed flow ($P > .05$). Transient ischemic attack occurred in 20 patients (2.7%). Local complications were encountered in 17 of 579 CAS (2.9%), comprising 15 hematomas and two patients with transient laryngeal palsy.

Conclusions.—CAS with the transcervical approach is a safe procedure with low incidence of stroke and complications. It can be used as an alternative to femoral access in patients with unfavorable aortoiliac or aortic arch anatomy.

▶ With the increasing life expectancy in the United States, there is a corresponding increase in the number of older persons needing hemodialysis. Unfortunately, there may not be a suitable vein for creation of an autogenous fistula, and prosthetic material implantation is necessary. The morbidity and mortality associated with grafts and catheters are well known mainly because of infectious complications. This study is a large database analysis of infectious and noninfectious complications over time in an international cohort of dialysis patients. The risk of any complication is much higher in the first 3 to 6 months after access placement. The risks are obviously higher in those with a catheter or graft, but, even so, risk of infection declines over time and, in this study, was independent of individual comorbid conditions or geographical location. Thrombosis risk also declined over time with all forms of access. The main recommendation to be gleaned from this interesting study is that special and close attention should be given to newly formed accesses of all types. Preventative measures, such as early interventions in fistulae failing to mature or aggressive wound care and meticulous technique in those with grafts and catheters, should be instituted.

R. L. Bush, MD, JD, MPH

Carotid Restenosis After Endarterectomy and Stenting: A Critical Issue?

Setacci F, Sirignano P, Galzerano G, et al (Univ of Siena, Italy)

Ann Vasc Surg 27:888-893, 2013

Background.—Carotid artery stenting (CAS) is currently considered a valid alternative to carotid endarterectomy (CEA) for the prevention of stroke in high-risk patients. One of the most important issues for both of these techniques is carotid restenosis. The aim of our study was to evaluate the incidence of post-CEA and post-CAS restenosis in a large cohort of patients in a single high-volume center.

Methods.—Between December 2000 and December 2010, 2453 CEA and 2628 CAS procedures were performed in the Vascular and Endovascular Surgery Unit at our institution. The mean age of patients was 73.8 years (range 55–89 years), 78% of whom were men. Indications for carotid revascularization were: presence of symptomatic carotid artery stenosis of >70%, or asymptomatic stenosis of at least 80%, especially in patients with vulnerable plaques.

Results.—Mild and long-term results after CEA and CAS were similar. The overall perioperative neurologic complication rate (minor and major stroke) was similar in the 2 groups. At 1-year follow-up the restenosis rate after CEA was 1.58%. In-stent restenosis after CAS occurred in 1.67% of the procedures. All but 3 arteries had been treated for postsurgical restenosis. All lesions were approached secondarily with endovascular procedures. Statistical analysis demonstrated that post-CEA restenosis was the most important predictive factor for the development of in-stent restenosis after CAS.

Conclusions.—This review of our 10-year experience confirms that patients who develop restenosis after CEA are also prone to developing in-stent restenosis after CAS.

▶ This is an interesting study from the University of Siena, Italy, reviewing more than 5000 carotid revascularization procedures over a 10-year span. In this single-center study, the authors evaluate the incidence of recurrent carotid stenosis with both carotid endarterectomy (CEA) and carotid artery stenting (CAS). I found it unusual that more than 50% of the procedures were CAS as opposed to CEA. In any event, the rate of restenosis was low for either procedure (CEA, 1.58% and CAS, 1.67%). All restenoses were treated with angioplasty and possible stent placement. More than 50% of their cohort was asymptomatic, in line with most studies of carotid procedures. The authors do comment on the meaningfulness of vulnerable plaques in asymptomatic patients. However, later in the discussion section they state that "even if a stenosis represents a stable, asymptomatic, non-emboligenic lesion, it can evolve." This is a purely speculative comment for which there are no data. So the question remains about the utility of plaque characteristics. Do we continue to try to recognize a vulnerable plaque or just proceed with the premise that it may evolve? These authors present valuable data to guide the treatment of restenosis and also raise some very important and unanswered questions.

R. L. Bush, MD, JD, MPH

United Kingdom Carotid Artery Stent Registry: Short- and Long-Term Outcomes

Goode SD, Cleveland TJ, Gaines PA (Northern General Hosp, Sheffield, UK)
Cardiovasc Intervent Radiol 36:1221-1231, 2013

Background.—Carotid artery stenting (CAS) has evolved to treat carotid artery disease with the intention of prevent stroke. The British Society of Interventional Radiologists developed a voluntary registry to monitor the practice of this novel procedure. We present the data from the United Kingdom (UK) CAS registry for short and long-term outcomes for symptomatic and asymptomatic carotid disease.

Methods.—The UK CAS registry collected data from 1998 to 2010 from 31 hospitals across the UK for 1,154 patients. All interventions were enrolled in the registry for both asymptomatic and symptomatic patients. Initial entry forms were completed for each patient entered with data including indications, demographic data, CAS data (including stents and protection device details) and 30-day outcomes. Complications were documented. Follow-up data were collected at yearly intervals.

Results.—Nine hundred fifty-three (83 %) symptomatic and 201 (17 %) asymptomatic patients were enrolled into the registry. The 30-day all stroke and death rates for symptomatic patients were 5.5 and 2.2 % for those with asymptomatic disease. The 30-day mortality rate was 1.7 % for symptomatic and 0.6 % for asymptomatic patients. For symptomatic patients undergoing CAS, the 7-year all-cause mortality rate was 22.2 % and for asymptomatic patients 18.1 %. The 7-year all-cause mortality and disabling stroke rates were 25.3 and 19.4 %, respectively.

Conclusion.—These data indicate that outside of the tight constraints of a randomised trial, CAS provides effective prophylaxis against stroke and death.

▶ It is important to understand the differences in practice patterns between specialties and between countries. This article exemplifies both of these concepts. The practice of carotid artery stenting (CAS) performed by interventional radiologists in the United Kingdom is a perfect example. The British Society of Interventional Radiologists maintains a CAS registry, which is voluntary and has not been validated. There is no standardization of data collection and entry or variable definition that I can glean from this article, and follow-up was not rigorously performed. Thus, it is difficult to ascertain meaningful results from the data, but one can certainly look at practice patterns, which differ from those in the United States. This registry covers dates from 1998 to 2010, much longer than CAS performance in the United States. Also, more than 80% of the entries are from patients with symptomatic carotid disease compared with registries in the United States, which have about 60% to 70% asymptomatic persons. Furthermore, in the asymptomatic group, the British registry results state that the most common reason for CAS is previous cardiac surgery (61% of registry cohort). This is dissimilar from the rationale in the United States, as multiple studies have shown no indication for carotid intervention in patients with concomitant coronary and asymptomatic carotid disease. The article also states that most patients are referred for CAS if they are unsuitable for endarterectomy (CEA), but the criteria for unsuitability are not given. The take-home message is that although the rationale for CAS seems divergent from some of the current literature, the performance of CEA is still the gold standard in the United Kingdom. I would recommend a more robust registry so that accurate and validated long-term data can be analyzed from this registry.

R. L. Bush, MD, JD, MPH

Accuracy of administrative data versus clinical data to evaluate carotid endarterectomy and carotid stenting

Bensley RP, Yoshida S, Lo RC, et al (Beth Israel Deaconess Med Ctr and Harvard Med School, Boston, MA)

J Vasc Surg 58:412-420, 2013

Objective.—Administrative data have been used to compare carotid endarterectomy (CEA) and carotid artery stenting (CAS). However, there are limitations in defining symptom status, Centers for Medicare and Medicaid Services high-risk status, as well as complications. Therefore, we did a direct comparison between administrative data and physician chart review as well as between data collected for the National Surgical Quality Improvement Program (NSQIP) and physician chart review for CEA and CAS.

Methods.—We performed an outcomes analysis on all CEA and CAS procedures from 2005 to 2011. We obtained International Classification of Diseases, Ninth Revision diagnosis codes from hospital discharge records regarding symptom status, high-risk status, and perioperative stroke. We also obtained data on all CEA patients submitted to NSQIP over the same time period. One of the study authors (R.B.) then performed a chart review of the same patients to determine symptom status, high-risk status, and perioperative strokes and the results were compared.

Results.—We identified 1342 patients who underwent CEA or CAS between 2005 and 2011 and 392 patients who underwent CEA that were submitted to NSQIP. Administrative data identified fewer symptomatic patients (17.0% vs 34.0%), physiologic high-risk patients (9.3% vs 23.0%), and anatomic high-risk patients (0% vs 15.2%). Although administrative data identified a similar proportion of perioperative strokes (1.9% vs 2.0%), this was due to the fact that these data identified eight false positive and nine false negative perioperative strokes. NSQIP data identified more symptomatic patients compared with chart review (44.1% vs 30.3%), fewer physiologic high-risk patients (13.0% vs 18.6%), fewer anatomic high-risk patients (0% vs 6.6%), and a similar proportion of perioperative strokes (1.5% vs 1.8%, only one false negative stroke and no false positives).

Conclusions.—Administrative data are unreliable for determining symptom status, high-risk status, and perioperative stroke and should not be used to analyze CEA and CAS. NSQIP data do not adequately identify high-risk patients, but do accurately identify perioperative strokes and to a lesser degree, symptom status.

▶ Patients undergoing carotid endarterectomy (CEA) generally do very well with the operation with most able to go home on the first postoperative day. Thus, most large administrative datasets only capture complications or events that happen in the few hours between surgery and hospital discharge. The 30-day event rates after carotid revascularization are not clear, with wide ranges being reported in the literature. How then does a surgeon counsel his or her patients appropriately before CEA so that the patient and family are well informed as to the risks involved? This important study analyzes a large dataset, the National Surgical Quality Improvement Project, which contains preoperative, intraoperative, and postoperative data extending to 30 days. The authors found that of almost 36 000 persons having a CEA, although the combined stroke, death, and cardiac event rate was low at 2.9%, 38% of events occurred after the patient was discharged. Interestingly, there was no difference in asymptomatic and symptomatic carotid patients. Significant predictors for these events were female gender, renal failure, and chronic obstructive pulmonary disease. These findings should help inform practitioners when choosing the best intervention for a patient and discussing options. Perhaps if the patient is at very high risk with multiple predictors of adverse events, the best course may be continued surveillance with no intervention. I recommend this article to persons performing carotid interventions and encourage them to also be realistic and exact about their own data and outcomes.

R. L. Bush, MD, JD, MPH

The current national criteria for carotid artery stenting overestimate its efficacy in patients who are symptomatic and at high risk

Yoshida S, Bensley RP, Glaser JD, et al (Beth Israel Deaconess Med Ctr and Harvard Med School, Boston, MA)
J Vasc Surg 58:120-127, 2013

Background.—The Centers for Medicare and Medicaid Services (CMS) have established guidelines that outline patients who are considered "high risk" for complications after carotid endarterectomy (CEA) for which carotid artery stenting (CAS) may provide benefit. The validity of these high-risk criteria are yet unproven. In this study, we stratified patients who underwent CAS or CEA by CMS high-risk criteria and symptom status and examined their 30-day outcomes.

Methods.—A nonrandomized, retrospective cohort study was performed by chart review of all patients undergoing CEA or CAS from January 1, 2005, to December 31, 2010, at our institution. Demographic data and data pertaining to the presence or absence of high-risk factors were collected. Patients were stratified using symptom status and high-risk status as variables, and 30-day adverse events (stroke, death, myocardial infarction [MI]) were compared.

Results.—A total of 271 patients underwent CAS, with 30-day complication rates of stroke (3.0%), death (1.1%), MI (1.5%), stroke/death (3.7%), and stroke/death/MI (5.2%). A total of 830 patients underwent CEA with 30-day complication rates of stroke (2.0%), death (0.1%), MI (0.6%), stroke/death (1.9%), and stroke/death/MI (2.7%). Among symptomatic patients, physiologic high-risk status was associated with increased stroke/death (6 of 42 [14.3%] vs 2 of 74 [2.7%]; $P < .01$), and anatomic high-risk status was associated with a trend toward increased stroke/death (5 of 31 [16.1%] vs 0 of 20 [0.0%]; $P = .14$) in patients who underwent CAS vs CEA. Analysis of asymptomatic patients showed no differences between the two groups overall, except for a trend toward a higher rate of MI after CAS than after CEA (3 of 71 [4.2%] vs 0 of 108 [0.0%]; $P = .06$) in those who were physiologically at high risk. Among symptomatic patients who underwent CAS, patients with physiologic and anatomic high-risk factors had a higher rate of stroke/death than non-high-risk patients (6 of 42 [14.3%] vs 0 of 24 [0.0%] and 5 of 31 [16.1%] vs 0 of 24 [0.0%], respectively; both $P \leq .05$).

Conclusions.—Physiologic high-risk status was associated with increased stroke/death, whereas anatomic high-risk status showed a trend toward increased stroke/death in symptomatic patients undergoing CAS compared with non-high-risk patients undergoing CAS or physiologically high-risk patients undergoing CEA. Our results suggest that the current national criteria for CAS overestimate its efficacy in patients who are symptomatic and at high risk.

▶ This is a must-read for those who have been monitoring the data concerning the indications, efficacy, and outcomes of carotid artery stenting (CAS) compared with the traditional gold standard, carotid endarterectomy (CEA). Practitioners who follow the criteria set forth for reimbursement by the Centers for Medicare and Medicaid Services will restrict their practice for CAS to the approved indications, age, symptomatology, and risk status. Two different levels of risk status are discussed, those of physiologic risk and those of anatomic risk. The authors used a unique 2-tiered stratification for their statistical analysis, including high risk and symptom status. The results and conclusions are somewhat surprising and may lead to further discussion and controversy. As would be expected, those who were symptomatic and had physiologic high risk had worse outcomes with CAS. The authors thus conclude that perhaps CAS should be reserved for those patients who are healthier and asymptomatic. Physiologic high-risk patients had better outcomes with CEA. The discussion section includes a good overview of the carotid stent vs carotid endarterectomy trials and the risk stratification in each study. Of course, the authors mention that perhaps reimbursement criteria should be revisited, although this will take future studies of comparative effectiveness and costs. I do hope that this talented group of investigators takes the lead in improving patient selection for this type of carotid revascularization.

R. L. Bush, MD, JD, MPH

13 Vascular Trauma

Patient-based outcomes and quality of life after salvageable wartime extremity vascular injury

Scott DJ, Arthurs ZM, Stannard A, et al (Lackland Air Force Base, San Antonio, TX; U.S. Army Inst of Surgical Res, Fort Sam Houston, TX; et al)

J Vasc Surg 59:173-179.e1, 2014

Objective.—To date, contemporary studies on wartime vascular trauma have focused on acute management strategies and early results, with no characterization of enduring functional limb salvage or its relation to quality of life. The objective of this study was to describe long-term, patient-based quality of life and function after extremity vascular injury (EVI).

Methods.—The Joint Theater Trauma Registry was queried for U.S. troops with EVI. Injury and management data was obtained and the Medical Outcomes Study Short Form 36 (SF-36) Health Survey administered after patient contact and consent. Demographic, injury, and management variables were analyzed and examined for correlation with the primary end points of favorable or unfavorable outcome defined by SF-36 Mental (MCS) or Physical Component Summary (PCS) scores of >42 or <42 (effect size ≥0.8).

Results.—Surveys were completed by 214 patients, who were a median age of 25 years (range, 19-52 years). The Injury Severity Score was 15.3 ± 8.6 and the Mangled Extremity Severity Score was 5.65 ± 1.4. Amputation-free survival was 84% at mean follow-up of 61 ± 24 months. Overall SF-36 PCS and MCS scores were 43.0 ± 9.2 and 46.6 ± 12.4, respectively, with 92 respondents (43%) reporting favorable outcomes on both MCS and PCS. On multivariate analysis, older age, severe extremity injury (Mangled Extremity Severity Scores ≥7), and chronic pain were predictive of unfavorable physical outcomes ($P < .05$). Presence of pain, nerve injury, and junior rank (<E7) were predictive of unfavorable MCS scores ($P < .05$). Higher educational background (baccalaureate or above) was associated with favorable outcome ($P < .05$).

Conclusions.—This study reports the first long-term patient-centered outcomes data after wartime EVI. At 5 years after injury, quality-of-life measures are reduced compared with national norms. Understanding high-risk characteristics, both demographic- and injury-specific, that are associated with unfavorable outcomes will help guide future acute management and long-term recovery strategies.

▶ An increased incidence of vascular injury has been witnessed in the recent American wars in Iraq and Afghanistan compared with other previous reports from combat. This increase is likely because of improvements in body armor and modern wounding mechanisms such as improvised explosive device detonation. Until now, there have never been any meaningful long-term data reported on outcomes after extremity vascular injury relating to severity of injury or method of repair.

Patients were appropriately identified and then contacted, consented, and surveyed. Respondents were predominantly male (98%), junior rank (73% < E7), and young, with a median age of 25 years (range, 19–52). Patients with a college degree had more favorable outcomes ($P < .05$).

One of the most unique features of this report was the validation of the mangled extremity severity score (MESS).[1] Although originally developed for predicting amputation in severely injured lower extremities, the MESS was used as an objective scale to define and compare injury severity of any afflicted limb. When used in this manner, the MESS was significantly predictive of an unfavorable outcome. When a conventional cutoff of greater than 7 was used, elevated MESS was associated with a 2-fold increased risk for an unfavorable long-term physical outcome. This is the first study of its kind to describe this over the long term.

The authors conclude that quality of life after wartime extremity vascular injury is reduced globally compared with population norms. The most influential factors contributing to a patient's quality of life depend on the patient's particular demographic status, socioeconomic background (preinjury and postinjury), and mental health.

B. W. Starnes, MD

Reference

1. Johansen K, Daines M, Howey T, Helfet D, Hansen ST Jr. Objective criteria accurately predict amputation following lower extremity trauma. *J Trauma*. 1990;30: 568-572.

Early management of pediatric vascular injuries through humanitarian surgical care during U.S. military operations

Dua A, Via KC, Kreishman P, et al (Univ of Texas Med Ctr, Houston; Walter Reed Army Med Ctr, Bethesda, MD; et al)
J Vasc Surg 58:695-700, 2013

Background.—The objective of this report is to describe our experience of pediatric vascular injuries in a U.S. military combat support hospital in Baghdad, Iraq. A retrospective study was designed using Joint Theater Trauma Registry (JTTR) records in order to evaluate the pediatric (age < 18 years) population presenting with vascular trauma to a combat hospital in Baghdad, Iraq between April 2006 and August 2008. Demographic data comprised casualty, age, gender, and mechanism of injury. Physiologic data included presenting vital signs (rectal temperature, blood pressure, and heart rate), arterial pH, base deficit, hemoglobin (g/dL), and international normalized ratio.

TABLE 2.—Summary of Median Transfusion requirements for 25 Transfused Children with Vascular Injuries

Blood Component	24-Hour Totals
Total blood products (range),[a] mL/kg	47 (0-119)
FFP (range), mL/kg	14 (0-68)
Plasma:RBC ratio	1:1.5
6 pk platelets, mean ± standard deviation	1.2 ± 3.68 units
Crystalloid (range), mL/kg	102 (19-253)
% Receiving rFVIIa (No.)	12 (3/25)

FFP, Fresh frozen plasma or thawed plasma; *RBC*, red blood cell; *rFVIIa*, recombinant factor VIIa.
[a]Packed RBCs.

Results.—Twenty-five children, median age 14 years (range, 5-17 years), median weight 48 kg (range, 15-80 kg) sustained 18 (72%) blast and 7 (28%) gunshot wounds. The mean Injury Severity Score was 25 ± 16.2. The median operative time for the vascular repairs was 189 minutes (range, 41-505 minutes). Patients were tachycardic (mean ± standard deviation, 136 ± 29 bpm), hypotensive (109/63 ± 29/19 mm Hg), and acidemic (pH 7.26 ± 0.07; BD −5.57 ± 5.1 mEq/L) on arrival to the emergency department and were physiologically improved upon admission to the intensive care unit 3 hours later. Repair techniques were ligation (14; 39%), saphenous graft (11; 31%), lateral suture (7; 19%), end anastomosis (2; 5%), patch (1; 3%), and thrombectomy (1; 3%). Twenty-four hour mean transfusion requirements included crystalloid 102 mL/kg (range, 19-253), transfused blood 47 mL/kg (range, 0-119), fresh frozen plasma 14 mL/kg (range, 0-68), and apheresis platelets (1.2 ± 3.68 units). Over a follow-up of 22 ± 5.5 days, the amputation-free survival was 80%.

Conclusions.—This is the largest reported wartime series to demonstrate in children that damage control resuscitation despite high injury severity permits simultaneous limb salvage (Table 2).

▶ One of the most stark realizations for any surgeon deploying to war is that children are inevitably caught in the middle of modern combat operations. Penetrating trauma has been the predominant mechanism of traumatic injury among pediatric patients during US Military operations in Iraq. Recent wartime publications have reported a penetrating arterial incidence ranging from 72% to 83%.[1,2] This report details a 2-year experience from senior military surgeons managing pediatric vascular injuries.

There are certain important lessons from this report that are transferable into civilian practice.

1 Arterial spasm and the potential for early thrombosis are much more common in pediatric vascular trauma—use of vasodilators such as papaverine or nitroglycerin may be helpful.

2 Vascular anastomoses should be performed using interrupted suture repair. Continuous suture repair will lead to narrowing as the patient grows.

3 Judicious use of tourniquets and temporary shunts may be helpful during transport—especially in austere conditions.
4 Early recognition and correction of shock and coagulopathy with a "damage control resuscitation" strategy (Table 2) in children seems to permit the additional operating time necessary for limb salvage.

B. W. Starnes, MD

References

1. Matos RI, Holcomb JB, Callahan C, Spinella PC. Increased mortality rates of young children with traumatic injuries at a US army combat support hospital in Baghdad, Iraq, 2004. *Pediatrics*. 2008;122:e959-e966.
2. Spinella PC, Borgman MA, Azarow KS. Pediatric trauma in an austere combat environment. *Crit Care Med*. 2008;36:S293-S296.

Early management of pediatric vascular injuries through humanitarian surgical care during U.S. military operations

Dua A, Via KC, Kreishman MP, et al (Univ of Texas Med Ctr, Houston; Walter Reed Army Med Ctr, Fort Sam Houston, TX; et al)
J Vasc Surg 58:695-700, 2013

Background.—The objective of this report is to describe our experience of pediatric vascular injuries in a U.S. military combat support hospital in Baghdad, Iraq. A retrospective study was designed using Joint Theater Trauma Registry (JTTR) records in order to evaluate the pediatric (age <18 years) population presenting with vascular trauma to a combat hospital in Baghdad, Iraq between April 2006 and August 2008. Demographic data comprised casualty, age, gender, and mechanism of injury. Physiologic data included presenting vital signs (rectal temperature, blood pressure, and heart rate), arterial pH, base deficit, hemoglobin (g/dL), and international normalized ratio.

Results.—Twenty-five children, median age 14 years (range, 5-17 years), median weight 48 kg (range, 15-80 kg) sustained 18 (72%) blast and 7 (28%) gunshot wounds. The mean Injury Severity Score was 25 ± 16.2. The median operative time for the vascular repairs was 189 minutes (range, 41-505 minutes). Patients were tachycardic (mean ± standard deviation, 136 ± 29 bpm), hypotensive (109/63 ± 29/19 mm Hg), and acidemic (pH 7.26 ± 0.07; BD −5.57 ± 5.1 mEq/L) on arrival to the emergency department and were physiologically improved upon admission to the intensive care unit 3 hours later. Repair techniques were ligation (14; 39%), saphenous graft (11; 31%), lateral suture (7; 19%), end anastomosis (2; 5%), patch (1; 3%), and thrombectomy (1; 3%). Twenty-four hour mean transfusion requirements included crystalloid 102 mL/kg (range, 19-253), transfused blood 47 mL/kg (range, 0-119), fresh frozen plasma 14 mL/kg (range, 0-68), and apheresis platelets (1.2 ± 3.68 units). Over a follow-up of 22 ± 5.5 days, the amputation-free survival was 80%.

Conclusions.—This is the largest reported wartime series to demonstrate in children that damage control resuscitation despite high injury severity permits simultaneous limb salvage.

▶ Reports on vascular care of pediatric patients are not common. Even less common are large reports on surgeons caring for the child with a vascular injury. Most vascular surgeons have little experience with this problem and remain somewhat pessimistic and intimidated by performing vascular operations on children. This report by Dua et al reports on a relatively large series of children with vascular injuries associated with military munitions. The age of children treated in this series ranged from 5 to 17 years with weight ranging from 15 to 80 kg. All patients were severely injured with average injury severity score of 25 ± 16. There were 36 vascular injuries in this group associated with blast (72%) GSW (28%). Arterial injuries were reported in 61% and venous injuries were reported in 39 percent. Vessels injured included carotid-subclavian (11%), pelvic (6%), upper extremity (25%), and lower extremity (58%). Vascular interventions were ligation (39%), saphenous vein graft (31%), lateral suture (19%), end-to-end anastomosis (5%), patch angioplasty (5%), and thrombectomy (3%). Fasciotomy was performed liberally (28%), and emergency tourniquets were used in prehospital resuscitation in half (52%). Temporary shunts were used in 12%. At a mean follow-up of 22 ± 5 days amputation-free survival was 80%. In the 4 patients with amputation, all sustained popliteal artery injury. One of these popliteal artery injuries was managed with ligation and 3 with bypass that thrombosed. The survival of this patient cohort was 96% overall. From this excellent report, you can take away that overall the techniques you use to care for adults is translatable to children. One can consider interrupted sutures when performing end-to-end repairs or vascular bypass, especially in small children. The principles of damage control resuscitation, however, remain valid and life saving.

D. L. Gillespie, MD, RVT, FACS

Diagnostic Performance of Computed Tomography Angiography in Peripheral Arterial Injury due to Trauma: A Systematic Review and Meta-analysis

Jens S, Kerstens MK, Legemate DA, et al (Academic Med Ctr, Amsterdam, The Netherlands)

Eur J Vasc Endovasc Surg 46:329-337, 2013

Objectives.—To evaluate the diagnostic accuracy of computed tomography angiography (CTA) in detecting arterial lesions in patients with suspected arterial injury of the upper or lower extremity due to trauma.

Methods.—A systematic review and meta-analysis was carried out. Medline and Embase were searched on August 13, 2012, for studies comparing CTA with surgery, digital subtraction angiography (DSA), or follow-up, which allowed extraction of data into two-by-two tables.

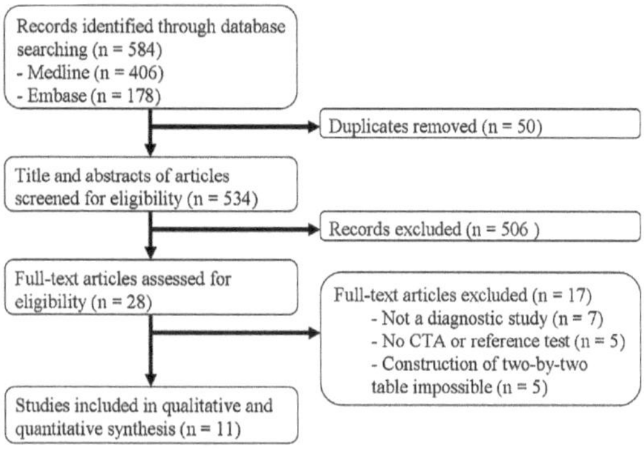

FIGURE 1.—Flow diagram of search and study selection. CTA = computed tomography angiography. (Reprinted from Jens S, Kerstens MK, Legemate DA, et al. Diagnostic performance of computed tomography angiography in peripheral arterial injury due to trauma: a systematic review and meta-analysis. *Eur J Vasc Endovasc Surg.* 2013;46:329-337, with permission from European Society for Vascular Surgery.)

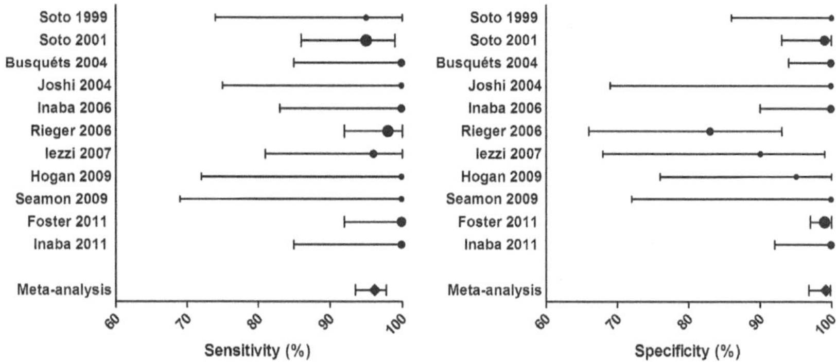

FIGURE 4.—Summary estimate and per study sensitivity and specificity of all included studies. (Reprinted from Jens S, Kerstens MK, Legemate DA, et al. Diagnostic performance of computed tomography angiography in peripheral arterial injury due to trauma: a systematic review and meta-analysis. *Eur J Vasc Endovasc Surg.* 2013;46:329-337, with permission from European Society for Vascular Surgery.)

The methodological quality of included studies was assessed using the QUADAS tool. Summary estimates of sensitivity and specificity of CTA in identifying or excluding arterial lesions were obtained using a bivariate model.

Results.—This review included 11 studies making up a total of 891 trauma patients. The included studies were of moderate methodological quality and at risk of misclassification and verification bias. Some 4.2% of all CTA studies were non-diagnostic. The summary estimates of sensitivity and specificity of CTA were 96.2% (95% CI 93.5–97.8%) and 99.2% (95% CI 96.8–99.8%), respectively.

Conclusion.—Despite methodological flaws, the excellent estimates of sensitivity and specificity indicate that CTA is an accurate modality for

TABLE 1.—Study Characteristics of Included Studies

Source	Design	Number of Patients	Number of Males (%)	Age, Mean (SD) or (Range)	Extremity Injury	Number of Slices CT Scanner	Slice Thickness	Reconstructions Done	Reference Standard when CTA Positive	Reference Standard when CTA Negative	Assessment of Lesion (per Patient/per Lesion)
Soto 1999[9]	Prospective	45	42 (93)	26.2 (16–56)	Upper and lower	1	1.0 mm	MIP and SSD	DSA	DSA	Per patient
Soto 2001[10]	Prospective	139	120 (86)	28.6 (16–77)	Upper and lower	1	1.0 mm	MIP, VRT, MPR and SSD	Surgery, DSA	Surgery, FU	Per-lesion
Busquéts 2004[11]	Retrospective	95[a]	82 (86)	31.0 (5.6)	Upper and lower	NA	1.0 mm	MIP, VRT, CPR and SSD	Surgery, DSA	DSA, FU	Both
Joshi 2004[12]	Retrospective	23	NA	NA	Upper and lower	4	2.5 mm	MIP, VRT and SSD	Surgery	FU	Per patient
Inaba 2006[13]	Retrospective	59[a]	51 (86)	37.0 (10–79)	Lower	4	1.6 mm	3D reconstruction	Surgery, DUS, FU	DSA, DUS, FU	Both
Rieger 2006[14]	Retrospective	87	71 (82)	37.0 (NA)	Upper and lower	4	0.8 mm	VRT and MPR	Surgery, DSA	Surgery, FU	Per lesion
Iezzi 2007[15]	Retrospective	47	29 (62)	38.6 (18–78)	Upper and lower	4	1.5 mm	MIP, VRT and MPR	Either surgery, DSA, FU	Either surgery, DSA, FU	Per patient
Hogan 2009[16]	Retrospective	32	NA	NA (0–18)	Upper and lower	4	1.6 mm	3D reconstruction	Either Surgery, imaging or FU	Either Surgery, imaging or FU	Per patient
Seamon 2009[17]	Prospective	21	19 (90)	26.1 (18–50)	Upper and lower	64 or 16	0.75 mm	3D reconstruction	Surgery, DSA	Surgery, DSA	Per lesion
Foster 2011[18]	Retrospective	284	217 (76)	40.0 (16–89)	Lower	64	0.625 mm	MPR	Surgery, DSA, FU	FU	Per patient
Inaba 2011[19]	Prospective	73	64 (88)	30.3 (12.7)	Upper and lower	64	1.0 mm	MIP, VRT and CPR	Surgery, FU	DSA, FU	Both

Note. CPR = curved-planar reformation; CTA = computed tomography angiography; DSA = digital subtraction angiography; DUS = duplex ultrasound; FU = follow-up; MIP = maximum intensity projection; MPR = multiplanar reformation; NA = not available; SSD = shaded surface display; VRT = volume-rendered technique.

Editor's Note: Please refer to original journal article for full references.

[a]Ten (Busquéts et al.[11]) and four (Inaba et al.[13]) patients did not have a reference test.

evaluating arterial lesions in patients with extremity trauma and can replace DSA (Figs 1 and 4, Table 1).

► Penetrating and blunt trauma can cause severe arterial injuries to the extremities, and these injuries require immediate diagnostic workup to prevent severe disability and possible limb loss. The aim of this study was to perform a systematic review with assessment of methodologic quality and a meta-analysis to obtain the best possible estimates of the diagnostic performance of computed tomography angiography (CTA) in patients with peripheral arterial injury in an emergency setting.

Eleven of 584 studies were chosen for methodologic quality and finally included in this review (Fig 1). One of the interesting things I found was that 7 of the 11 studies had old-generation computed tomography scanners (4-slice or less), further bolstering the eventual conclusions of the article that CTA should be the diagnostic study of choice for peripheral arterial injury (Table 1).

This meta-analysis shows that CTA compared with the reference standard of digital subtraction angiography, surgery or follow-up, is an accurate diagnostic tool for detecting arterial injury of the extremities due to trauma, with a sensitivity of 96.2% and a specificity of 99.2% (Fig 4). Having worked at a major US Trauma Center for the past 8 years, I can personally attest to the data presented herein. The fact that imaging has continuously improved over the past 2 decades leads me to believe that not only will this be the modality of choice for diagnosing these injuries, it will only become faster over time. The main advantage of performing CTA instead of digital subtraction angiography is the time gained to adequate treatment.

B. W. Starnes, MD

Diagnostic Performance of Computed Tomography Angiography in Peripheral Arterial Injury due to Trauma: A Systematic Review and Meta-analysis

Jens S, Kerstens MK, Legemate DA, et al (Academic Med Ctr, Amsterdam, The Netherlands)

Eur J Vasc Endovasc Surg 46:329-337, 2013

Objectives.—To evaluate the diagnostic accuracy of computed tomography angiography (CTA) in detecting arterial lesions in patients with suspected arterial injury of the upper or lower extremity due to trauma.

Methods.—A systematic review and meta-analysis was carried out. Medline and Embase were searched on August 13, 2012, for studies comparing CTA with surgery, digital subtraction angiography (DSA), or follow-up, which allowed extraction of data into two-by-two tables. The methodological quality of included studies was assessed using the QUADAS tool. Summary estimates of sensitivity and specificity of CTA in identifying or excluding arterial lesions were obtained using a bivariate model.

Results.—This review included 11 studies making up a total of 891 trauma patients. The included studies were of moderate methodological quality and at risk of misclassification and verification bias. Some 4.2% of all CTA studies were non-diagnostic. The summary estimates of sensitivity and specificity of CTA were 96.2% (95% CI 93.5–97.8%) and 99.2% (95% CI 96.8–99.8%), respectively.

Conclusion.—Despite methodological flaws, the excellent estimates of sensitivity and specificity indicate that CTA is an accurate modality for evaluating arterial lesions in patients with extremity trauma and can replace DSA.

▶ The evaluation of vascular trauma presents many challenges to the clinician. Eric Frykberg clearly demonstrated the value of physical examination in detecting vascular injuries in the early 1990s. As technology continues to develop, the number of useful diagnostic and therapeutic tools available to the clinician has increased. Advanced imaging in particular has shown increasing utility. This excellent meta-analysis reviews recent studies on the use of computed tomography angiography (CTA) in diagnosing peripheral vascular injuries. The authors performed a thorough search of the literature and carefully chose the studies they included in their review to reduce heterogeneity and ensure the inclusion of only high-quality articles.

Their analysis confirms the high sensitivity and specificity of CTA in detecting vascular injuries. As the authors suggest, CTA should replace purely diagnostic catheter-directed digital subtraction angiography (DSA) in most trauma patients. In the future, I expect that DSA will be limited to use in conjunction with endovascular therapeutic procedures.

A limitation of this article was the limited number of studies using multidetector row CTA. Most of the included studies used 4-slice or less CT scanners. Interestingly, the authors found that despite the improved image quality of multidetector row scanners, the rate of nondiagnostic studies had increased.

P. White, MD, FACS

Histologic analysis of stent graft oversizing in the thoracic aorta

Sincos IR, da Silva ES, Belczak SQ, et al (Hosp Israelita Albert Einstein, São Paulo, Brazil; et al)

J Vasc Surg 58:1644-1651.e4, 2013

Objective.—To elucidate the histologic changes after stent graft oversizing in nonatherosclerotic aortas using an experimental porcine model. We previously reported that the diameter and angulation of the aorta in this model are similar to those in young individuals who undergo stent graft repair for blunt aortic injuries. The lack of commercially available stent grafts specific for repairing blunt aortic injuries, particularly for small and angulated aortas, may be related to the high rate of endograft complications in this population.

Methods.—Twenty-five pigs were randomized into one control group (without stent graft implantation) and four oversized groups (A: 10%-19%, B: 20%-29%, C: 30%-39%, and D: >40%). Three circumferential fragments were collected from the aorta for histologic and immunohistochemical studies. Morphometric analyzes were performed using an inflow system and image analysis software (Quantimet 500; Leica Cambridge Ltd, Cambridge, UK).

Results.—Collagen expression in the aortic wall was not significantly different among the five groups ($P = .5604$). There were significantly fewer muscle fibers in the aortic wall in the oversized groups compared with the control group ($P = .000198$). The proportion of elastic fibers in the aortic wall was significantly smaller in the oversized groups compared with the control group ($P = .0000001$). Immunohistochemical analysis showed that α-actin expression in the aortic wall was significantly decreased in the oversized groups compared with the control group ($P = .002031$). There were no significant differences in either the number of muscle fibers or α-actin expression among the four oversized groups.

Conclusions.—Histologic and immunohistochemical studies confirmed the structural disarrangement of the aortic wall after insertion of an endoprosthesis, including reduced number of muscle and elastic fibers.

▶ The majority of patients who experience traumatic aortic injury are usually younger and have a smaller aortic diameter (19 mm) than those who have aneurysms. Most commercially available stent grafts are specifically designed for the repair of aortic aneurysms, and the lack of availability of smaller stent grafts for repairing blunt aortic injuries may explain the high rates of endograft complications in this population. These complications include endoleak, stroke, and graft collapse. An international consensus suggests that oversizing > 20% should not be used after trauma in young individuals because the prothesis can collapse and obstruct the aorta. The present study evaluated the histologic changes after stent graft oversizing in nonatherosclerotic aortas using an experimental porcine model. The authors' results demonstrated a tendency for a reduction in the force supported by the aortic wall with increasing endograft oversizing and a loss of elasticity of the aortic wall with any degree of oversizing. Their histologic and immunohistochemical studies revealed that implantation of an endoprosthesis caused structural disarrangement of the aortic wall, particularly decreased amounts of muscle and elastic fibers. This is the first study to examine the effects of oversizing of a thoracic endoprosthesis on structural changes of the aortic wall. Although only 1 type of stent graft was used, it clearly demonstrates that oversizing can lead to a reduction in force supported by the aortic wall. These results highlight the importance of accurate graft sizing not only in patients who experience traumatic aortic injury but in all cases that require stent grafts.

J. Cullen, PhD

Intentional coverage of the left subclavian artery during endovascular repair of traumatic descending thoracic aortic transection

Antonello M, Menegolo M, Maturi C, et al (Univ of Padua, Italy)

J Vasc Surg 57:684-690.e1, 2013

Objective.—This single-center, prospective study aimed to investigate the technical success and outcome of intentional coverage of the left subclavian artery (LSA) in patients undergoing thoracic endovascular aortic repair (TEVAR) for traumatic rupture of the aortic isthmus at a tertiary care medical center.

Methods.—From January 2005 to June 2011, patients who presented with traumatic aortic transection underwent TEVAR with coverage of the LSA when the distance between the artery and the rupture was <2 cm. At 12, 24, and 72 hours postoperatively, clinical and neurologic evaluation including transcranial Doppler insonation of the brachial artery was performed. A decrease in peak systolic velocity (PSV) >60% with respect to the contralateral one was considered relevant. Functional status of the left arm was evaluated using a provocative test. Thoracoabdominal computerized tomographic angiography was performed postoperatively at 3-, 6-, and 12-month follow-up.

Results.—Thirty-one patients (mean age 35 years) underwent emergency TEVAR for traumatic aortic transection with intentional LSA coverage during the study period. In four cases (12.9%) coverage was partial. Two patients (6.4%) died during the postoperative period due to associated lesions. No signs of vertebrobasilar insufficiency, stroke, or paraplegia were observed in any of the patients. Nine patients (36%) had severe arm claudication (ischemic pain within 60 seconds of beginning arm exercise and decrease of PSV between 50% and 60%). Risk factors for the condition were left vertebral artery diameter < 3 mm ($P < .0001$). A significant correlation was found between the degree of PSV reduction and left arm symptoms ($P < .0001$). There was an improvement in ischemic arm symptoms ($P < .0001$) during mean follow-up of 36 months (range, 6-65 months), with only one patient (4.2%) presenting with severe claudication. Freedom from reintervention at 48 months was 93.5%. No signs of endoleaks or graft migrations were detected on computerized tomographic angiography control scans.

Conclusions.—Coverage of the LSA during TEVAR for traumatic aortic injuries appears to be a feasible, safe method for extending the endograft landing zone without increasing the risk of paraplegia, stroke, or left arm ischemia. Left vertebral artery diameter can be used to identify patients at risk for postoperative left arm ischemia.

▶ The authors prospectively set out to examine the consequences of covering the left subclavian artery when performing an endovascular repair of traumatic aortic injuries. The absence of severe neurologic or upper extremity ischemic complications in the short-term in this series of about 30 patients indicates that in an emergent situation, coverage of the left subclavian artery is a useful option to stabilize the patient and minimize operating times in the acute period. The authors claim that 93% of their patients did not require revascularization of the left subclavian artery during the follow-up period and propose duplex US criteria for guiding this decision. This seems more the result of a refusal to treat upper extremity claudication than anything else. Nearly 40% of patients at discharge and 25% of patients at 6-month follow-up had moderate or severe upper extremity claudication. This report adds further evidence that coverage of the left subclavian artery is safe and feasible in the acute setting, but its claim that left subclavian revascularization can be avoided in most patients falls short. Many more patients would probably benefit from electable subclavian revascularization at a later date.

P. White, MD, FACS

A 14-year experience with blunt thoracic aortic injury

Watson J, Slaiby J, Garcia Toca M, et al (The Warren Alpert Med School of Brown Univ, Providence RI)

J Vasc Surg 58:380-385, 2013

Objective.—This study reviewed the natural history of blunt thoracic aortic trauma (BTAT) over a 14-year period at our level 1 trauma center and compared open vs endovascular treatment.

Methods.—All patients with BTAT presenting to a level 1 trauma center from 1998 to 2011 were included in a retrospective analysis. Multiple data points and short-term and midterm outcomes were ascertained through a retrospective record review.

Results.—We identified 129 patients with BTAT. Of these, 32 (25%) were dead on arrival, 38 (29%) underwent a resuscitative thoracotomy and died, 33 (26%) underwent open repair, 14 (11%) underwent endovascular repair, 9 (7%) underwent simultaneous procedures, and 3 (2%) were managed nonoperatively. Mean Injury Severity Scores and Revised Trauma Scores were similar ($P = .484$, $P = .551$) between the open repair group ($n = 36$) and the endovascular repair group ($n = 14$). In the open repair group, there were 14 deaths (42%) ≤30 days of injury, 3 strokes (9%), 2 patients (6%) with paralysis, 2 myocardial infarctions (MIs; 6%), and 3 patients (9%) who required hemodialysis. In the endovascular group, there was 1 death (7%) ≤30 days of injury, 1 (7%) stroke, and 1 (7%) stent collapse. No paralysis, MI, or renal failure requiring hemodialysis was noted in the endovascular group. The average length of stay was 15 days for patients treated with endovascular repair vs 24 days for those treated with open repair ($P = .003$).

Conclusions.—The incidence of BTAT is low but the mortality associated with it is significant. During the 14-year period studied, there was a clear change in management preference from open repair to endovascular repair at our level 1 trauma center. Outcomes, including stroke, MI, renal failure, paralysis, length of stay, and death, appear to be reduced in the endovascular group.

▶ This retrospective review provides an interesting historical perspective on the transition from open therapy to endovascular therapy for blunt thoracic aortic trauma (BTAT) at a single institution. It adds to the growing body of evidence that endovascular repair most likely offers a better option for addressing these devastating injuries. This report highlights several important aspects of managing vascular trauma in the endovascular era. First, endovascular therapy is often more compatible with damage control surgery than open repair. In this series, endovascular cases were shorter, had less blood loss, and concluded with a warmer, more stable patient. Considering the differences in the physiologic insult between open and endovascular surgery, this makes perfect sense. Second, delaying surgical therapy for advanced imaging (ie, for a computed tomography [CT] scan) might not deserve the condemnation it once received. In this series, nearly every patient who was too unstable to receive a chest CT died. The fact that advanced imaging potentiates less-invasive endovascular therapies probably more than makes up for a delay in therapy. The authors of this report provided an interesting review of the historical adoption of endovascular repair for BTAT while emphasizing the advantages that led them to completely replace open repair with endovascular repair.

P. White, MD, FACS

Changing presentation of knee dislocation and vascular injury from high-energy trauma to low-energy falls in the morbidly obese

Georgiadis AG, Mohammad FH, Mizerik KT, et al (Henry Ford Hosp, Detroit, MI)

J Vasc Surg 57:1196-1203, 2013

Objective.—Reports in the literature of low-energy (LE) knee dislocation (KD) in obese patients have been increasing. This study was undertaken to define the risk factors for KD by LE mechanisms and the outcomes of these patients compared with those with high-energy (HE) trauma.

Methods.—All patients with a complete KD presenting to the emergency department of a large urban level I trauma center were reviewed. Patient information collected included age, sex, weight, height, body mass index (BMI), injury mechanism, neurovascular and orthopedic injuries, and operations performed to treat vascular injuries. Risk factors for KD and concomitant injuries were compared between HE traumatic dislocations and LE dislocations in obese patients (BMI >30 kg/m^2), including stratification for increasing levels of obesity.

Results.—Between January 1995 and April 2012, 53 patients with KD were identified. The mechanism of injury was HE in 28 (53%) and LE in 25 (47%). Of the LE KDs, 18 (72%) were related to obesity (BMI >30 kg/m^2). Obese patients with LE trauma were more likely to have associated nerve injuries (50% vs 6%; $P < .001$), vascular injuries requiring intervention (33% vs 9%; $P = .048$), and vascular surgical repairs (28% vs 6%; $P = .038$) than patients with HE traumatic dislocations. These rates were highest in the patients with a BMI >40 kg/m^2. Although all LE KDs in the obese involved an isolated extremity, the hospital lengths of stay were comparable to those with HE KDs who frequently had multisystem trauma (8.7 vs 11.4 days). During a 17-year period, LE KDs in the obese represented an increasing proportion, from 17% in 1995 to 2000 up to 53% in 2007 to 2012, and the eventual majority of all KDs at our institution ($P = .024$).

Conclusions.—LE KDs in obese patients are becoming increasingly prevalent. These patients are more likely to have nerve and vascular injuries and are more likely to undergo vascular repair than patients with HE trauma. The epidemic of obesity in the United States presents unique challenges in the identification and treatment of patients with LE KD and their associated injuries.

▶ The obesity epidemic in the United States has been well described, and this article highlights one of the consequences of this epidemic. Complex knee dislocations (KD) can often have devastating results, and, as this article points out, seemingly minor falls or injuries are much more likely to cause KD in the morbidly obese. Over the course of their series, the authors found that these injuries are now more frequently occurring from falls in the obese than from severe trauma. Obesity further complicates these injuries because associated nerve injuries are also more common, operative repair is more difficult, and postoperative complications are more frequent. As the radiographs in the figure show, the physiologic stress placed on the notoriously fragile knee joint by excessive bodyweight should not be underestimated, and, because prompt intervention is often required for the vascular injuries associated with complex KD, emergency department physicians, orthopedic surgeons, and vascular surgeons need increased vigilance in treating the morbidly obese.

P. White, MD, FACS

14 Venous Thrombosis and Pulmonary Embolism

Isolated calf muscular vein thrombosis is associated with pulmonary embolism and a high incidence of additional ipsilateral and contralateral deep venous thrombosis

Kret MR, Liem TK, Mitchell EL, et al (Oregon Health and Science Univ, Portland)

J Vasc Surg Venous Lymphat Disord 1:33-38, 2013

Objective.—Little is known about the natural history of isolated gastrocnemial and soleal vein thrombosis (IGSVT), and recommendations for treatment and follow-up are therefore anecdotal. This study sought to determine the rates of venous thromboembolism (VTE) progression and resolution and the effect of antithrombotic therapy in patients with IGSVT.

Methods.—A vascular laboratory database was queried from January 2002 to December 2006 to identify patients with duplex-diagnosed IGSVT and follow-up duplex scan studies. Duplex scan examinations were reviewed to determine rates of resolution and development of new ipsilateral and contralateral VTE. Records were reviewed for comorbid conditions, VTE risk factors, anticoagulation therapy, the effect of anticoagulation on resolution of IGSVT, and diagnosis of pulmonary embolism (PE) confirmed by computed tomographic angiography.

Results.—Patients with at least one follow-up duplex scan study were included in our analysis. Sixty-five limbs with isolated IGSVT were identified in 57 patients with follow-up duplex scans (mean, 2.75 studies per patient; mean follow-up, 113 days). Twenty patients (35%) received therapeutic anticoagulation after the IGSVT diagnosis. There were seven PEs, two on the same day as initial IGSVT diagnosis, and two within 1 week of diagnosis. IGSVT resolution rates by Kaplan-Meier analysis at 1 and 3 months were 20% and 41%, respectively. Eleven patients (19%) developed additional ipsilateral deep venous thrombosis (DVT; three axial calf vein thromboses and five proximal DVT) or contralateral DVT (one axial calf vein thrombosis [CVT], one IGSVT, and one proximal DVT) during follow-up. Of the eight patients who developed additional ipsilateral DVT, five also developed concurrent contralateral DVT. Overall, 14% of patients developed contralateral DVT. Median time to development of additional DVT was 10 days. Therapeutic anticoagulation was associated with DVT resolution. However, VTE recurrence was not significantly affected by age, gender, anticoagulation, oral contraceptives, known hypercoagulable states, or comorbidities (smoking, cancer, trauma, postsurgical status, renal failure, hyperlipidemia, diabetes, or cardiopulmonary abnormalities; $P > .05$).

Conclusions.—Isolated calf muscular vein thrombosis is associated with PE and a significant incidence of VTE progression. Therapeutic anticoagulation is associated with DVT resolution, but its effect on VTE recurrence was not demonstrated. Untreated patients with IGSVT should receive follow-up bilateral lower extremity venous duplex scans within 10 days of diagnosis.

▶ Management of isolated calf vein thrombosis remains controversial. Although there is growing evidence supporting benefit of therapeutic anticoagulation in patients with isolated tibial and peroneal vein thrombosis, recommendations for isolated muscular calf vein thrombosis (IGSVT) involving gastrocnemius and soleal veins remain unclear in large part because of a lack of understanding of natural history and role of anticoagulation therapy. Although this study shows that IGSVT has a significant rate of thrombus propagation, new thrombosis of the contralateral lower extremity veins, and incidence of pulmonary embolism, these observations are based on retrospective analysis of a sample population with IGSVT only. Only those patients with IGSVT who had at least one follow-up ultrasound scan were included, but timing of serial imaging was not controlled. Contrary to the observation of benefit regarding venous thrombosis resolution in patients receiving therapeutic anticoagulation, because there was no controlled-use anticoagulation, any additional therapeutic recommendations regarding anticoagulation use is indeterminate and should be reserved for properly conducted randomized, controlled investigation.

M. A. Passman, MD

Analysis of venous thromboembolic events after saphenous ablation

Benarroch-Gampel J, Sheffield KM, Boyd CA, et al (Univ of Texas Med Branch, Galveston)

J Vasc Surg Venous Lymphat Disord 1:26-32, 2013

Background.—Venous thromboembolic events after saphenous vein ablation procedures for varicose veins have been reported. Current knowledge of these events is based on single-institution studies or studies with small numbers of patients.

Methods.—The National Surgical Quality Improvement Program (NSQIP) database (2005-2009) was used to identify 3874 patients who underwent radiofrequency ablation (RFA) or endovenous laser ablation (EVLA) of the saphenous veins with or without stab phlebectomy. Outcome variables included documented postoperative deep vein thrombosis (DVT) or pulmonary embolism (PE). Bivariate and multivariate logistic regression analyses were performed to identify factors associated with venous thromboembolic events after ablation procedures.

Results.—Procedures for lower extremity varicose veins included RFA in 2897 patients (74.8%) and EVLA in 977 (25.2%). Patients who underwent RFA were more likely to be older, obese, diabetic, hypertensive, and to have undergone procedures involving more than one vein (24% vs 4%; $P < .0001$). Patients who underwent EVLA were more likely to have received general anesthesia (56.9% vs 40.8%; $P < .0001$) and to have undergone concomitant stab phlebectomy (44.9% vs 31.7%; $P < .0001$). The incidences of DVT (1.74% vs 1.52%; $P = .63$) and pulmonary embolus (0.07% vs 0%; $P > .99$) were similar between EVLA and RFA. No significant predictors of DVT in the postoperative period were identified on bivariate or multivariate analyses. In the subgroup of 2514 patients who underwent ablation procedures without stab phlebectomy, those undergoing EVLA showed a trend toward a higher incidence of DVT (2.6% vs 1.4%; $P = .057$). After adjusting for patient demographics, DVT was 2.4 times more likely to develop in patients presenting with lower extremity ulcers than in those without ulcers (odds ratio, 2.4; 95% confidence interval, 1.01-6.11; $P = .04$). Although not statistically significant, the multivariate model found that when only ablation procedures were performed, EVLA was associated with an 83% increase in odds of DVT compared with RFA (odds ratio, 1.83; 95% confidence interval, 0.95-3.52; $P = .06$).

Conclusions.—The incidence of venous thromboembolic events after saphenous ablation is low. However, given that patients with lower extremity ulcers experienced an increased risk of DVT, care should be taken to ensure that the ablation catheter is positioned an appropriate distance from the saphenofemoral or sapheno-popliteal junction and that periprocedural preventative measures, such as anticoagulation prophylaxis, early ambulation, and lower extremity compression, are emphasized. The finding of a trend toward increased venous thromboembolic events in patients undergoing EVLA warrants further investigation in a large patient population.

▶ Although this study uses the multicenter National Surgical Quality Improvement Program (NSQIP) and confirms a low incidence of thromboembolic events in patients undergoing endovenous ablation procedures for lower-extremity venous insufficiency, it is important to note that the sample population was inpatient based and included only those procedures performed by general and vascular surgeons at institutions participating in NSQIP. Because many endovenous ablation procedures are performed in outpatient centers and may include specialties other than general and vascular surgery, it is difficult to extrapolate these results to these other settings. Furthermore, as a multicenter national database, there are several additional limitations, including lack of procedural details for radiofrequency or endovenous laser, no specific data on venous thrombosis such as differentiation of deep venous thrombosis (DVT) or endothermal heat-induced thrombosis, prior DVT risk profiles, and other more granular data.

M. A. Passman, MD

Analysis of venous thromboembolic events after saphenous ablation

Benarroch-Gampel J, Sheffield KM, Boyd CA, et al (Univ of Texas Med Branch, Galveston)

J Vasc Surg Venous Lymphat Disord 1:26-32, 2013

Background.—Venous thromboembolic events after saphenous vein ablation procedures for varicose veins have been reported. Current knowledge of these events is based on single-institution studies or studies with small numbers of patients.

Methods.—The National Surgical Quality Improvement Program (NSQIP) database (2005-2009) was used to identify 3874 patients who underwent radiofrequency ablation (RFA) or endovenous laser ablation (EVLA) of the saphenous veins with or without stab phlebectomy. Outcome variables included documented postoperative deep vein thrombosis (DVT) or pulmonary embolism (PE). Bivariate and multivariate logistic regression analyses were performed to identify factors associated with venous thromboembolic events after ablation procedures.

Results.—Procedures for lower extremity varicose veins included RFA in 2897 patients (74.8%) and EVLA in 977 (25.2%). Patients who underwent RFA were more likely to be older, obese, diabetic, hypertensive, and to have undergone procedures involving more than one vein (24% vs 4%; $P < .0001$). Patients who underwent EVLA were more likely to have received general anesthesia (56.9% vs 40.8%; $P < .0001$) and to have undergone concomitant stab phlebectomy (44.9% vs 31.7%; $P < .0001$). The incidences of DVT (1.74% vs 1.52%; $P = .63$) and pulmonary embolus (0.07% vs 0%; $P > .99$) were similar between EVLA and RFA. No significant predictors of DVT in the postoperative period were identified on bivariate or multivariate analyses. In the subgroup of 2514 patients who underwent ablation procedures without stab phlebectomy, those undergoing EVLA showed a trend toward a higher incidence of DVT (2.6% vs 1.4%; $P = .057$). After adjusting for patient demographics, DVT was 2.4 times more likely to develop in patients presenting with lower extremity ulcers than in those without ulcers (odds ratio, 2.4; 95% confidence interval, 1.01-6.11; $P = .04$). Although not statistically significant, the multivariate model found that when only ablation procedures were performed, EVLA was associated with an 83% increase in odds of DVT compared with RFA (odds ratio, 1.83; 95% confidence interval, 0.95-3.52; $P = .06$).

Conclusions.—The incidence of venous thromboembolic events after saphenous ablation is low. However, given that patients with lower extremity ulcers experienced an increased risk of DVT, care should be taken to ensure that the ablation catheter is positioned an appropriate distance from the saphenofemoral or sapheno-popliteal junction and that periprocedural preventative measures, such as anticoagulation prophylaxis, early ambulation, and lower extremity compression, are emphasized. The finding of a trend toward increased venous thromboembolic events in patients undergoing EVLA warrants further investigation in a large patient population.

▶ This article, a retrospective review of the National Surgical Quality Improvement Program (NSQIP) data analyzing venous thromboembolic events (VTE) after endovenous ablation, is an excellent example of how a quality improvement database can verify results from smaller, prospective studies. That the rate of VTE following endovenous ablation is low (~1.5% incidence of deep venous thrombosis and less than 0.1% incidence of pulmonary embolism) is reassuring. Several shortcomings with the NSQIP data do exist, however. The authors convey no data on the timing of VTE, although they do describe their standard practice of obtaining a postoperative duplex ultrasound between 48 and 72 hours after surgery. This is my practice as well, but similar confirmation about the timing of VTE after endovenous ablation from a large series of patients would be valuable. The authors also found that the only risk factor for VTE appeared to be the presence of venous ulcers. The authors recommend perioperative VTE prophylaxis with low molecular weight heparin in conjunction with perioperative and postoperative compression stockings. It would be interesting to compare this treatment avenue with preoperative compression therapy until the ulcers are healed followed by endovenous ablation to prevent recurrence. Overall, this article offers useful confirmation of the low VTE incidence after endovenous ablation.

P. White, MD, FACS

Ultrasound-accelerated catheter-directed thrombolysis in acute iliofemoral deep venous thrombosis

Strijkers RHW, Grommes J, Arnoldussen CWKP, et al (Maastricht Univ Med Centre, The Netherlands; Univ Hosp RWTH Aachen, The Netherlands)
J Vasc Surg Venous Lymphat Disord 1:225-230, 2013

Background.—Iliofemoral deep venous thrombosis (DVT) is associated with a high incidence of the post-thrombotic syndrome. The current CHEST guidelines suggest that catheter-directed thrombolysis can be used for patients with acute iliofemoral DVT and severe leg complaints. Current literature shows that catheter-directed thrombolysis increases patency of the affected tract and may reduce post-thrombotic complications, but treatment time and bleeding complications are high. Ultrasound-accelerated catheter-directed thrombolysis (UACDT) uses ultrasound waves to enhance clot lysis, which should lower treatment time and bleeding complications with the same or higher patency rates. We report our clinical experience with UACDT on patency and complications in patients with acute iliofemoral DVT.

Methods.—Patients treated with UACDT for acute iliofemoral DVT were included in our analyses. Diagnosis of iliofemoral DVT was confirmed using duplex sonography and magnetic resonance venography. In addition to thrombolysis, stents were placed or an arteriovenous fistula was created to ensure patency of the treated vein, if indicated. The main outcome is patency after 1 year. Secondary outcome measures are treatment time, bleeding complications, and pulmonary embolism. Patency was assessed using duplex sonography.

Results.—In total, 37 patients (average age at intervention, 42 years; range, 5-76 years) were included. The DVT location was unilateral in 33 patients (20 left side, 13 right side), and four were bilateral. The average treatment time was 43 ± 17 hours. The success rate of thrombolysis was 95% (n = 35); re-thrombosis occurred in 11 (30%) patients. Major bleeding occurred in one patient (3%), and three minor bleedings occurred at the insertion side of the catheter (8%). One pulmonary embolism was encountered (3%). One patient had fever with positive blood cultures for *Staphylococcus aureus*. Additional procedures were required in 54% (n = 20) of patients. Primary patency was 70% at 1 year; secondary patency was 87% after 1-year follow up.

Conclusions.—UACDT of acute iliofemoral DVT is feasible and safe. Supplementary percutaneous transluminal angioplasty and stenting play an important role in preventing re-thrombosis.

▶ Although removal of clot in patients with iliofemoral deep venous thrombosis (DVT) may be beneficial in decreasing potential for postthrombotic morbidity, timing and most optimal method for removal have yet to be determined. This study shows that ultrasound-accelerated catheter-directed thrombolysis is feasible, safe, and effective in thrombus removal, and, like other studies on iliofemoral DVT, catheter therapy confirms that at least 50% of patients will have an underlying lesion that will need further treatment with angioplasty/stenting. However, in the absence of comparison with other options for catheter-directed clot removal, how this technology fits into the armamentarium of other options of pharmacologic thrombolysis and mechanical thrombectomy or prevents progression to postthrombotic syndrome remains unclear.

M. A. Passman, MD

Technical and Patient-related Characteristics Associated with Challenging Retrieval of Inferior Vena Cava Filters

Avgerinos ED, Bath J, Stevens J, et al (Univ of Pittsburgh Med Ctr, PA)

Eur J Vasc Endovasc Surg 46:353-359, 2013

Objective.—To identify patient-related and device-specific predictors of challenging and failed inferior vena cava (IVC) filter retrievals.

Methods.—Retrospective single center review of consecutive retrievable IVC filters placed between 2004 and 2009. Retrieval was defined as challenging when it was unsuccessful owing to reported technical failure or when adjunctive endovascular maneuvers or access sites were recruited. Data regarding patient- and filter-specific information were collected. Logistic regression models were used to identify predictors of the reported outcomes. Statistical significance was set at $p < .05$.

Results.—Four hundred and one patients underwent retrievable IVC filter placement—the majority indicated for prophylaxis (67%). Two hundred and fifty-nine retrievals were attempted and 237 filters were successfully retrieved (overall retrieval rate: 59.1%). Eleven out of 259 (4.2%) attempts were aborted owing to significant thrombus within the filter and 11 (4.2%) were technically unsuccessful. In 142 patients no attempt for filter retrieval was made—the major reason being physician oversight (44.3%). Thirty-eight out of 248 (15.3%) non-aborted filter retrievals were recorded as challenging. Failed retrievals were predicted by prolonged dwell time (96.9 ± 111.9 vs. 29.5 ± 25.1 days, odds ratio [OR] 1.034, 95% confidence interval [CI] 1.016–1.053, $p < .001$), therapeutic indication (OR 5.197, 95% CI 1.200–22.511, $p = .028$), and filter wall apposition (OR 11.857, 95% CI 2.069–67.968, $p = .006$). Challenging retrievals were predicted by dwell time (51.1 ± 69.8 vs. 29.1 ± 24.5 days, OR 1.017, 95% CI 1.005–1.029, $p = .007$), filter tilt (OR 2.607, 95% CI 1.045–6.508, $p = .040$) and filter wall apposition (OR 6.149, 95% CI 2.398–15.763, $p = < .001$).

Conclusions.—Physician oversight leads to poor IVC filter retrieval rates. Retrievals can be challenging or fail when the dwell time is >50 days and >90 days, respectively, and when the filter hook apposes the caval wall. Filter tilt increases retrieval difficulty but not failure rates.

▶ Inferior vena cava (IVC) filters have been receiving increased US Food and Drug Administration (FDA) scrutiny in recent years because of increasingly observed events reported to the FDA and poor retrieval rates. As a single-center study on IVC filters practice, filter retrieval rate was still low (59.1%) and attributed to physician oversights, thereby reinforcing the need for active retrieval protocol to decrease lost follow-up. Even when patients underwent filter retrieval, technical challenges were increased greater than 50 days, and success of retrieval greater than 90 days, which corresponds with other reports. Overall, this study supports the need for an active protocol for patients after filter placement and the need to remove IVC filters as soon as possible based on clinical status.

M. A. Passman, MD

Biomarkers for post-thrombotic syndrome

Bouman AC, Atalay S, ten Cate H, et al (Maastricht Univ Med Centre, The Netherlands; Flevohospital, Almere, The Netherlands)
J Vasc Surg Venous Lymphat Disord 2:79-88, 2014

Background.—Post-thrombotic syndrome (PTS) is a serious condition that occurs in 20%-50% of patients following deep venous thrombosis

(DVT). Biomarkers can be of use in further exploring the etiology as well as in developing risk stratification tools for PTS. The relationship between PTS and specific biomarkers may help guide prevention and therapy based on a patient's individual risk profile. This review gives an overview of the current knowledge on biomarkers in relation to PTS.

Methods.—A systematic search was executed in three databases (Pubmed, Embase/Medline, Cochrane) to identify all publications on biomarkers in relation to PTS. Where possible, results of studies were pooled and a meta-analysis was performed using Review Manager 5.1 (The Cochrane Collaboration).

Results.—Twenty-four papers were included in this review. In patients after DVT, increased D-dimer appeared to be associated with the development of PTS (odds ratio [OR], 2.04; 95% confidence interval [CI], 1.02-4.08; $P = .04$). Neither prothrombin G20210A (OR, 0.95; 95% CI, 0.53-1.69; $P = .86$, nor increased factor VIII (OR, 1.78; 95% CI, 0.88-3.57; $P = .11$) were associated with PTS. For factor V Leiden (FVL), conflicting results were found. FVL was not associated with PTS within a population of patients with a history of DVT (OR, 0.98; 95% CI, 0.74-1.29; $P = .88$), but FVL was positively associated with post-thrombotic ulceration in severe PTS, in patients compared with healthy individuals without a history of DVT (OR, 11.42; 95% CI, 6.37-20.48; $P < .00001$). A meta-analysis could not be performed for markers of inflammation and tissue remodelling in relation to PTS.

Conclusions.—Increased D-dimer levels are associated with a twofold increased risk for PTS. Inherited hypercoagulability, including FVL is not associated with PTS in general. In contrast, FVL is strongly associated with post-thrombotic ulceration in severe PTS. The role of inflammation in the etiology of PTS still has to be elucidated.

▶ Postthrombotic syndrome (PTS) is a chronic, and the most common, complication that can develop in patients who have suffered a deep vein thrombosis (DVT), with nearly half of these patients having the complication. There are multiple symptoms and signs of PTS including itching, cramps, tingling, heaviness, edema, and pain, and because PTS is considered to be a syndrome, there are no standard diagnostic tests available. It is thought that the symptoms of PTS arise as a result of venous stasis disturbing the microcirculation and blood supply to the lower limb; however, its pathology and pathogenesis have not been well characterized. This article is a review of all publications on biomarkers in relation to PTS, with the potential of identifying biomarkers that can be of use in further exploring the etiology, as well as in developing risk stratification tools, for PTS. Their analysis demonstrated that increased D-dimer levels are associated with a 2-fold increased risk for PTS. Inherited hypercoagulability, including factor V Leiden (FVL) is not associated with PTS in general. However, in contrast, FVL is strongly associated with postthrombotic ulceration in severe PTS. It is interesting that D-dimer, a marker intertwined in coagulation and fibrinolysis, suggests a role for hypercoagulation in these patients, whereas the other results did not indicate a significant role of hypercoagulability in the etiology of PTS. Although their systematic search of the literature reveals some interesting information on the increased D-dimer levels, it is difficult to perform such an analysis on multiple studies that do not have standardized methods and the same biomarker profiles.

J. Cullen, PhD

Factors affecting Cook Gunther Tulip and Cook Celect inferior vena cava filter retrieval success

Glocker RJ, Novak Z, Matthews TC, et al (Univ of Alabama at Birmingham)
J Vasc Surg Venous Lymphat Disord 2:21-25, 2014

Objective.—Success rates vary for the retrieval of inferior vena cava filters (IVCFs). The optimal retrieval time and factors influencing retrieval success remain unproven. This study aims to determine optimal time and evaluate factors related to successful IVCF retrieval.

Methods.—An institutional prospectively maintained database was reviewed for all IVCF retrieval attempts from 2006 to 2012. Patient demographics, comorbidities, indications for procedure, placement technique, IVCF type, presence of angulation, and time to retrieval were evaluated with respect to success or failure of retrieval. Statistical analyses (*t*-test, χ^2, correlations, and Kaplan-Meier plots) were performed comparing successful and unsuccessful retrievals.

Results.—Of 121 attempted IVCF retrievals, 92 (76%) were successful and 29 (24%) were unsuccessful. There were no significant differences between the successful and unsuccessful attempts in terms of patient demographics, comorbidities, indications for procedure, placement technique, or IVCF type, which included 93 Celect (77%) and 28 Gunther Tulip (23%). Time since IVCF placement was significantly different ($P = .025$) between the successful and unsuccessful retrieval groups (medians were 105 [7-368] and 162 [43-379] days, respectively). Time since IVCF placement greater than 117 days correlated significantly with unsuccessful IVCF retrieval (R = 0.218; $P = .017$; odds ratio, 2.88; $P = .02$). Angulation greater than 20 degrees on anteroposterior radiograph was noted in seven of 29 (24%) unsuccessful retrievals compared with seven of 92 (8%) successful retrievals and was significant ($P = .012$).

Conclusions.—Cook Gunther Tulip and Celect IVCF retrieval is most likely to be successful within 3 to 4 months of placement. Unsuccessful retrieval attempts are more likely to occur when IVCF position is angulated.

▶ The use of inferior vena cava (IVC) filters to prevent death from pulmonary embolism in our patients who cannot receive standard anticoagulation has arguably improved the care of these patients. The use of retrievable IVC filters is more controversial. On this note, the rate of successful retrieval of these filters has varied considerably. In this article from the vascular surgeons at University of Alabama at Birmingham, they attempt to detail factors affecting successful retrieval of the Cook Gunther-Tulip and Celect filters. The authors reviewed their prospectively collected data over a 6-year period. Of note the authors standardized their method of insertion, follow-up, indications for removal, and removal technique. They recorded retrieval technique, success, and other procedural details such as operating time. With this methodology, they achieved an admirable retrieval rate of 76%. This included filters placed using venography (40%) and those placed using other imaging methods such as intravascular ultrasound (40%). Factors associated with a failure to retrieve included inability to engage the retrieval hook on the apex of the filter and inability to disengage the filter from the IVC wall once the hook was successfully snared. Further analysis of these cases revealed angulation > 20 degrees on AP radiograph (24 vs 8%) and the need to use adjunctive retrieval methods such as balloon angioplasty, or a double snare technique (41 vs 3%). In addition, they had only 3 successful retrievals of 15 (20%) attempts when choosing to use these adjunctive techniques. The authors recommend the use of active follow-up methods to increase the rate of retrievability.

D. L. Gillespie, MD, RVT, FACS

The effect of matrix metalloproteinase 2 and matrix metalloproteinase 2/9 deletion in experimental post-thrombotic vein wall remodeling

Deatrick KB, Luke CE, Elfline MA, et al (Univ of Michigan Med School, Ann Arbor; et al)

J Vasc Surg 58:1375-1384.e2, 2013

Background.—Vein wall fibrotic injury following deep venous thrombosis (VT) is associated with elevated matrix metalloproteinases (MMPs). Whether and by what mechanism MMP2 contributes to vein wall remodeling after VT is unknown.

Methods.—Stasis VT was produced by ligation of the inferior vena cava and tissue was harvested at 2, 8, and 21 days in MMP2 –/– and genetic wild type (WT) mice. Tissue analysis by immunohistochemistry, enzyme-linked immunosorbent assay, real-time polymerase chain reaction, and zymography was performed.

Results.—Thrombus resolution was less at 8 days in MMP2 –/– compared with WT, evidenced by a 51% increase in VT size ($P < .01$), and threefold fewer von Willebrand's factor positive channels ($P < .05$). In MMP2 –/– mice, the main phenotypic fibrotic differences occurred at 8 days post-VT, with significantly less vein wall collagen content ($P = .013$), fourfold lower procollagen III gene expression ($P < .01$), but no difference in procollagen I compared with WT. Decreased inflammation in MMP2 –/– vein walls was suggested by ~ threefold reduced TNFα and IL-1β at 2 days and 8 days post-VT ($P < .05$). A fourfold increase in vein wall monocytes ($P = .03$) with threefold decreased apoptosis ($P < .05$), but no difference in cellular proliferation at 8 days was found in MMP2 –/– compared with WT. As increased compensatory MMP9 activity was observed in the MMP2 –/–mice, MMP2/9 double null mice had thrombus induced with VT harvest at 8 days. Consistently, twofold larger VT, a threefold decrease in vein wall collagen, and a threefold increase in monocytes were found (all $P < .05$). Similar findings were observed in MMP9 –/– mice administered an exogenous MMP2 inhibitor.

Conclusions.—In stasis VT, deletion of MMP2 was associated with less midterm vein wall fibrosis and inflammation, despite an increase in monocytes. Consideration that VT resolution was impaired with MMP2 (and MMP2/9) deletion suggests direct inhibition will likely also require anticoagulant therapy.

▶ After the formation of a deep vein thrombosis, thrombus resolution by our own intrinsic fibrinolytic mechanism is an important aspect of deep venous recanalization. The time to complete recanalization (or lysis) is important in maintaining valve function and reducing reflux-related symptoms.[1] The pathways and mechanisms involve many elements in the inflammatory, proteinases, adhesion molecules, selectins, microparticles, NETS, chemokines and cytokines, and the coagulation and the fibrinolytic cascades. Matrix metalloproteinases (MMPs), which are zinc-dependent endopeptidases and able to metabolize nearly all components of the extracellular matrix,[2] have been determined to play a critical role in experimental venous thrombus resolution.[3] In this beautiful, well-designed, and elegant study, the authors sought to determine the role of MMP-2 and MMP-9, also known as the gelatinases, in their regulation and mechanism of venous thrombus resolution, vein wall fibrosis and inflammatory remodeling, in a genetic gelatinase knockout mouse model of inferior vena cava ligation. The main findings of this study in the MMP knockout mice compared with wild-type mice at days 2 and 8, but not day 21, analyses were the following: (1) venous thrombus was greater; (2) decreased von Willebrand's factor consistent with reduction in vascular channels during venous thrombus resolution; (3) decreased vein wall collagen, specifically decreased procollagen III gene expression, and decreased tropoelastin gene expression precursor to elastin; (4) Decreased apoptosis, but no difference in cellular proliferation; (5) decreased vein wall inflammatory cytokines—specifically tumor necrosis factor and interleukin—but significant increase in vein wall monocytes; and (6) similar findings as for the MMP-2 knockout mouse were seen for double knockout MMP-2/9 or knockout MMP-9. What I find fascinating about this study's results is that in one respect, to achieve better venous thrombus resolution, MMP-2 and MMP-9 are required; however, during the remodeling phase and vein wall inflammation, the gelatinases lead to increased vein wall fibrosis (increased collagen and cytokines). More interesting, and sort of an enigma, is that the MMP genetic knockouts have a significantly higher 4-fold population of monocytes in the vein wall that are known to produce cytokines, chemokines, and MMP! However, this may also depend on the type of macrophage present, M1 (inflammatory) and/or M2 (anti-inflammatory), which future studies will assess. That there are more monocytes but yet less vein wall inflammation is striking. I see 2 important phases that are required in this model: (1) the venous luminal thrombus resolution and (2) reduction of vein wall inflammation and fibrosis. Further work in this active area of research is necessary to determine timing and appropriateness of MMP inhibitors, anticoagulation strategies, administration of inflammatory modulators, and modulation of adhesion molecule/selectins/microparticle/NETS. The ultimate goal is to decrease the morbidity associated with clinical deep venous thrombosis and the postthrombotic syndrome.

J. D. Raffetto, MD

References

1. Meissner MH, Manzo RA, Bergelin RO, Markel A, Strandness DE Jr. Deep venous insufficiency: the relationship between lysis and subsequent reflux. *J Vasc Surg.* 1993;18:596-605.
2. Raffetto JD, Khalil RA. Matrix metalloproteinases in venous tissue remodeling and varicose vein formation. *Curr Vasc Pharmacol.* 2008;6:158-172.
3. Deatrick KB, Eliason JL, Lynch EM, et al. Vein wall remodeling after deep vein thrombosis involves matrix metalloproteinases and late fibrosis in a mouse model. *J Vasc Surg.* 2005;42:140-148.

A population-based case-control study on the association between rheumatoid arthritis and deep vein thrombosis

Kang J-H, Keller JJ, Lin Y-K, et al (Taipei Med Univ Hosp, Taiwan; Taipei Med Univ, Taiwan)
J Vasc Surg 56:1642-1648, 2012

Objective.—Chronic inflammation has been associated with endothelial dysfunction and altered coagulation status. However, at the present time, the data regarding the risk for developing deep vein thrombosis (DVT) in patients with rheumatoid arthritis (RA) is still scanty and conflicted. This study aimed to explore the frequency and association of DVT with RA using a population-based dataset.

Methods.—This was a case-control study conducted in Taiwan. A total of 5193 patients with DVT were identified from the Longitudinal Health Insurance Database 2000 (LHID2000) database. In total, 20,772 controls matched with cases in terms of gender, age, and year of index date were randomly selected. We used conditional logistic regression to calculate the odds ratio (OR) for having been previously diagnosed with RA between cases and controls.

Results.—Of the total 25,965 sampled subjects, 235 (0.9%) had been previously diagnosed with RA. Seventy-seven of these previous diagnoses were found among cases (1.5%) and 158 among controls (0.8%). Conditional logistic regression analysis revealed that cases were more likely to have had prior RA than controls (OR, 1.92; 95% confidence interval [CI], 1.46-2.53; $P < .001$). After adjusting for hospitalization history, pregnancy, fracture, surgery, cancer, inflammatory bowel disease, heart failure, hypertension, diabetes, coronary heart disease, hyperlipidemia, and renal disease, there was still a significant association between DVT and prior RA (OR, 1.88; 95% CI, 1.42-2.58; $P < .001$).

Conclusions.—We found RA to be significantly associated with DVT. Appropriate management should be taken to minimize the risk of DVT in patients with RA. Further study is needed to confirm our findings.

▶ From the basic science laboratory it is clear that deep venous thrombosis (DVT) involves a complex signaling cascade with leukocytes attaching to endothelial cells, rolling, and activating with transmigration and inflammation in the venous wall. Simultaneously, endothelial prothrombotic molecules are exposed because of stasis or injury with increased circulating microparticles and tissue factor, platelets activated, and fibrin deposition beginning with thrombosis of the vessel. Several conditions are recognized to be associated with a higher risk of developing DVT, including heart failure, malignancy, fracture, major surgery, and brief periods of immobilization. Several inflammatory diseases have systemic manifestations; however, the association of inflammatory conditions and DVT is not well studied. The attribution of rheumatoid arthritis to increasing the risk of DVT is not actually known, but chronic systemic inflammatory conditions cause endothelial and coagulation dysfunction. In this large-scale, population-based, case-control study, the authors aim to determine the frequency and association of DVT with patients afflicted with rheumatoid arthritis. The study design included data obtained from the Longitudinal Health Insurance Database 2000. The database consists of all the original claims data and registration files of 1 000 000 individuals randomly sampled from the 2000 Registry for Beneficiaries of the Taiwan National Health Insurance. Cases were selected from DVT, Deep vein thrombosis; ICD-9-CM, International Classification of Disease, 9th Revision (ICD-9-CM). A total of 5193 patients, age 18 years with a first-time diagnosis of DVT who had received at least 2 diagnoses of DVT, and 20 772 controls matched with the cases in terms of gender and age in intervals of 10 years, were identified in the study. Rheumatoid arthritis cases were identified on the ICD-9-CM code 714.0, and the diagnosis of rheumatoid arthritis was made by a rheumatologist, with at least 2 diagnoses of rheumatoid arthritis on at least one antirheumatoid drug that preceded the diagnosis of DVT. There were 1.6% of patients with rheumatoid arthritis before the index date diagnosis of DVT, and 0.8% of controls with rheumatoid arthritis. After adjusting for 12 confounding variables, the association of prior rheumatoid arthritis with DVT was strong with an odds ratio of 1.88 (95% confidence interval, 1.42–2.58; $P < .001$). Interestingly, there were no adjustments for body mass index, smoking status, thrombophilia, family history of DVT or pulmonary embolism, and contraceptive use, which, the authors admit, is a limiting factor. Although there are adjustments for surgery, it is not known whether the surgery was minor or major, what the specialty of surgery was, and what the complications of the surgery were, which all have an impact in the risk of DVT development. This may be a limitation of the sampling of the health insurance database, an administrative database that is subject to coding inaccuracy and in which certain information may not be captured or is incomplete. The implications of this study are that the presence of rheumatoid arthritis increases the risk of DVT, at least in the Han Chinese population, indicating that careful prophylaxis and treatment needs to be considered. Future prospective studies, with carefully controlled variables and different ethnicities, will be required to validate this interesting retrospective case-control ICD-9-CM—based study and to determine the best prophylactic and therapeutic treatment strategies.

J. D. Raffetto, MD

Midterm results of percutaneous endovascular treatment for acute and chronic deep venous thrombosis

Stanley GA, Murphy EH, Plummer MM, et al (Univ of Texas Southwestern Med School, Dallas, TX; Univ of Pennsylvania, Philadelphia; et al)
J Vasc Surg Venous Lymphat Disord 1:52-58, 2013

Background.—Treatment of deep venous thrombosis (DVT) with therapeutic anticoagulation has been increasingly challenged by aggressive percutaneous treatment using ultrasound-accelerated catheter-directed thrombolysis (US-CDT) or percutaneous pharmacomechanical thrombectomy (PMT). These techniques have been promoted to improve thrombus removal, prolong venous patency, prevent venous insufficiency, and reduce postthrombotic syndrome. This study reviews midterm results using these endovascular techniques for both acute and chronic DVT.

Methods.—A retrospective chart review was performed on patients treated for acute or chronic DVT with US-CDT and/or PMT. Charts were reviewed for patient demographics, medical history and treatment, operative details, and postoperative outcomes. Intraoperative venography and intravascular ultrasound quantified clot response to therapy. Duplex ultrasound defined the pre- and postoperative extent of venous thrombosis, venous patency, and valvular function.

Results.—Between October 1, 2002 and September 30, 2010, 80 patients were treated for iliofemoral (n = 48), iliofemoropopliteal (n = 15), or femoropopliteal (n = 17) venous thrombosis. Mean age was 45.8 years (range, 15-78 years), and 24 patients (30%) had a documented history of hypercoagulable state. Intravascular ultrasound confirmed May-Thurner syndrome in 34 patients (42.5%). Fifty-two patients (65%) were treated for acute DVT; the mean time to intervention from symptom onset was 8.7 ± 4.5 days (range, 1-14 days). The remaining 28 patients (35%) had chronic symptoms and were treated at a mean of 8.6 ± 10.9 months (range, 1.5-36 months) after DVT diagnosis was made. Patients were treated with PMT (n = 43, 53.8%), US-CDT (n = 14, 17.5%), or both (n = 32, 28.7%). Clot lysis (>90%) was achieved in 72 of 80 patients (90%). Tenecteplase was used for all cases, and the mean dose was 8.6 ± 4.3 mg. Adjunctive procedures, including angioplasty with or without stent placement, were required in 90% (n = 47) of acute patients and in 96% (n = 27) of chronic patients (*P* = .33). Three patients (3.8%) had postoperative bleeding events requiring blood transfusion; there were no occurrences of intracranial hemorrhage or clinically significant pulmonary embolism. At a mean follow-up of 3.8 years (range, 1-8.9 years), venous patency was present in 49 of 52 acute patients (94%) and in 23 of 28

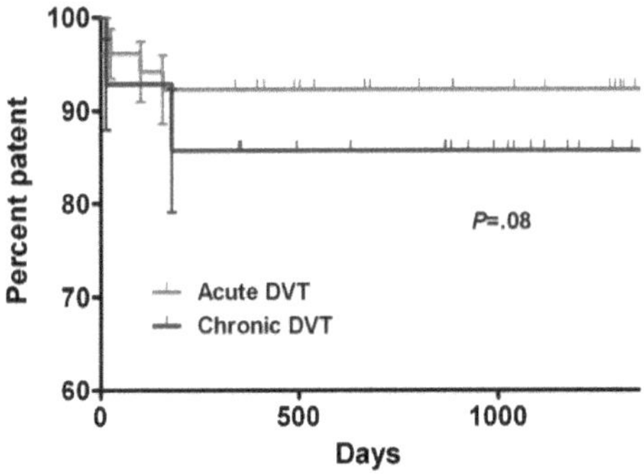

Time (days)	0	365	730	1095
Number at risk				
Acute DVT	52	48	41	37
Chronic DVT	28	23	21	12

FIGURE 2.—Kaplan-Meier life-table analysis of the vein patency after endovascular thrombus removal in patients with acute and chronic deep venous thrombosis (*DVT*). (Reprinted from Stanley GA, Murphy EH, Plummer MM, et al. Midterm results of percutaneous endovascular treatment for acute and chronic deep venous thrombosis. *J Vasc Surg Venous Lymphat Disord.* 2013;1:52-58, with permission from the Society for Vascular Surgery.)

chronic patients (82%) ($P = .12$). Valve function was preserved in 41 of 52 (79%) acute patients vs 11 of 28 (39%) chronic patients ($P < .001$).

Conclusions.—US-CDT and PMT can effectively remove acute and chronic thrombus in the lower extremity deep venous system. Vein patency and valvular function is better preserved at midterm follow-up after treatment for acute DVT, however intervention should be considered in patients with chronic DVT as well (Fig 2).

▶ Iliofemoral and femoropopliteal deep vein thrombosis can lead to the postthrombotic syndrome. The risk is much higher with iliofemoral vein thrombosis. Traditional treatment has been with anticoagulation, but more aggressive approaches with pharmacomechanical thrombolysis endovenous interventions, catheter-based interventions, and endovenous stenting with the goal of early thrombus removal and correcting the underlying intraluminal pathology or extraluminal venous compression may result in decreased postthrombotic syndrome, better functional outcome, and improved quality of life.[1] In this retrospective study, the authors evaluated their experience of endovenous treatment of acute and chronic deep venous thrombosis (DVT), with the primary end points of thrombus clearance, venous patency, and valvular function. There were 80 patients assessed, with 65% treated for acute presentation of the DVT. In this study, successful thrombus lysis, defined as greater than 90% thrombus removal, was achieved in 90% of patients, by using a combination of pharmacomechanical thrombolysis and/or ultrasound-assisted catheter-directed thrombolysis. A significant number of patients required adjunctive interventions with balloon angioplasty and/or stents (acute 90%, chronic 96%). At a mean follow-up of 3.8 years, vein patency was maintained in the acute DVT cohort in 49 of 52 patients (94%), compared with 23 of 28 patients (82%) with chronic DVT ($P = .12$; Fig 2). As one would expect, valvular patency was significantly better for patients presenting with acute thrombus than patients with chronic thrombus (79% vs 39%, $P < .001$). I find this article interesting because in their series, 35% of patients presented with chronic DVT with a mean time to presentation of 8.6 ± 10.9 months, but by applying endovenous therapies, the authors achieved very respectable results with patency; however, valvular patency was significantly worse than that of patients presenting with acute DVT. This indicates that you can also treat symptomatic patients with a history of DVT using more aggressive treatments, and these should be offered to such patients. Factors that were not clarified include Villalta scores at follow-up, patient quality of life, how many patients progressed in CEAP clinical class and Venous Clinical Severity Score, and whether the patients with chronic DVT had improved symptoms despite decreased valvular function. In fairness, though, these concerns were not the primary objectives of this study. Further research for patients with chronic venous thrombosis that will determine patient-derived outcomes is warranted, and, for acute DVT, the ATTRACT trial will hopefully help guide therapy and have a positive impact on reducing the postthrombotic syndrome with early aggressive endovenous interventions.

J. D. Raffetto, MD

Reference

1. Meissner MH, Gloviczki P, Comerota AJ, et al. Society for Vascular Surgery, American Venous Forum. Early thrombus removal strategies for acute deep venous thrombosis: clinical practice guidelines of the Society for Vascular Surgery and the American Venous Forum. *J Vasc Surg*. 2012;55:1449-1462.

Prediction of postdischarge venous thromboembolism using a risk assessment model

Iannuzzi JC, Young KC, Kim MJ, et al (Univ of Rochester Med Ctr, NY)
J Vasc Surg 58:1014-1020.e1, 2013

Objective.—The risk of postdischarge venous thromboembolism (VTE) (either deep vein or pulmonary embolism) is increasingly recognized yet the prescription of postdischarge thromboprophylaxis is inconsistent. There is a paucity of information to aid clinicians in identifying surgical patients who are at increased risk for postdischarge VTE. This study aimed to determine the incidence and risk factors associated with symptomatic postdischarge VTE and develop a risk score to identify patients who may benefit from extended duration thromboprophylaxis.

Methods.—This was a retrospective study. All nonorthopedic cases in which the patient was discharged alive without inpatient VTE were selected from the 2005-2009 National Surgical Quality Improvement Program database. A multivariate logistic regression was used to create a risk score for postdischarge VTE prediction. The dataset was split into two-thirds for risk score development and validated in the remaining one-third.

TABLE 3.—Risk Score Multivariate Model for Postdischarge VTE

	OR (95% CI)	*P* Value
Age, ≥58 years	1.38 (1.25-1.52)	<.0001
Operative time, ≥100 minutes	1.48 (1.33-1.65)	<.0001
Steroid use	2.08 (1.74-2.48)	<.0001
Functional status, dependent	1.39 (1.13-1.7)	<.0005
BMI ≥30	1.39 (1.27-1.53)	<.0001
Smoker, yes	0.84 (0.74-0.95)	<.01
Malignancy	1.29 (1.15-1.44)	<.0001
	Beta	
Postoperative major complication, 1 vs 0	0.879	<.005
Days from operation to discharge		<.0001
0	Reference	
1-3	0.3371	
4-6	1.1092	
7-8	1.3766	
9-14	1.479	
LOS* major complication		<.0001
0	Reference	
1-3	0.5705	
4-6	0.763	
7-8	−0.3384	
9-14	−0.6832	

BMI, Body mass index; *CI*, confidence interval; *LOS*, length of stay; *OR*, odds ratio; *VTE*, venous thromboembolism.

TABLE 4.—Point Scores for Postdischarge VTE

Independent Variables	Points to Add	Points for Individual Patient
Steroid use	4	
Age ≥58 years	2	
Operative time ≥ 100 minutes	2	
Dependent functional status	2	
BMI ≥30	2	
Current smoker	−1	
Days from Operation to Discharge	Major Complication	
0-1	Yes	5
	No	0
1-3	Yes	10
	No	2
4-6	Yes	12
	No	6
7-8	Yes	11
	No	8
9-14	Yes	10
	No	8
Total postdischarge risk score (sum of final column)		

BMI, Body mass index; *VTE*, venous thromboembolism.
Mark relevant points in right-hand column; final cell equals sum of the right-hand column.

Results.—The overall incidence of early postdischarge VTE for 2005-2009 National Surgical Quality Improvement Program was 0.3%. The risk score stratified patients into low, moderate, and high risk for postdischarge VTE with the incidence based on the risk score ranging from 0.07% to 2.2%. The risk score had good predictive ability with c-statistic = 0.72 for model development and c-statistic = 0.71 in the validation dataset. Factors associated with postdischarge VTE on multivariate analysis included race, increasing age, steroid use, body mass index ≥30, malignancy, higher American Society of Anesthesiologists class, increasing operative time, length of postsurgical stay, and major postoperative complication.

Conclusions.—This novel postdischarge VTE prediction score utilizes patient, operative, and early outcome factors to accurately identify patients at increased risk of a postdischarge thromboembolic event. The development of a patient-specific postdischarge VTE risk profile may help address the challenge of determining postdischarge prophylaxis requirements (Tables 3 and 4).

▶ Venous thromboembolism (VTE) is a national problem in the United States, and in September 2008, the Surgeon General had a call to action, given the high morbidity and mortality associated with VTE. The action was to highlight public awareness about the risk factors, triggering events, and symptoms of venous thrombosis and pulmonary embolism and encourage the development of evidence-based practices for screening, prevention, diagnosis, and treatment of venous thrombosis and pulmonary embolism.[1] With that theme in mind, in this important study, the authors performed a retrospective analysis using the National Surgical Quality Improvement Program data set evaluating all nonorthopedic procedures performed between 2005 to 2009 in patients discharged alive without VTE; they then analyzed patients having a VTE after discharge from the hospital and the risk factors associated with the event. The types of procedures studied were grouped as follows: (1) general surgery-intermediate cases (cholecystectomy, any hernia surgery not involving a concomitant bowel resection), (2) vascular surgery, (3) urology or gynecology, (4) thoracic surgery, (5) cardiac surgery, (6) colorectal surgery, (7) integumentary/maxillofacial/ear/nose/throat, (8) breast or endocrine, (9) upper gastrointestinal, (10) hepatobiliary/pancreas, (11) neurosurgery, and (12) spleen/lymphatics. The importance of this is that it has become apparent that the risk of VTE extends well beyond in-hospital care, and a significant number of VTE events occur after discharge. In fact several randomized clinical trials have demonstrated a reduction in VTE events with extended thromboprophylaxis use beyond the hospital period in patients at high risk for VTE.[2] The study found important predictors responsible for postdischarge VTE (Table 3), and, based on risk factors, a weighted point system was formulated to predict the probability of risk in the development of a postdischarge VTE (Table 4). They then validated within the data set one-third of the population studied. Because in this model there was poor correlation/precision with the type of surgical procedure as a variable, the type of procedure was not considered in the final model. Cancer was an independent predictor for the likelihood of postdischarge VTE, and certainly oncologic procedures would carry higher risks. Using a postdischarge VTE risk score identifies the subset of patients in whom extended postdischarge prophylaxis should be strongly considered. An advantage of this particular scoring system is that it is simple and easy to use clinically with only 8 total factors.

With any intervention, it is imperative to identify the population that will benefit from it, weigh risks versus benefits, determine the cost-effectiveness of such a treatment, and determine how many individuals need to be treated to prevent 1 postdischarge VTE. Future randomized trials may be required to answer these questions.

J. D. Raffetto, MD

References

1. Wakefield TW, McLafferty RB, Lohr JM, Caprini JA, Gillespie DL, Passman MA, Executive Committee of the American Venous Forum. Call to action to prevent venous thromboembolism. *J Vasc Surg*. 2009;49:1620-1623.
2. Bergqvist D, Agnelli G, Cohen AT, et al. Duration of prophylaxis against venous thromboembolism with enoxaparin after surgery for cancer. *N Engl J Med*. 2002;346:975-980.

The role of urokinase plasminogen activator and plasmin activator inhibitor-1 on vein wall remodeling in experimental deep vein thrombosis

Baldwin JF, Sood V, Elfline MA, et al (Univ of Michigan Med School, Ann Arbor)

J Vasc Surg 56:1089-1097, 2012

Objective.—Deep vein thrombosis (DVT) resolution instigates an inflammatory response, resulting in vessel wall damage and scarring. Urokinase-plasminogen activator (uPA) and its inhibitor, plasminogen activator inhibitor-1 (PAI-1), are integral components of the fibrinolytic system, essential for venous thrombosis (VT) resolution. This study determined the vein wall response when exposed to increased and decreased plasmin activity.

Methods.—A mouse inferior vena cava (IVC) ligation model in uPA −/− or PAI-1 −/− and their genetic wild types (B6/SvEv and C57/BL6, respectively) was used to create stasis thrombi, with tissue harvest at either 8 or 21 days. Tissue analysis included gene expression of vascular smooth muscle cells (alpha smooth muscle actin [αSMA], SM22) and endothelial marker (CD31), by real-time polymerase chain reaction, enzyme-linked immunosorbent assay, matrix metalloproteinase (MMP)-2 and -9 activity by zymography, and vein wall collagen by picro-Sirius red histologic analysis. A $P < .05$ was considered significant.

Results.—Thrombi were significantly larger in both 8-day and 21-day uPA −/− as compared with wild type (WT) and were significantly smaller in both 8-day and 21-day PAI-1 −/− as compared with WT. Correspondingly, 8-day plasmin levels were reduced in half in uPA −/− and increased three-fold in PAI-1 −/− when compared with respective WT thrombi ($P < .05$; $n = 5\text{-}6$). The endothelial marker CD31 was elevated two-fold in PAI-1 −/− mice at 8 days, but reduced 2.5-fold at 21 days in uPA −/− as compared with WT ($P = .02$; $n = 5\text{-}6$), suggesting less endothelial preservation. Vein wall vascular smooth muscle cell (VSMC) gene expression showed that 8-day and 21-day PAI-1 −/− mice had 2.3- and 3.8-fold more SM22 and 1.8- and 2.3-fold more αSMA expression than respective WT ($P < .05$; n = 5-7), as well as 1.8-fold increased αSMA (+) cells ($P \leq .05$; n = 3-5). No significant difference in MMP-2 or -9 activity was found in the PAI-1 −/− mice compared with WT, while 5.4-fold more MMP-9 was present in 21-day WT than 21-day uPA −/− ($P = .03$; n = 5). Lastly, collagen was ~two-fold greater at 8 days in PAI-1 −/− IVC as compared with WT ($P = .03$; n = 6) with no differences observed in uPA −/− mice.

Conclusions.—In stasis DVT, plasmin activity is critical for thrombus resolution. Divergent vein wall responses occur with gain or loss of plasmin activity, and despite smaller VT, greater vein wall fibrosis was associated with lack of PAI-1.

▶ Deep venous thrombus (DVT) and pulmonary embolism (PE), known together as venous thromboembolism (VTE), affect up to 900 000 individuals per year in the United States, with an estimated 300 000 deaths per year. In addition, DVT has significant consequence when the postthrombotic syndrome develops, which can affect up to one-third of patients with DVT. The understanding of DVT and VTE from a basic science perspective is complex and multifaceted. DVT resolution is dependent on many factors, which involves inflammatory cells, thrombus neovascularization, enzymatic action by metalloproteinases, cytokine and chemokine function, and vein wall remodeling. The importance of plasmin and antiplasmin activities during the sentinel events in DVT resolution is poorly understood. Currently, both the mechanism of thrombus formation and the length of contact time between the thrombus and the vein wall are believed to influence the vessel wall response and remodeling. The major plasminogen activator found in circulation is urokinase-plasminogen activator (uPA), and the major inhibitor of plasminogen activators is plasminogen activator inhibitor-1 (PAI-1). In this study, the authors hypothesized that greater plasmin activity (PAI-1 −/−) would be associated with less vein wall fibrosis, and less plasmin activity (uPA −/−) would be associated with greater fibrosis in an inferior vena cava mouse thrombosis stasis model. The major findings of this study involving uPA −/− mice vs PAI −/−, were the following in uPA −/−: (1) elevated thrombus weight at 8 and 21 days, (2) decreased plasmin level, and (3) decreased CD31 (indicator of endothelial cell presence, not injured). In PAI-1 −/−, the following were observed: (1) increased vascular smooth muscle cells (VSMC) expression and proliferation and (2) increased procollagen 1 and 3 gene expression with increased collagen content in the vein wall (indicating increased wall fibrosis). Both uPA −/− and PAI-1 −/− mice at 21 days had increased infiltration of monocytes in the vein wall compared with wild type, but no differences were observed between the 2 genetic knockout mice. These findings suggest plasmin has a critical role in thrombus formation/resolution, and that vein wall fibrosis ensues despite less thrombus formation and higher plasmin activity. What is surprising is that a larger thrombus formation, from an experimental animal stasis model, is not associated with greater vein wall damage. The explanation for this is unknown, but likely involves other factors, namely, the inflammatory response, the cytokines released, the proteinases produced, local shear stress, distension of the vein wall, and cellular elements unique in the venous thrombus. Less thrombin (as measured by TAT [thrombin-antithrombin] complex) was also observed in the uPA −/− thrombi, and thrombin has profibrotic effects. Further, less fibrinogen, per weight of thrombus, was also found in the uPA −/− thrombi, and fibrinogen may stimulate leukocyte pro-inflammatory and secondary profibrotic activities. In addition, increased VSMC proliferation occurs with lack of PAI-1 and may be caused by the known effect of PAI-1 on thrombin inhibitory activity; therefore, inhibiting PAI-1 (PAI-1 −/− model) has the adverse effect of increasing VSMC proliferation, vein wall fibrosis, and damage. Although the initial hypothesis was found to be actually the reverse (greater plasmin activity in PAI-1 −/− mice was actually associated with increased, and not decreased vein wall fibrosis), the data are extremely valuable suggesting that the thrombosis mechanism (stasis vs nonstasis model) is likely more important than the size of the thrombus itself in the vein wall injury response, and that having the same amount of monocytes in the vein wall (as determined in this study) is not the sole factor in determining vein wall damage. Thus, although PAI-1 inhibition appears attractive to reduce thrombus load, alone it is not sufficient to prevent venous wall damage (increased fibrosis), but it is important in preserving endothelial viability. To gain the full benefit of decreased thrombus and integrity of vein wall may require not only PAI-1 inhibitors but also the addition of anticoagulants such as thrombin inhibitors, as this study suggests. Further research in this fascinating disease process will be required to fully understand the magnitude and multitude of pathways in DVT formation and resolution. I congratulate this group on their tireless work to provide a better understanding of the pathophysiology of DVT with respect to the complex biologic and chemical factors involved. Further study is required to determine optimal treatment strategies, and to apply what has been learned in the basic sciences to clinical practice in an effort to reduce the morbidity and mortality associated with DVT and VTE.

J. D. Raffetto, MD

15 Chronic Venous and Lymphatic Disease

Comparing endovenous laser ablation, foam sclerotherapy, and conventional surgery for great saphenous varicose veins

Biemans AAM, Kockaert M, Akkersdijk GP, et al (Erasmus Med Ctr, Rotterdam, The Netherlands; et al)

J Vasc Surg 58:727-734, 2013

Background.—Many case series have been published on treatments of varicose veins, but comparative randomized controlled trials remain sparse.

Objective.—To compare the anatomic success rate, frequency of major complications, and quality-of-life improvement of endovenous laser ablation (EVLA), ultrasound-guided foam sclerotherapy (UGFS), and conventional surgery (CS), after 1-year follow-up.

Methods.—A total of 240 consecutive patients with primary symptomatic great saphenous vein reflux were randomized to EVLA, UGFS, or CS, consisting of high ligation and short stripping. Primary outcome was anatomic success defined as obliteration or absence of the treated vein on ultrasound examination after 1 year. Secondary outcomes were complications, improvement of the "C" class of the CEAP classification, and improvement of disease-specific (Chronic Venous Insufficiency Quality-of-Life Questionnaire) and general (EuroQol 5) quality-of-life scores.

Results.—More than 80% of the study population was classified as C2 or C3 venous disease. After 1 year, the anatomic success rate was highest after EVLA (88.5%), followed by CS (88.2%) and UGFS (72.2%) ($P < .001$). The complication rate was low and comparable between treatment groups. All groups showed significant ($P < .001$) improvement of EuroQol 5 and Chronic Venous Insufficiency Quality-of-Life Questionnaire scores after therapy; 84.3% of all treated patients showed an improvement of the "C" of the CEAP classification.

Conclusions.—After 1-year follow-up, EVLA is as effective as CS and superior to UGFS according to occlusion on ultrasound duplex. Quality of life improves after treatment in all groups significantly.

▶ As a randomized controlled trial, endovenous ablation was as effective as conventional high ligation and stripping and superior to ultrasound-guided foam sclerotherapy for the treatment of great saphenous vein (GSV) reflux based on primary end points of anatomic success defined as complete obliteration of the GSV confirmed by ultrasound at 1 year. Secondary outcomes including complications, clinical CEAP, and disease-specific quality of life assessment were improved in all groups. Although postoperative neovascularization at saphenofemoral junction was assessed, no further analysis was provided and may be part of a later follow-up study. Overall, although there may be a difference in anatomic endpoints, clinical outcomes were equivalent, which ultimately correlates with other trials showing reasonable clinical outcomes and patient satisfaction for all 3 therapies.

M. A. Passman, MD

Comparing endovenous laser ablation, foam sclerotherapy, and conventional surgery for great saphenous varicose veins

Biemans AAM, Kockaert M, Akkersdijk GP, et al (Erasmus Med Ctr, Rotterdam, The Netherlands; et al)

J Vasc Surg 58:727-734, 2013

Background.—Many case series have been published on treatments of varicose veins, but comparative randomized controlled trials remain sparse.

Objective.—To compare the anatomic success rate, frequency of major complications, and quality-of-life improvement of endovenous laser ablation (EVLA), ultrasound-guided foam sclerotherapy (UGFS), and conventional surgery (CS), after 1-year follow-up.

Methods.—A total of 240 consecutive patients with primary symptomatic great saphenous vein reflux were randomized to EVLA, UGFS, or CS, consisting of high ligation and short stripping. Primary outcome was anatomic success defined as obliteration or absence of the treated vein on ultrasound examination after 1 year. Secondary outcomes were complications, improvement of the "C" class of the CEAP classification, and improvement of disease-specific (Chronic Venous Insufficiency Quality-of-Life Questionnaire) and general (EuroQol 5) quality-of-life scores.

Results.—More than 80% of the study population was classified as C2 or C3 venous disease. After 1 year, the anatomic success rate was highest after EVLA (88.5%), followed by CS (88.2%) and UGFS (72.2%) ($P < .001$). The complication rate was low and comparable between treatment groups. All groups showed significant ($P < .001$) improvement of EuroQol 5 and Chronic Venous Insufficiency Quality-of-Life Questionnaire scores after therapy; 84.3% of all treated patients showed an improvement of the "C" of the CEAP classification.

Conclusions.—After 1-year follow-up, EVLA is as effective as CS and superior to UGFS according to occlusion on ultrasound duplex. Quality of life improves after treatment in all groups significantly.

▶ Endovenous ablative techniques using thermal energy, chemical sclerosant, and mechanochemical ablation, are common practice in the treatment of symptomatic patients with refluxing varicose great saphenous vein. The gold standard in treating the varicose great saphenous vein is high ligation and stripping; however, this technique is seldom used in modern venous clinical practice. If as clinicians we are to embrace the newer less-invasive ablative techniques in treating varicose veins, it is imperative that evidence-based trials are performed to show equivalency, safety, durability, and patient-reported outcomes. Slowly, investigators are starting to populate the literature with randomized, controlled clinical trials, by evaluating the effectiveness and patient-reported outcomes between the traditional open surgery versus endovenous methods in the treatment of varicose veins.[1] In this study, 240 patients are randomly assigned to laser ablation (ELA), ultrasound-guided foam sclerotherapy (USGFS), or conventional surgery with high ligation and stripping (CS). Most (82.3%) patients studied were of C2 (varicose veins) and C3 (edema caused by venous disease). The study primary outcome was success rate of ablative segment of the great saphenous vein at 1 year. Secondary outcomes were improvement in clinical class based on Clinical, Etiology, Anatomy, Pathophysiology (CEAP) classification, and improvement on the Chronic Venous Insufficiency quality of life (QoL) questionnaire (CIVIQ). At 1 year, the anatomic success rate was highest for ELA (88.5%) and CS (88.2%), and significantly lower for USGFS (72.7%), which is consistent with other published studies. As expected, all treatment modalities led to improvement in symptoms with 84.3% of patients improving their CEAP "C" clinical class, and there were no differences among treatment groups. Finally, treatment groups led to the improvement of their CIVIQ QoL. With regard to complications, there were no deep venous thrombosis, pulmonary emboli, or deaths; however, and as previously reported in other trials, there were increased wound complications in the CS group. A randomized, controlled trial comparing recurrences, VCSS, and QoL in patients treated with either endovenous laser ablation or ligation and stripping showed no difference in these outcomes at 2-year mid-term follow-up.[2] The 5-year long-term results are awaiting publication. A limiting factor with many of these studies is the duration of follow-up. Much of this is driven because of the novelty of using different endovenous ablative techniques, but certainly this is not an excuse to not perform trials comparing effective therapy and patient-reported outcomes. Certainly, we expect to have more data in the next 5 years that will show durability as well as patient satisfaction with newer treatment modalities for symptomatic varicose veins.

J. D. Raffetto, MD

References

1. Rasmussen LH, Lawaetz M, Bjoern L, Vennits B, Blemings A, Eklof B. Randomized clinical trial comparing endovenous laser ablation, radiofrequency ablation, foam sclerotherapy and surgical stripping for great saphenous varicose veins. *Br J Surg*. 2011;98:1079-1087.
2. Rasmussen LH, Bjoern L, Lawaetz M, Lawaetz B, Blemings A, Eklöf B. Randomised clinical trial comparing endovenous laser ablation with stripping of the great saphenous vein: clinical outcome and recurrence after 2 years. *Eur J Vasc Endovasc Surg*. 2010;39:630-635.

Increasing ablation distance peripheral to the saphenofemoral junction may result in a diminished rate of endothermal heat-induced thrombosis

Sadek M, Kabnick LS, Rockman CB, et al (New York Univ Langone Med Ctr)

J Vasc Surg Venous Lymphat Disord 1:257-262, 2013

Objective.—The treatment of venous insufficiency using endovenous laser ablation or radiofrequency ablation may result in endothermal heat-induced thrombosis (EHIT), a form of deep venous thrombosis. This study sought to assess whether increasing the ablation distance peripheral to the deep venous junction would result in a reduction in the incidence of EHIT II.

Methods.—This study was a retrospective review of a prospectively maintained database from April 2007 to December 2011. Consecutive patients undergoing great saphenous vein (GSV) or small saphenous vein (SSV) ablation were evaluated. Previous to February 2011, all venous ablations were performed 2 cm peripheral to the saphenofemoral or saphenopopliteal junction (group I). Subsequent to February 2011, ablations were performed greater than or equal to 2.5 cm peripheral to the respective deep system junction (group II). The primary outcome was the development of EHIT II or greater (ie, thrombus protruding into the deep venous system but comprising less than 50% of the deep vein lumen). Secondary outcomes included procedure-site complications such as thrombophlebitis and hematomas. χ^2 tests were performed for all discrete variables, and unpaired Student's *t*-tests were performed for all continuous variables. $P < .05$ was considered statistically significant.

Results.—A total of 4223 procedures were performed among group I (n = 3239) and group II (n = 984). Patient demographics were similar between the two groups; however, the CEAP classification was higher by a small margin in group II, and the result was significant (group I: 2.6% ± 0.9% vs group II: 2.8% ± 1.0%; $P = .006$). The incidence of EHIT II was 76 in group I and 13 in group II. This represented a trend toward diminished frequency in group II as compared with group I (group I: 2.3% vs group II: 1.3%; $P = .066$). There were no reported cases of EHIT III or IV in this patient cohort. Patients who developed an EHIT II in group I were treated using anticoagulation 54% of the time, and patients who developed an EHIT II in group II were treated using anticoagulation 100% of the time.

Conclusions.—This study suggests that changing the treatment distance from 2 cm to greater than or equal to 2.5 cm peripheral to the deep venous junction may result in a diminished incidence of EHIT II. Ongoing evaluation is required to validate these results and to affirm the long-term durability of this technique.

▶ Endothermal heat-induced thrombosis (EHIT) after endovenous laser or radiofrequency ablation is infrequent, but there is concern that EHIT II (extension into deep venous system < 50%) can lead to propagation to complete deep venous thrombosis. Although the formation of EHIT may be multifactorial, this study show a trend that increasing distance of ablation catheter from 2.0 to 2.5 cm from the saphenofemoral junction can reduce incidence of EHIT II, although this effect was not statistically significant. Although these preliminary results are of interest, as a retrospective analysis, it is difficult to determine whether increased distance is the sole factor or whether there are other considerations, and further prospective validation is needed.

M. A. Passman, MD

Minimally invasive treatment of chronic iliofemoral venous occlusive disease

de Wolf MAF, Arnoldussen CW, Grommes J, et al (Maastricht Univ Med Centre, The Netherlands; Aachen Univ Hosp, Germany)

J Vasc Surg Venous Lymphat Disord 1:146-153, 2013

Background.—As one of the primary etiologies of the postthrombotic syndrome, chronic venous occlusion is a huge burden on patient quality of life and medical costs. In this study, we evaluate the short-term and mid-term results of endovenous recanalization by angioplasty and stenting in chronic iliofemoral deep venous occlusions.

Methods.—This is a retrospective observational study set in a tertiary medical referral center. Patients with venous claudication or C4-6 venous disease combined with duplex and magnetic resonance-confirmed iliofemoral or caval occlusion were included. Patients with recent deep vein thrombosis (<1 year) were excluded. The intervention was endovascular deep venous recanalization, followed by angioplasty and stenting. Safety and feasibility were clinically evaluated during the procedure and during follow-up. Reocclusions and other treatment failures were evaluated during a maximum followup of 31 months by ultrasound imaging and venography.

Results.—Seventy-five procedures were performed in 63 patients (average age, 44 years; range, 18-75 years), of whom 86% had a history of deep venous thrombosis. The mean time between the initial deep venous thrombosis and treatment with PTA and stenting was 12 years (maximum, 31 years). May-Thurner syndrome was present in 57%. Forty-two procedures were performed in the left, six in the right, and 11 in both lower extremities. The vena cava inferior was partially stented in 25 patients. An average of 2.6 stents (median, 2) were used per procedure. Primary patency was 74% after 1 year. Assisted primary and secondary patency rates were 81% and 96%, respectively, at 1 year. Secondary procedures included restenting, catheter-directed thrombolysis, endophlebectomy of the common femoral vein, and creation of an arteriovenous fistula. No clinically evident pulmonary emboli were noted. A bleeding complication occurred after six procedures and was deemed major in two. No patients died. Relief or significant improvement of symptoms of chronic venous occlusive disease was achieved in 81% of patients.

Conclusions.—Endovenous recanalization by angioplasty and stenting of chronically occluded iliofemoral vein segments is a safe and effective treatment with good short-term results, even when treatment takes place decades after the initial deep venous thrombosis. Most reocclusions can be adequately treated by a secondary procedure.

▶ Postthrombotic iliofemoral venous occlusion can result in significant clinical venous obstructive–type complaints. Minimally invasive catheter-based techniques have been expanded and are becoming the preferred treatment for patients with significant venous disability from chronic iliofemoral venous occlusion. This retrospective study shows that endovenous recanalization followed by angioplasty and stent placement can be performed safely and result in effective relief and improvement in most patients. Although these results are short-term, they compare favorably to other published evidence and help support further aggressive catheter management as a first-line therapy in properly selected patients.

M. A. Passman, MD

Multicenter assessment of the repeatability and reproducibility of the revised Venous Clinical Severity Score (rVCSS)

Marston WA, Vasquez MA, Lurie F, et al (Univ of North Carolina, Chapel Hill; State Univ of New York at Buffalo; Jobst Vascular Inst, Toledo, OH; et al)
J Vasc Surg Venous Lymphat Disord 1:219-224, 2013

Background.—The Venous Clinical Severity Score (VCSS) was designed and validated as an objective measure of disease severity in patients with chronic venous disease (CVD). Recently, a revision of the VCSS (rVCSS) was performed to resolve ambiguity in the clinical descriptors and improve clarity and ease of use. This new revised VCSS requires validation to determine its repeatability and reproducibility in clinical evaluation of patients with varying levels of CVD.

Methods.—A prospective multicenter protocol was designed to enroll patients undergoing evaluation for CVD at venous practices with experience using the original VCSS. At the time of initial evaluation, two clinicians independently assessed both lower extremities to determine the rVCSS and the CEAP clinical score. Between 1 and 6 weeks, patients returned and received repeat assessment of the rVCSS by the same two clinicians independently. Patients were excluded if any venous intervention occurred between the two separate evaluation visits. Scores were compared to determine inter- and intra-observer variability overall and within each CEAP clinical class.

Results.—Seven centers enrolled a total of 136 limbs yielding 248 paired evaluations for interobserver variability and 258 paired evaluations for intraobserver variability. The mean interobserver rVCSS difference was 1.4 ± 1.7 and the mean intraobserver variability was 1.3 ± 1.6. Statistical assessment with weighted kappa yielded good repeatability ($\kappa = 0.68$; $P < .0001$) and good reproducibility ($\kappa = 0.72$; $P < .000001$) for the rVCSS. The rVCSS correlated well with the CEAP clinical class with significant differences between rVCSS in increasing classes. ($P < .0001$).

Conclusions.—In this multicenter evaluation, the rVCSS was demonstrated to be a reliable and reproducible instrument for documentation of the severity of symptoms in patients with lower extremity venous insufficiency.

▶ With development of the Venous Clinical Severity Score (VCSS) in 2000 as a supplement to the Clinical, Etiology, Anatomy, Pathophysiology (CEAP) classification system, came a more descriptive and dynamic system for severity of venous disease with subsequent published validation. However, because of inconsistencies in the original VCSS limiting its overall utilization, a revised VCSS (rVCSS) was proposed in 2010, with the purpose of updating terminology, simplifying application, and eliminating ambiguities. While the new system was proposed based on the expert opinion of the American Venous Forum Ad Hoc Outcomes Working Group, this is the first evidence-based validation of rVCSS. Based on this prospective multicenter study, both inter- and intraobserver variability were good thereby showing reliability and reproducibility of rVCSS. Although replacement of the original VCSS can be recommended based on the parameters in this study, additional validation is still required on the responsiveness of rVCSS to identify changes in venous clinical severity over time or based on treatment, before wider dissemination of rVCSS can be fully recommended.

M. A. Passman, MD

Clinical and anatomic outcomes of endovenous radiofrequency ablation performed on symptomatic small-diameter great saphenous veins

Perrins S, Cha A, Qaqish R, et al (Danbury Hosp, CT)
J Vasc Surg Venous Lymphat Disord 1:245-249, 2013

Objective.—The efficacy of radiofrequency ablation (RFA) for symptomatic varicose veins is well established. Alternatively, there is less consensus and little data on outcomes when treating great saphenous veins (GSV) of small diameter (≤5 mm). The purpose of this study is to assess clinical and anatomical outcomes of RFA on symptomatic patients withsmall GSV.

Methods.—A retrospective analysis was performed on our symptomatic patients who received RFA of incompetent GSV without any concomitant adjunctive procedures between January 2008 and December 2011. Limbs with GSV thigh diameter ≤5 mm and >5 mm on duplex while standing were subject to review. Clinical success was defined as an improvement in Venous Clinical Severity Score (VCSS) at 3 months. Anatomic success was defined as absence of venousflow ≤3 cm distal to the saphenofemoral junction on duplex ultrasound examination. Changes in CEAP class were noted.

Results.—In 307 patients, 55 limbs in 44 patients met inclusion criteria. Baseline median VCSS was 4 (interquartile range [IQR], 4, 5) for those patients with diameter ≤5 mm. Clinical success was seen in 83% of limbs at 3 months with a median VCSS change of −2 (IQR, −3, −1). None of the treated limbs had phlebectomy for symptomatic refluxing GSV varicosities prior to 3-month follow up. One phlebectomy was performed for cosmesis at 78 days postprocedure. Anatomic success was achieved in 96% of limbs at 3 months. Baseline median CEAP was 2 (IQR, 2, 2). The median CEAP change at 3 months was 0 (IQR, −1, 0). One patient experienced thrombus extension into the saphenofemoral junction at 4 days.

Conclusions.—In our experience, RFA of symptomatic small-diameter GSV provides comparable clinical and anatomic outcomes to that of current published data. Our findings suggest that these patients benefit clinically from RFA.

▶ Although increased-size saphenous veins have a higher propensity for reflux, there is a subpopulation of patients with small saphenous veins who still may have clinically significant reflux. Although current evidence-based guidelines for endovenous ablation suggest great saphenous veins (GSV) less than 0.2 mm as inappropriate for treatment, some insurance carriers have tried to limit coverage to patients with GSVs greater than 0.5 m. In this study, patients with documented reflux in small GSVs (0.3–0.5 mm) had comparable results with radiofrequency ablation to those with larger-diameter GSVs (>0.5 mm) based on venous outcome measures. Although there are some limitations in this retrospective analysis, this study does support the notion that endovenous ablation should not be denied by insurance carriers based on GSV diameter alone and that other clinical factors and documentation of reflux should be factored into the decision algorithm.

M. A. Passman, MD

Popliteal vein compression syndrome pathophysiology and correlation with popliteal compartment pressures

Dijkstra ML, Khin NY, Thomas SD, et al (Macquarie Univ Hosp, North Ryde, New South Wales, Australia; Macquarie Univ, North Ryde, New South Wales, Australia; Royal North Shore Hosp, St. Leonards, New South Wales, Australia; et al)

J Vasc Surg Venous Lymphat Disord 1:181-186, 2013

Objective.—The link between obesity and popliteal vein compression syndrome (PVCS) has been documented, but the pathophysiological mechanism is unclear. The aim of this study is to understand the pathogenesis of PVCS by assessing popliteal compartment pressures (PCP).

Methods.—Twenty-three limbs (15 patients) were included. Eleven limbs were ultrasonically diagnosed with PVCS and underwent popliteal vein decompression. The control group consisted of 12 limbs with functional popliteal artery entrapment. Perioperatively, PCP measurements were obtained. The body mass index (BMI) was calculated and the clinical symptoms were documented (CEAP).

Results.—The median BMI for the PVCS group was 32 (range, 26-45.8) compared with 28 (range, 19-31) for the control group ($P = .05$). In PVCS, the popliteal vein internal diameter was 9.4 mm (range, 8.0-20.0 mm) upon knee flexion, compared with 0 mm (range, 0.0-0.1 mm) upon knee extension. Upon knee flexion, there was no difference in pressure (PVCS 10.0 [range, 4-20] vs control 11.5 [range, 3-22]; $P = .95$). Upon knee extension, the median PCP in the PVCS group was 53 cm H_2O (range, 38-76 cm H_2O) compared with 26 cm H_2O (range, 17-43 cm H_2O) in the control group ($P < .001$).

Conclusions.—PVCS is associated with high popliteal compartment pressures compared with controls. The pathophysiology of popliteal obstruction, in the absence of anatomical abnormalities, is related to an increase in popliteal compartment pressure while standing due an increase of the popliteal fat pad, related to high BMI.

▶ Although an association between obesity and venous disease has been previously suggested, the role of popliteal vein compression syndrome and its correlation with popliteal compartment pressures is unclear. This small study provides some connection between popliteal vein compression observed on duplex ultrasound and increased intraoperative-measured popliteal compartment pressures, but the connection to increased popliteal fat pad related to obesity in the absence of anatomic abnormalities causing compression is soft and based on intraoperative findings during popliteal operative decompression, not physiologic evaluation. Although this study highlights an underappreciated potential syndrome, with absence of specific diagnostic criteria or physiologic venous correlation for popliteal venous compression syndrome, the clinical significance of the syndrome and the potential for treatment remain unclear.

M. A. Passman, MD

Endovenous management of venous leg ulcers

Raju S, Kirk OK, Jones TL (Rane Ctr, Jackson, MS; Univ of Florida, Gainesville)

J Vasc Surg Venous Lymphat Disord 1:165-172, 2013

Background.—Compression is the current "standard" in the treatment of venous leg ulcers, and corrective surgery is ancillary. The emergence of safe and effective minimally invasive corrective techniques prompts a reappraisal of this paradigm.

Methods.—Among 192 consecutive limbs with venous leg ulcers, 189 were treated by (1) endovenous laser ablation (n = 30), (2) iliac vein stent placement (n = 89), or (3) both (n = 69). Residual deep reflux was *not* treated. No specialized wound care was used, and 38% of patients did not use stockings. Outcome measures were time to heal the ulcer and cumulative long-term healing.

Results.—Sixty percent of the limbs were post-thrombotic. The median reflux segment score was 3 (range, 0-7). Thirty-seven percent had deep axial reflux. Median intravascular ultrasound-detected stenosis was 70% (range, 0%-100%) in stented patients. Sensitivity of venography to iliac vein obstruction was 52%. Postprocedural mortality was 0%, and 2% had deep venous thrombosis (<30 days). By 14 weeks, 81% of the small ulcers approximately ≤1 inch in diameter had healed. Larger ulcers were slower in healing ($P < .001$). Postthrombotic etiology, presence of uncorrected deep reflux, demographic factors, or stocking use had no bearing on healing time. Long-term cumulative healing at 5 years overall was 75%. Healing was better in nonthrombotic limbs compared with postthrombotic limbs (87% vs 66% at 5 years; $P < .02$) but was similar among the various demographic subsets, procedures, and whether or not patients used compression. Quality-of-life measures improved significantly. Cumulative long-term healing was unaffected by residual axial reflux and was unrelated to hemodynamic severity (air plethysmography, ambulatory venous pressure). However, longterm ulcer healing was inferior in limbs with reflux segment score of ≥3 ($P < .03$). Post-thrombotic limbs with a reflux score of ≥3 had the lowest cumulative healing among cohorts, but even in this category, 60% of limbs had durable healing with very few recurrences.

Conclusions.—Most venous leg ulcers in this consecutive series achieved long-term healing with the described minimally invasive algorithm. Uncorrected residual reflux was not an impediment to ulcer healing. Ulcers sized ≤1 inch required no specialized or prolonged wound care. Compression was not necessary to achieve or maintain healing after interventional correction.

▶ Management of venous leg ulcers requires a multimodal approach that includes primary topical ulcer wound care, compression, and more recent evolution of endovenous treatment options along with more traditional operative therapies. Although this is a retrospective study on consecutive patients, there is an underlying clinical decision algorithm that involves assessment of obstructive and reflux components and application of appropriate endovenous management: For patients with isolated iliac vein obstruction, iliac vein stenting was the primary therapy; for patients with isolated superficial saphenous vein reflux, endovenous laser ablation was performed; and for patients with both, iliac vein stenting was combined with endovenous laser. Using the described minimally invasive algorithm, most venous leg ulcers achieved healing. However, use of compression and wound dressing care was not controlled. Although uncorrected residual deep reflux did not impede ulcer healing, because the authors' algorithm did not include any primary deep venous operative treatment, this study is also somewhat limited to the endovenous perspective. As a result, the role of these endovenous techniques in a more global algorithm that includes multimodal wound care, compression, and deep and perforator venous operative therapies remains unclear.

M. A. Passman, MD

First human use of cyanoacrylate adhesive for treatment of saphenous vein incompetence

Almeida JI, Javier JJ, Mackay E, et al (Miami Vein Ctr, FL; Vein Ctr at Physicians Regional, Naples, FL; Mackay Vein Inst, St Petersburg, FL; et al)

J Vasc Surg Venous Lymphat Disord 1:174-180, 2013

Objective.—The primary objective of this study was to assess the feasibility of an endovenous cyanoacrylate (CA) adhesive implant, delivered with a catheter-based administration system engineered with a nonstick surface, for the treatment of incompetent great saphenous veins (GSVs). The primary safety end point was the rate of serious adverse events related to the procedure. The primary efficacy end point was vein occlusion during follow-up. Secondary end points included the rate of all adverse events and the change in Venous Clinical Severity Scores (VCSSs).

Methods.—Thirty-eight incompetent GSVs in 38 symptomatic patients were treated by catheter deployment of CA under ultrasound guidance via a repetitive bolus injection algorithm. By protocol design, perivenous tumescent anesthesia and compression stockings were omitted. Duplex ultrasound imaging and clinical follow-up were performed immediately after the procedure, at 48 hours, and 1, 3, 6, and 12 months.

Results.—The mean total volume of endovenous CA delivered was 1.3 ± 0.4 mL (range, 0.6-2.3 mL). Immediately after the procedure and at the 48-hour follow-up, the 38 patients (100%) demonstrated complete closure of the GSV. One complete and two partial recanalizations were observed during follow-up at 1, 3, and 6 months, respectively. Kaplan-Meier analysis yielded an occlusion rate of 92% at 12 months of follow-up. Side effects were generally mild and self-limited, most frequently, phlebitis in six patients (15.8%) requiring nonsteroidal anti-inflammatory drugs for an average of 5.7 days. Eight patients (21.1%) showed thread-like thrombus extensions into the common femoral vein of a mean length of 12.6 mm (range, 3.5-35 mm), which resolved spontaneously without anticoagulation. VCSS improved in all patients from a mean of 6.1 ± 2.7 at baseline to 1.5 ± 1.4 at 12 months ($P < .0001$). Edema improved in 34 legs (89%) at the 48-hour follow-up. At the 12-month follow-up, and without additional adjunctive treatment, 18 legs (50%) were free from visible varicosities and an additional eight legs (25%) showed limited varicosities.

Conclusions.—The first human use of endovenous CA for closure of insufficient GSVs proved to be feasible, safe, and effective. Endovenous delivery of CA may prove to be an alternative for the correction of saphenous incompetence and may be used without tumescent anesthesia and medical compression stockings.

▶ With the objective of assessing the feasibility of catheter-based administration of cyanoacrylate adhesive for treatment of incompetent great saphenous vein, this study achieved the primary end point of vein occlusion (92% at 1 year) and low secondary end points of adverse events. With feasibility, safety, and efficacy documented, use of endovenously delivered cyanoacrylate adhesive as an alternative to currently available endothermal ablation options may offer advantages of avoiding the need for tumescent anesthesia, avoiding thermal-related injuries to adjacent structures, and less potential for postoperative pain and neuropathic complaints. However, as a single-arm feasibility-designed study, additional comparative effectiveness showing at least equivalence if not superiority would need to be shown before determining the clinical role and further expansion of this technique.

M. A. Passman, MD

First human use of cyanoacrylate adhesive for treatment of saphenous vein incompetence

Almeida JI, Javier JJ, Mackay E, et al (Miami Vein Ctr, FL; Vein Ctr at Physicians Regional, Naples, FL; Mackay Vein Inst, St Petersburg, FL; et al)
J Vasc Surg Venous Lymphat Disord 1:174-180, 2013

Objective.—The primary objective of this study was to assess the feasibility of an endovenous cyanoacrylate (CA) adhesive implant, delivered with a catheter-based administration system engineered with a nonstick surface, for the treatment of incompetent great saphenous veins (GSVs). The primary safety end point was the rate of serious adverse events related to the procedure. The primary efficacy end point was vein occlusion during follow-up. Secondary end points included the rate of all adverse events and the change in Venous Clinical Severity Scores (VCSSs).

Methods.—Thirty-eight incompetent GSVs in 38 symptomatic patients were treated by catheter deployment of CA under ultrasound guidance via a repetitive bolus injection algorithm. By protocol design, perivenous tumescent anesthesia and compression stockings were omitted. Duplex ultrasound imaging and clinical follow-up were performed immediately after the procedure, at 48 hours, and 1, 3, 6, and 12 months.

Results.—The mean total volume of endovenous CA delivered was 1.3 ± 0.4 mL (range, 0.6-2.3 mL). Immediately after the procedure and at the 48-hour follow-up, the 38 patients (100%) demonstrated complete closure of the GSV. One complete and two partial recanalizations were observed during follow-up at 1, 3, and 6 months, respectively. Kaplan-Meier analysis yielded an occlusion rate of 92% at 12 months of follow-up. Side effects were generally mild and self-limited, most frequently, phlebitis in six patients (15.8%) requiring nonsteroidal anti-inflammatory drugs for an average of 5.7 days. Eight patients (21.1%) showed thread-like thrombus extensions into the common femoral vein of a mean length of 12.6 mm (range, 3.5-35 mm), which resolved spontaneously without anticoagulation. VCSS improved in all patients from a mean of 6.1 ± 2.7 at baseline to 1.5 ± 1.4 at 12 months ($P < .0001$). Edema improved in 34 legs (89%) at the 48-hour follow-up. At the 12-month follow-up, and without additional adjunctive treatment, 18 legs (50%) were free from visible varicosities and an additional eight legs (25%) showed limited varicosities.

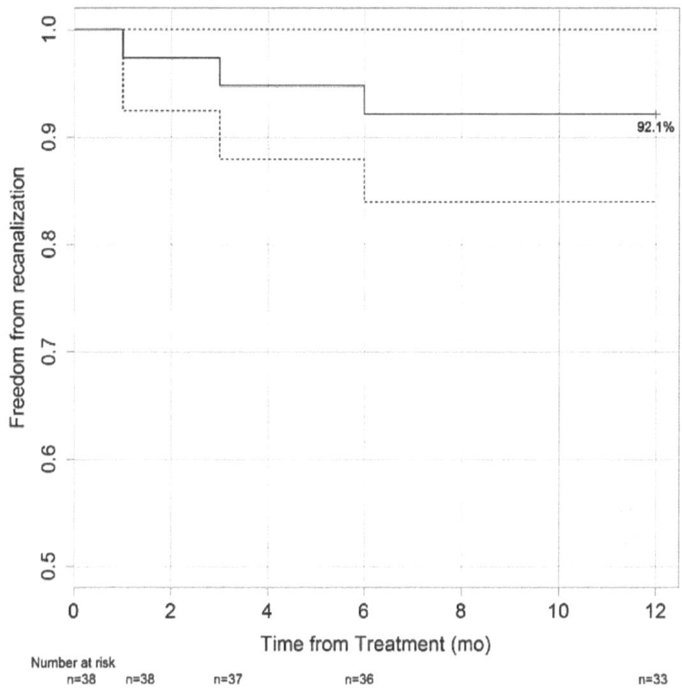

FIGURE 2.—Life-table analysis shows (**A**) freedom from any recanalization of great saphenous veins after successful cyanoacrylate embolization. The *dotted lines* show the 95% confidence intervals. Patients at risk are given below the time axis. Standard error was <5% at all times. (Reprinted from Almeida JI, Javier JJ, Mackay E, et al. First human use of cyanoacrylate adhesive for treatment of saphenous vein incompetence. *J Vasc Surg Venous Lymphat Disord.* 2013;1:174-180, with permission from the Society for Vascular Surgery.)

Conclusions.—The first human use of endovenous CA for closure of insufficient GSVs proved to be feasible, safe, and effective. Endovenous delivery of CA may prove to be an alternative for the correction of saphenous incompetence and may be used without tumescent anesthesia and medical compression stockings (Fig 2A).

▶ Endovenous ablative procedures for great saphenous vein (GSV) insufficiency are a common practice. Common procedures include endovenous laser ablation (EVLA), radiofrequency ablation (RFA), ultrasound-guided foam sclerotherapy (USGFS), and mechanochemical ablation (MOCA). Both USGFS and MOCA are tumescentless techniques, having the advantage of not requiring perivenous infiltration of locally administered anesthetic as well as a means to dissipate the heat produced by the thermal catheters. The current modalities involve thermal energy to cause endothelial-wall injury with protein denaturation with occlusion (EVLA, RFA), endothelial and wall injury by detergents acting on the wall (USGFS), or combining detergent with a mechanical component to allow further penetration of the injury into the vein wall (MOCA). Now a new treatment involves using glue—namely, endovenous administration of cyanoacrylate (CA), without the need for tumescent anesthetic. This trial is an open-label prospective clinical study, evaluating the safety and efficacy of CA.

Thirty-eight symptomatic patients underwent GSV endovenous ablation. Some important aspects from this study were that nearly half of the patients had advanced disease (C4–C6). The average preprocedure Venous Clinical Severity Score was 6.0 ± 2.7 (range, 2–17), and the mean preprocedural diameter of the GSV at the saphenofemoral junction in the standing position was 8.0 ± 2.2 mm (range, 4.1–12.0 mm). As per protocol no compression was used periprocedurally. There were 9 (21%) adverse events, including phlebitis, cellulitis, and hyperpigmentation, all of which were self-limiting. At 12-month follow-up (36 of 38 patients), the GSV occlusion rate was 92.1% (Fig 2A). Importantly, the VCSS improved in the 36 patients who were seen at 12 months with an average improvement from 6.1 ± 2.7 at baseline to 1.5 ± 1.4 ($P < .0001$). One possible advantage of the new tumescentless endovenous ablative techniques (USGFS, MOCA, CA) is that treatment of the entire refluxing GSV is possible, with negligible risk of nerve injury because no thermal energy is required. Further study with randomized trials, longer-duration follow-up, and patient-derived outcomes (quality-of-life disease-specific questionnaires) will be required, before CA can be considered a standard-of-care treatment for chronic venous disease.

J. D. Raffetto, MD

On the existence of helical flow in veins of the lower extremities

Lurie F, Kistner RL (Univ of Hawaii, Honolulu)

J Vasc Surg Venous Lymphat Disord 1:134-138, 2013

Purpose.—Helical flow has been shown to be present in the heart and arteries, but its existence in veins has not been demonstrated before. This study aimed to investigate if helical flow is present in the venous system and if the venous valves contribute to development of this flow pattern.

Methods.—Color and spectral Doppler were used to calculate the true velocity vectors at five cross-sectional planes of the femoral and common femoral veins in 10 healthy individuals and eight patients with chronic venous disease.

Results.—This study demonstrated that helical flow is a normal finding in the segments of veins that are in close proximity and downstream from a venous valve and a venous junction. This flow pattern is more prevalent when the calf muscle pump is active. Incompetence of the proximal great saphenous vein affects the outflow pattern, so that the helical flow is no longer present and is replaced by disorganized turbulent flow.

Conclusions.—These findings suggest that helical flow is detectable, may have a physiological role in venous circulation, and the absence of it may be a feature of venous disease.

▶ Although venous flow was previously assumed to be laminar in most models, diameter changes, curvatures, and junctions in venous tributaries can change laminar flow patterns, and evidence on the influence of valves on venous flow pattern is limited. This study identifies the existence of a helical flow pattern in normal vein segments that are in close proximity and downstream from the femoral vein valve and saphenofemoral junction. Prior evidence from the same authors has shown that the terminal and subterminal valves of the GSV are positioned at an angle to each other,[1] but the observation in this study of absent helical flow when the proximal valve in the great saphenous vein is incompetent suggests that the geometric shape of the saphenofemoral junction as well as the presence of a competent terminal valve at this location may be necessary to generate helical flow. The significance of these findings and whether the presence of helical flow offers some physiologic benefit has yet to be determined, but this study offers some insight into its existence, which may not only be important in understanding of the effect of venous flow disturbance but may also be useful in the future development of implantable venous valves.

M. A. Passman, MD

Reference

1. Lurie F, Kistner RL. The relative position of paired valves at venous junctions suggests their role in modulating three-dimensional flow pattern in veins. *Eur J Vasc Endovasc Surg*. 2012;44:337-340.

The relationship between increased body mass index and primary venous disease severity and concomitant deep primary venous reflux

Vines L, Gemayel G, Christenson JT (Univ of Geneva, Switzerland)

J Vasc Surg Venous Lymphat Disord 1:239-244, 2013

Background.—The role of overweight in chronic venous disease is still controversial. The aim of this study was to evaluate the impact of overweight and obesity in chronic primary venous disease in relation to disease severity, using the CEAP and the Venous Clinical Severity Score (VCSS) as well as well as body weight on the presence of concomitant primary deep venous reflux.

Material.—Between October 2005 and September 2010, 1445 consecutive patients (2023 limbs) presenting with duplex ultrasound-confirmed chronic primary venous disease and planned for intervention were evaluated from a database. The patients were classified according to CEAP, the VCSS, and body mass index (BMI; kg/m^2), using the World Health Organization definition. Concomitant primary deep venous reflux was evaluated and re-examined following eradication of the superficial reflux.

Results.—There were 636 normal weight patients (890 limbs; BMI < 25), 526 overweight patients (740 limbs; BMI 25 to 29.9), and 283 obese patients (393 limbs; BMI $\geq$ 30 kg/m^2). Overweight patients had more incompetent perforators ($P < .001$), hypertension ($P < .001$), and diabetes ($P = .019$) than normal weight patients and higher C class (CEAP classification) and VCSS ($P < .001$). Obese patients had more incompetent perforators ($P < .001$), hypertension ($P < .001$), diabetes ($P = .004$), and primary deep insufficiency ($P < .001$) than overweight patients as well as higher C class and VCSS ($P < .001$). Correlation between the C class and the VCSS was found excellent ($r = 0.80$). Obese patients had more axial reflux than the two other groups. There was no relationship between disease duration, body weight, and severity within each group. After eradication of superficial reflux, abolition of the deep reflux was lowest among obese patients (13.7%) compared with overweight patients (22.5%).

Conclusions.—There was a close relation between body weight and clinical severity of primary venous disease. Both overweight and obesity appear to be a separate risk factor for increased severity in patients with chronic primary venous disease without correlation to disease duration. CEAP and VCSS seem to accurately evaluate disease severity with an excellent correlation between the two scores. Concomitant primary deep venous reflux is more often observed in the obese patients, withless abolishment following eradication of the superficial reflux than observed for normal weight and overweight patients.

▶ This study adds to a growing body of evidence suggesting a relationship between obesity and venous disease with correlation of increased body mass index and clinically significant venous disease severity reflected by venous outcomes scoring and the presence of venous reflux on venous duplex ultrasound. However, the underlying cause of this association, whether from increased intra-abdominal pressure, decreased activity, dysfunctional calf muscle pump, or primary valvular dysfunction, remains unclear. Interestingly, after correction of underlying superficial venous reflux, deep reflux disappeared more so in normal weight patients than overweight or obese patients, implying that there is a component of persistent deep venous reflux that is independently related to the underlying increased body mass index. Although these observations are interesting, further investigation is needed to evaluate population-based association of obesity and venous disease and whether weight loss has any impact on improvement of clinically significant venous disease.

M. A. Passman, MD

Randomized clinical trial comparing endovenous laser ablation and stripping of the great saphenous vein with clinical and duplex outcome after 5 years

Rasmussen L, Lawaetz M, Bjoern L, et al (Danish Vein Ctrs, Naestved, Denmark)

J Vasc Surg 58:421-426, 2013

Objective.—This is the first randomized controlled trial with a 5-year follow-up comparing endovenous laser ablation (EVLA) with high ligation and pin-stripping in patients with great saphenous vein (GSV) incompetence.

Methods.—One hundred twenty-one consecutive patients (137 legs) with GSV incompetence were randomized to EVLA (980 nm bare fiber) or high ligation and stripping using tumescent local anesthesia with light sedation. Mini-phlebectomies were performed in all patients. The patients were examined with duplex scanning before treatment and after 12 days, and then after 1, 3, and 6 months, and yearly thereafter for up to 5 years. The primary end point was open refluxing GSV. Secondary end points were recurrent varicose veins, frequency of reoperations, Venous Clinical Severity Score, and quality of life scores (Aberdeen Varicose Vein Symptoms Severity Score and Short Form-36).

Results.—In the EVLA and stripping group, nine (Kaplan-Meier [KM] estimate, 17.9%) and four (KM estimate, 10.1%) of GSVs had open refluxing segments of 5 cm or more (ns). Clinical recurrence was recorded in 24 (KM estimate, 46.6%) and 25 (KM estimate, 54.6%), whereas reoperations were performed in 17 (KM estimate, 38.6%) and 15 (KM estimate, 37.7%) legs (ns). Venous Clinical Severity Score and Aberdeen Varicose Vein Symptoms Severity Score improved whereas Medical Outcomes Study Short Form-36 quality of life score improved in several domains in both groups with no difference between the groups.

Conclusions.—Five-year follow-up of our randomized controlled trial comparing EVLA with open surgery in patients with GSV incompetence did not show any significant difference between the two groups in primary or secondary end points, perhaps because of the small sample size. EVLA seems to be a valid alternative to open surgery.

▶ This randomized trial comparing endovenous laser ablation (EVLA) and stripping of the great saphenous vein was initiated in 2005 with previously published short-term results showing little difference in outcomes except for slightly less postoperative pain in the EVLA group,[1] and midterm results showing no difference in clinical or ultrasound recurrences.[2] Similarly, in this 5-year follow-up, there was no difference in the primary endpoint of open refluxing great saphenous vein or secondary endpoints of recurrent varicose veins, reoperations, and outcome scoring using Venous Clinical Severity Scoring and quality-of-life assessment. Combining the current study with those previously published from the same data set, a temporally related benefit can then be supported short-term, with merging of outcomes at the mid- and long-term intervals. Although this study has a small sample size and may not have been adequately powered for these long-term outcomes, the lack of difference in this study combined with the short- and mid-term reports, supports EVLA as an alternative to open stripping.

M. A. Passman, MD

References

1. Rasmussen LH, Bjoern L, Lawaetz M, Blemings A, Lawaetz B, Eklof B. Randomized trial comparing endovenous laser ablation of the great saphenous vein with high ligation and stripping in patients with varicose veins: short-term results. *J Vasc Surg*. 2007;46:308-315.
2. Rasmussen LH, Bjoern L, Lawaetz M, Lawaetz B, Blemings A, Eklöf B. Randomised clinical trial comparing endovenous laser ablation with stripping of the great saphenous vein: Clinical outcome and recurrence after 2 years. *Eur J Vasc Endovasc Surg*. 2010;39:630-635.

Compression stockings significantly improve hemodynamic performance in post-thrombotic syndrome irrespective of class or length

Lattimer CR, Azzam M, Kalodiki E, et al (Imperial College, London, UK; Ealing Hosp, Middlesex, UK)

J Vasc Surg 58:158-165, 2013

Background.—Graduated elastic compression (GEC) stockings have been demonstrated to reduce the morbidity associated with post-thrombotic syndrome. The ideal length or compression strength required to achieve this is speculative and related to physician preference and patient compliance. The aim of this study was to evaluate the hemodynamic performance of four different stockings and determine the patient's preference.

Methods.—Thirty-four consecutive patients (40 legs, 34 male) with post-thrombotic syndrome were tested with four different stockings (Mediven plus open toe, Bayreuth, Germany) of their size in random order: class 1 (18-21 mm Hg) and class II (23-32 mm Hg), below-knee (BK) and above-knee thigh-length (AK). The median age, Venous Clinical Severity Score, Venous Segmental Disease Score, and Villalta scale were 62 years (range, 31-81 years), 8 (range, 1-21), 5 (range, 2-10), and 10 (range, 2-22), respectively. The C of $C_{0\text{-}6}E_sA_{s,d,p}P_{r,o}$ was $C_0 = 2$, $C_2 = 1$, $C_3 = 3$, $C_{4a} = 12$, $C_{4b} = 7$, $C_5 = 12$, $C_6 = 3$. Obstruction and reflux was observed on duplex in 47.5% legs, with deep venous reflux alone in 45%. Air plethysmography was used to measure the venous filling index (VFI), venous volume, and time to fill 90% of the venous volume. Direct pressure measurements were obtained while lying and standing using the PicoPress device (Microlab Elettronica, Nicolò, Italy). The pressure sensor was placed underneath the test stocking 5 cm above and 2 cm posterior to the medial malleolus. At the end of the study session, patients stated their preferred stocking based on comfort.

Results.—The VFI, venous volume, and time to fill 90% of the venous volume improved significantly with all types of stocking versus no compression. In class I, the VFI (mL/s) improved from a median of 4.9 (range, 1.7-16.3) without compression to 3.7 (range, 0-14) BK (24.5%) and 3.6 (range, 0.6-14.5) AK (26.5%). With class II, the corresponding improvement was to 4.0 (range, 0.3-16.2) BK (18.8%) and 3.7 (range, 0.5-14.2) AK (24.5%). Median stocking pressure (mm Hg) as measured with the PicoPress in class I was 23 (range, 12-33) lying and 27 (range, 19-39) standing ($P < .0005$) and in class II was 28 (range, 21-40) lying and 32 (range, 23-46) standing ($P < .0005$). There was a significant but weak correlation (Spearman) between stocking interface pressure measured directly with the PicoPress and the VFI improvement (baseline VFI—compression VFI) at $r = .237$; $P = .005$. Twenty-one patients (legs) changed their preference of compression and 38% of these (8/21 patients, 9/21 legs) preferred an AK-GEC stocking.

Conclusions.—Compression significantly improved all hemodynamic parameters on air plethysmography. However, the hemodynamic benefit did not significantly change with the class or length of stocking. These results support the liberal selection of a GEC stocking based on patient preference.

▶ The value of graduated elastic compression stockings for reduced morbidity associated with postthrombotic syndrome, is not new. Yet, it is surprising how many patients are referred to vascular specialists after lower extremity deep venous thrombosis with postthrombotic complaints who are not wearing compression stockings either because they were never recommended by their primary providers or because of poor compliance by patients owing to not understanding their importance or improperly fitted or prescribed stockings. Part of this confusion may not only be lack of awareness among nonvascular providers of the importance of compression as soon as possible after deep venous thrombosis, which should extend into the chronic phase, but also confusion as to what constitutes proper graduated compression therapy. Although this study has a small sample population, the benefit of graduated elastic compression is clear across different class and lengths of stockings. This finding supports the notion that providers should not only recommend graduated compression therapy but may have more liberty to prescribe a compression stocking independent of class or length.

M. A. Passman, MD

Compression stockings significantly improve hemodynamic performance in post-thrombotic syndrome irrespective of class or length

Lattimer CR, Azzam M, Kalodiki E, et al (Imperial College, London, UK; Ealing Hosp, Middlesex, UK)

J Vasc Surg 58:158-165, 2013

Background.—Graduated elastic compression (GEC) stockings have been demonstrated to reduce the morbidity associated with post-thrombotic syndrome. The ideal length or compression strength required to achieve this is speculative and related to physician preference and patient compliance. The aim of this study was to evaluate the hemodynamic performance of four different stockings and determine the patient's preference.

Methods.—Thirty-four consecutive patients (40 legs, 34 male) with post-thrombotic syndrome were tested with four different stockings (Mediven plus open toe, Bayreuth, Germany) of their size in random order: class 1 (18-21 mm Hg) and class II (23-32 mm Hg), below-knee (BK) and above-knee thigh-length (AK). The median age, Venous Clinical Severity Score, Venous Segmental Disease Score, and Villalta scale were 62 years (range, 31-81 years), 8 (range, 1-21), 5 (range, 2-10), and 10 (range, 2-22), respectively. The C of $C_{0\text{-}6}E_sA_{s,d,p}P_{r,o}$ was $C_0 = 2$, $C_2 = 1$, $C_3 = 3$, $C_{4a} = 12$, $C_{4b} = 7$, $C_5 = 12$, $C_6 = 3$. Obstruction and reflux was observed on duplex in 47.5% legs, with deep venous reflux alone in 45%. Air plethysmography was used to measure the venous filling index (VFI), venous volume, and time to fill 90% of the venous volume. Direct pressure measurements were obtained while lying and standing using the PicoPress device (Microlab Elettronica, Nicolò, Italy). The pressure sensor was placed underneath the test stocking 5 cm above and 2 cm posterior to the medial malleolus. At the end of the study session, patients stated their preferred stocking based on comfort.

Results.—The VFI, venous volume, and time to fill 90% of the venous volume improved significantly with all types of stocking versus no compression. In class I, the VFI (mL/s) improved from a median of 4.9 (range, 1.7-16.3) without compression to 3.7 (range, 0-14) BK (24.5%) and 3.6 (range, 0.6-14.5) AK (26.5%). With class II, the corresponding improvement was to 4.0 (range, 0.3-16.2) BK (18.8%) and 3.7 (range, 0.5-14.2) AK (24.5%). Median stocking pressure (mm Hg) as measured with the PicoPress in class I was 23 (range, 12-33) lying and 27 (range, 19-39) standing ($P < .0005$) and in class II was 28 (range, 21-40) lying and 32 (range, 23-46) standing ($P < .0005$). There was a significant but weak correlation (Spearman) between stocking interface pressure measured directly with the PicoPress and the VFI improvement (baseline VFI−compression VFI) at $r = .237$; $P = .005$. Twenty-one patients (legs) changed their preference of compression and 38% of these (8/21 patients, 9/21 legs) preferred an AK-GEC stocking.

Conclusions.—Compression significantly improved all hemodynamic parameters on air plethysmography. However, the hemodynamic benefit did not significantly change with the class or length of stocking. These results support the liberal selection of a GEC stocking based on patient preference (Figs 3 and 4).

▶ Several studies have looked at the effects of compression stockings on the venous hemodynamics in the lower-extremity veins. Of interest, compression in

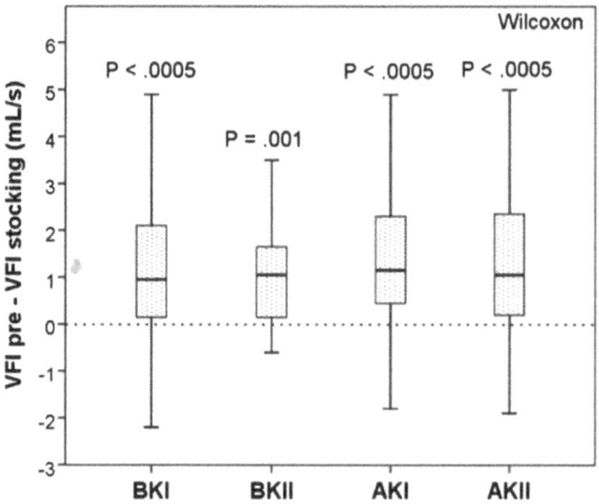

FIGURE 3.—Significant reductions in venous filling index (*VFI*) in relation to class and length of stocking. The *dashed line* represents no improvement. *AK*, Above knee; *BK*, below knee. (Reprinted from Lattimer CR, Azzam M, Kalodiki E, et al. Compression stockings significantly improve hemodynamic performance in post-thrombotic syndrome irrespective of class or length. *J Vasc Surg*. 2013;58:158-165, Copyright 2013, with permission from The Society for Vascular Surgery.)

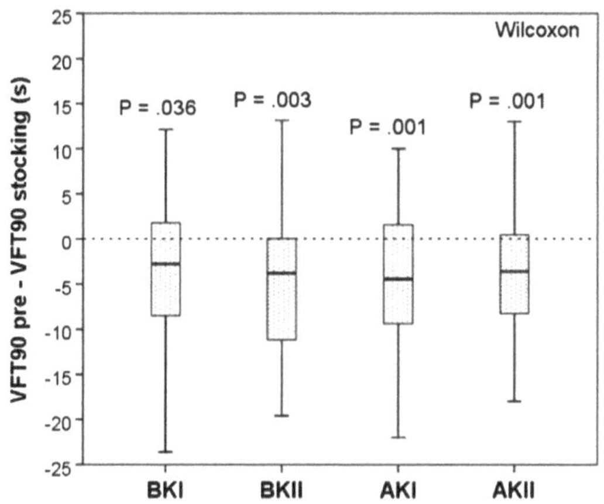

FIGURE 4.—Significant increases in venous filling time (VFT) in relation to class and length of stocking. The *dashed line* represents no improvement. AK, Above knee; BK, below knee. (Reprinted from Lattimer CR, Azzam M, Kalodiki E, et al. Compression stockings significantly improve hemodynamic performance in post-thrombotic syndrome irrespective of class or length. *J Vasc Surg*. 2013;58:158-165, Copyright 2013, with permission from The Society for Vascular Surgery.)

patients who have more advanced forms of chronic venous disease can reduce symptoms; reduce inflammation; increase venous flow; improve venous hemodynamics with respect to venous filling index, ejection fraction, and residual volume fraction as measured by air plethysmography (APG); improve calf muscle pump function; reduce edema; and reduce recurrence of venous ulceration.[1] Patients who have had deep venous thrombosis (DVT) are at risk for post-thrombotic syndrome (PTS), and many practitioners prescribe compression garments to prevent development of symptoms; several randomized trials have determined their effectiveness in reducing post-thrombotic symptoms.[2] However, the notion is that higher pressure and whole limb treated (above the knee or thigh high) may be better than lower pressure or partial limb treated (below the knee), and the effective pressure applied with compression and the type of garment (knee high or thigh high), has not been systematically evaluated in patients at risk or with PTS. In this study, the authors wanted to determine if type of compression stocking (below knee or above knee) and the dose of pressure (class I, 18–21 mm Hg or class II, 23–32 mm Hg) had an impact on venous hemodynamics measured by APG (the key parameter measured was reduction in reflux as determined by venous filling index [VFI]) and also determine the patient's preference of the type and pressure of the stocking worn. Thirty-four patients (40 limbs, 28 men) were enrolled, all of whom had DVT with postthrombotic syndrome, and 85% of limbs had advanced chronic venous disease (C4–C6). All patients had the opportunity to wear all 4 types of compression, and all had baseline hemodynamics performed without the compression and then with the compression for all types of compression stocking worn. The authors measured the applied pressure by the stocking (interface pressure) on the patients with a pressure transducer called a PicoPress that is placed near the tendinous insertion of the gastrocnemius muscle on the medial aspect of the leg, also known as the B1 position, a common place to measure stocking interface pressure on a given limb. The static stiffness index (SSI) is less than 10 (the pressure difference measured between standing and supine), which implies that the stocking is static, indicating that the pressure exerted does not change significantly from when the patients go from a supine to standing position and is a function of the textile properties of the material used in elastic compression garments. An elastic compression stocking is considered a static material as opposed to a short stretch bandage or inelastic compression garment in which the SSI would be greater than 10, indicating that the interface pressure would increase on standing. The interesting findings of this study were that the VFI improved significantly (Fig 3), and the venous filling time increased significantly (Fig 4) regardless of the type and pressure of the stocking, and there was a clear preference of the type of compression stocking. Importantly, there was no statistical difference between the magnitude of improvement between stockings. This indicated that stocking length and pressure applied were unrelated variables in reducing reflux. Interestingly, there was also a preference, in that 52.5% patients indicated they wanted to change their compression, and 38% of these preferred an above-the-knee stocking. When considering a compression stocking in patients with PTS, the adage that stronger compression and higher length will give the best hemodynamic results, appears not so true anymore, and a class I is equally effective as a class II, as knee high is as effective as thigh compression at improving venous hemodynamics! Finally, we should consider what the patient's preference is with regard to the length of the stockings preferred, because in reality, and based on the data presented in this report, there is no advantage of a full-length compression versus a partial knee-high compression.

J. D. Raffetto, MD

References

1. Christopoulos DG, Nicolaides AN, Szendro G, Irvine AT, Bull ML, Eastcott HH. Air-plethysmography and the effect of elastic compression on venous hemodynamics of the leg. *J Vasc Surg*. 1987;5:148-159.
2. Prandoni P, Lensing AW, Prins MH, et al. Below-knee elastic compression stockings to prevent the post-thrombotic syndrome: a randomized, controlled trial. *Ann Intern Med*. 2004;141:249-256.

Contemporary results after sapheno-popliteal bypass for chronic femoral vein occlusion

Coleman DM, Rectenwald JE, Vandy FC, et al (Univ of Michigan Cardiovascular Ctr, Ann Arbor)

J Vasc Surg Venous Lymphat Disord 1:45-51, 2013

Background.—Chronic occlusion of the femoral or the proximal popliteal vein responsible for venous obstruction and the constellation of clinical sequelae that ensue remains a surgical challenge that carries notable patient morbidity. Saphenopopliteal bypass (SPB) remains a surgical reconstructive option for select patients that demonstrate patency of the popliteal vein, great saphenous vein, saphenofemoral junction, and iliac veins. We sought to analyze our single-institution experience with this technique.

Methods.—A retrospective review of a single-center experience with SPB was performed. Preoperative risk factors and indications for intervention (ie, venous claudication, ulceration) were identified. Duration of follow-up and endpoints, including clinical improvement, wound healing, patency, and limb loss were assessed. A Kaplan-Meier analysis for primary and secondary patency was performed.

Results.—Seventeen patients underwent SPB for chronic lower extremity venous obstruction between July 1988 and August 2011. Median age at operation was 41 years (range, 23-69 years). There was a male predominance noted (n = 12; 71%). All patients had chronic edema and venous claudication. Five patients (29%) had evidence of venous ulceration preoperatively. Eight patients (47%) underwent a preceding venous intervention (ie, iliac stenting or venous thrombolysis). Three patients had a concomitant arteriovenous fistula, created at the time of bypass to enhance in-flow; three patients underwent concomitant femoral-femoral venous bypass. Four patients (24%) experienced hematoma postoperatively that required operative evacuation; in two patients, compression from this hematoma resulted in early graft occlusion. After a median follow-up of 103 months (range, 3-271 months), 82% of patients experienced near or complete resolution of venous claudication. Three of the five patients with venous ulceration healed their wounds (67%). Of the 16 patients that underwent Duplex scan follow-up, primary patency after a median follow-up of 103 months was 56%, primary-assisted patency was 69%, and secondary patency was 75%. One patient required amputation approximately 21 years after SPB and there were no deaths. This secondary patency rate exceeds previously published patency rates.

Conclusions.—SPB may be indicated for certain patients with chronic venous stasis disease secondary to femoral venous obstruction that have failed other standard therapies. SPB remains a satisfactory and reliable procedure that produces clinical improvement in a selected group of patients and should be considered in a contemporary venous surgical practice.

▶ Over the past decade, we have seen a resurgence of interest in the treatment of venous disease. This has occurred in the treatment of both superficial and deep venous disease. Percutaneous stenting for obstructive iliofemoral venous lesions is becoming commonplace and standard of care. It is tempting to apply the same logic and techniques to the femoral vein. Unfortunately, we have excellent data on how the profunda femoral vein becomes the major outflow tract for the lower extremity in cases of femoral vein occlusion, and we have few data on patients who are symptomatic. This small series from the University of Michigan provides some data on this exact population. This single-center retrospective review reports on 17 patient data collected over a 23-year period. All patients had chronic edema and venous claudication. In this case, all patients were treated using saphenopopliteal venous bypass. With 103 months of follow-up, the authors were able to show a primary patency rate of 56%, primary assisted patency rate of 69%, and a secondary patency rate of 75%. In addition, the authors report a 67% rate of ulcer healing. From these data, we can clearly see that some patients do not get enough outflow from their profunda vein alone to remain asymptomatic. We must await further reports to see if other studies can find a larger population of patients who are symptomatic from femoral vein occlusion to analyze the effects of percutaneous stenting. Clearly, however, femoral venous stenting at this time remains controversial.

D. L. Gillespie, MD, RVT, FACS

Analysis of the Association Between an Insertion/Deletion Polymorphism Within the 3′ Untranslated Region of *COL1A2* and Chronic Venous Insufficiency

Jin Y, Xu G, Huang J, et al (Suzhou Municipal Hosp, Jiangsu, China)
Ann Vasc Surg 27:959-963, 2013

Background.—Chronic venous insufficiency (CVI) is a common cause of leg pain and swelling and is commonly associated with varicose veins. It has significant socioeconomic consequences and is among the most common problems encountered in surgical practice. Although our current understanding of the pathogenesis of CVI is far from clear, there is a growing body of evidence suggesting a genetic contribution to the etiology of CVI.

Methods.—By analyzing 254 CVI cases and 508 healthy controls in a Chinese population, we used a candidate gene approach to evaluate the association between a 7–base pair insertion/deletion (indel) polymorphism (rs3917) in the 3′ untranslated region (3′UTR) of the alpha-2 type I collagen gene (*COL1A2*) and CVI susceptibility. Logistic regression was used to analyze the association between rs3917 and CVI risk, adjusted for sex and age. Computational modeling was used to predict potential molecular mechanisms underlying the association.

Results.—Logistic regression analysis revealed that subjects carrying indel or deletion/deletion genotypes had a significantly increased risk for CVI than individuals carrying insertion/insertion genotypes (adjusted odds ratio, 1.64; 95% confidence interval [CI], 1.10–2.45; $P = 0.010$). Carrying the 7–base pair deletion allele was associated with a 1.60-fold risk for CVI (95% CI, 1.11–2.31; $P = 0.008$). Computational modeling suggests that the rs3917 insertion allele lies within a predicted binding site (seed region) for microRNA-382 and that the deletion allele alters the affinity of microRNA–mRNA binding by disrupting the local structure of COL1A2 mRNA, presumably allowing for upregulated COL1A2 expression.

Conclusions.—Taken together, our data suggest that common genetic variations in *COL1A2* may influence CVI risk, possibly through microRNA-382–mediated regulation. Replication of our studies in other populations will strengthen our understanding of this association.

▶ Varicose veins, the most common manifestation of chronic venous insufficiency (CVI), represent one of the most common vascular conditions in the adult population and can affect 1 of 2 people aged 50 and older. Despite their prevalence and enormous burden on health, the mechanism of their formation remains unclear, and there are no effective therapies for preventing or healing them. Many lines of evidence suggest a genetic role in the etiology of CVI, and it has been estimated that the additive genetic component is approximately 17%. In addition, multiple studies have shown that alterations and remodeling of connective tissues occur in these patients. Vessel wall remodeling, associated with an increase in thick and disorganized collagen bundles and altered collagen synthesis by dermal fibroblasts, has been shown in patients with varicose veins. Based on the fact that a 7-base pair (bp) insertion/deletion (indel) polymorphism (rs3917) was identified in the 3′ untranslated region of *COL1A2*, which encodes for type I collagen and was shown to be associated with hepatocellular carcinoma susceptibility, the present study examined the association between the 7-bp indel polymorphism and CVI susceptibility. They analyzed 254 CVI cases and 508 healthy controls and demonstrated that carrying the 7-bp deletion allele was associated with a 1.60-fold greater risk for CVI. Although this study was conducted only on a Chinese population and there are significant genetic differences in different populations for different polymorphisms, the potential of using rs3917 as a target could be of potential use in the management of varicose veins.

J. Cullen, PhD

In vivo assessment of endothelial function in human lower extremity arteries

Kashyap VS, Lakin RO, Feiten LE, et al (Univ Hosps, Cleveland, OH; Cleveland Clinic, OH)
J Vasc Surg 58:1259-1266, 2013

Objective.—Endothelial function has been measured in preclinical studies in human brachial and coronary arteries but not in lower extremity arteries affected by atherosclerosis. We describe a novel, first-in-man evaluation of endothelial function of the superficial femoral arteries (SFAs) in patients with peripheral arterial disease (PAD).

Methods.—Enrolled were 25 patients with PAD requiring lower extremity angiography. Endothelial-dependent relaxation was measured using intravascular ultrasound (IVUS) imaging and a Doppler flow wire after the infusion of acetylcholine (Ach). IVUS-derived virtual histology of the same vessel was calculated. Endothelial-independent relaxation was measured with an infusion of nitroglycerin (200 μg). Levels of nitric oxide and serum nitric oxide metabolites were determined by laboratory analysis.

Results.—Patients (48% male; mean age, 62 years) had a history of hypertension (80%), coronary disease (36%), and diabetes (40%). The mean SFA diameter was 5.2 ± 1 mm (range, 3.2-6.9 mm). Patients tolerated Ach infusion with no adverse events. Endothelial-dependent relaxation increased over baseline for all patients with Ach infusion of 10^{-6} to 10^{-4}. At Ach 10^{-4}, diameter (0.5%) and area (1.8%) changes in the diseased SFAs were modest and insignificant; however, average peak velocity of blood flow significantly increased 26%, 46%, and 63% with an Ach 10^{-6} to 10^{-4} infusion. Calculations of limb volumetric flow (68% at Ach 10^{-4}) were significantly increased after Ach infusion. Lower extremity nitric oxide levels were slightly lower than systemic venous levels ($P = .04$). Nitroglycerin infusion indicated normal smooth muscle responsiveness (3% diameter, 9% area, and 116% velocity change over baseline). IVUS-virtual histology plaque stratification indicated predominantly fibrous morphology (46%; necrotic core, 29%; calcium, 18%). Atheroma burden was 14.9 ± 5.5 mm^3/cm and did not correlate with endothelial responsiveness.

Conclusions.—Endothelial function can be measured directly in human lower extremity arteries at the sites of vascular disease. Despite extensive atherosclerosis, endothelial function is still intact. These data support the application of regional endothelial-specific biologic therapies in patients with PAD.

▶ The vascular endothelium serves as an autocrine and paracrine organ that regulates vascular wall function by controlling vasomotor tone and preventing atherosclerosis and thrombosis. For years, endothelial function has been measured in human brachial and coronary arteries; however, given that peripheral artery disease (PAD) affects approximately 20% of Americans aged 65 and older, it is surprising that endothelial function in the lower extremity arteries has never been investigated. This article describes a novel assay using a combination of angiography, intravascular ultrasound, a flow wire, and infusion of endothelial agonists. This approach directly allows quantification of endothelial function and assessment of atherosclerosis in the same area and is the first-in-human approach to allow further understanding of endothelial dysfunction in patients with PAD by correlating endothelial function in vivo to the morphology of arterial plaque and systemic risk factors. Surprisingly, their results demonstrated that volumetric flow increases in the limb with acetylcholine infusion and nitric oxide are present despite extensive atherosclerosis and suggest that endothelial function does not correlate with degree of plaque burden or plaque morphology. Given the small number of patients in this trial and the surprising results, further studies are warranted using this novel in vivo approach to assessing endothelial function in lower extremities.

J. Cullen, PhD

Cyanoacrylate glue for the treatment of great saphenous vein incompetence in the anticoagulated patient

Lane TRA, Kelleher D, Moore HM, et al (Charing Cross Hosp, London, UK)
J Vasc Surg Venous Lymphat Disord 1:298-300, 2013

The Sapheon Venaseal Closure System (Sapheon Inc, Santa Rosa, Calif), using cyanoacrylate glue, has provided a new modality of treatment, with patients treated without both tumescent anesthesia and postoperative compression. We present the first case of great saphenous vein occlusion performed using glue while the patient was fully anticoagulated with warfarin. This was tolerated well, and the treated vein showed complete early occlusion at 8 weeks; however at 6 months, extensive recanalization was demonstrated on duplex imaging.

▶ Endovenous ablative procedures for great saphenous vein insufficiency are a common practice. These procedures include endovenous laser ablation (EVLA), radiofrequency ablation (RFA), ultrasound guided foam sclerotherapy (USGFS), and mechanochemical ablation (MOCA). Both USGFS and MOCA are nontumescent techniques, with the advantage of not requiring perivenous infiltration of locally administered anesthetic or a means to dissipate the heat produced by the thermal catheters. The current modalities involve thermal energy that creates endothelial wall injury and protein denaturation with occlusion (EVLA, RFA), endothelial and wall injury by detergents acting on the wall (USGFS), or combining the use of detergent with a mechanical component to allow further penetration of the injury into the vein wall (MOCA). Now a new treatment involves using glue—namely, cyanoacrylate.

This case report describes treatment of a patient with advanced varicose veins (C4bs, Venous Clinical Severity Score [VCSS] 14), significant reflux, and large-diameter (15 mm) great saphenous vein. The patient was on anticoagulation therapy for atrial fibrillation. Technically, the procedure described is not difficult; it requires infusion of the glue while maintaining occlusion of the proximal great saphenous vein 2 cm distal to the saphenofemoral junction by placement of the ultrasound probe. As with the other endovenous ablative techniques, the cyanoacrylate glue endovenous administration procedure can be performed while the patient remains on anticoagulation. At 8-week follow-up, and as expected, the patient's symptoms improved; his VCSS dropped to 7, and the vein remained occluded on ultrasound.

With any new technique, long-term follow-up is important to determine the effectiveness of the procedure. The authors did see this patient again at 6 months, and unfortunately, his symptoms recurred, with increased edema, increase of VCSS to 10, and recanalization and reflux of the great saphenous vein. The patient underwent another treatment, this time with foam sclerotherapy.

Before we can embrace endovenous cyanoacrylate ablation for treating varicose veins, additional randomized trials may be required, with patient-centered outcomes and the common surrogate end points. However, it may be difficult to justify a large-scale multicenter randomized controlled trial comparing cyanoacrylate glue to other accepted and well-established endovenous modalities because these ablation techniques have proven as effective as traditional ligation and stripping, showing midterm results with excellent patient-reported outcomes.[1]

J. D. Raffetto, MD

Reference

1. Rasmussen LH, Lawaetz M, Bjoern L, Vennits B, Blemings A, Eklof B. Randomized clinical trial comparing endovenous laser ablation, radiofrequency ablation, foam sclerotherapy and surgical stripping for great saphenous varicose veins. *Br J Surg*. 2011;98:1079-1087.

HMGB1 and TLR4 mediate skeletal muscle recovery in a murine model of hindlimb ischemia

Sachdev U, Cui X, Tzeng E (Univ of Pittsburgh Med Ctr, PA)
J Vasc Surg 58:460-469, 2013

Background.—We have previously shown that the danger signal high-mobility group box 1 (HMGB1) promotes angiogenesis when administered to ischemic muscle. HMGB1 signals through Toll-like receptor 4 (TLR4) as well as the receptor for advanced glycation end-products (RAGE). However, the actions of these receptors in ischemic injury and muscle recovery are not known. We hypothesize that TLR4 mediates tissue recovery and angiogenesis in response to ischemia.

Methods.—Femoral artery ligation was performed in control, TLR4 competent (C3H/HeOuJ) and incompetent (C3H/HeJ) mice, as well as RAGE knockout mice and their C57B6 control counterparts. In other experiments, control mice were pretreated with anti-HMGB1 neutralizing antibody before femoral artery ligation. After 2 weeks, limb perfusion was evaluated using laser Doppler perfusion imaging and reported as the ratio of blood flow in the ischemic to nonischemic limb. Muscle necrosis, fat replacement, and vascular density in the anterior tibialis muscle were quantified histologically. In vitro, TLR4 and RAGE expression was evaluated in human dermal microvascular endothelial cells in response to hypoxia. Human dermal microvascular endothelial cells treated with HMGB1 alone and in the presence of anti-TLR4 antibody were probed for phosphorylated extracellular signal-regulated kinase (ERK), a signaling molecule critical to endothelial cell (EC) angiogenic behavior.

Results.—Both anti-HMGB1 antibody as well as defective TLR4 signaling in HeJ mice resulted in prominent muscle necrosis 2 weeks after femoral artery ligation. Control HeOuJ mice had less necrosis than TLR4 incompetent HeJ mice, but a greater amount of fat replacement. In contrast to control C3H mice, control C57B6 mice demonstrated prominent muscle regeneration with very little necrosis. Muscle regeneration was not dependent on RAGE. While vascular density did not differ between strains, mice with intact RAGE and TLR4 signaling had less blood flow in ischemic limbs compared with mutant strains. In vitro, EC TLR4 expression increased in response to hypoxia while TLR4 antagonism decreased HMGB1-induced activation of extracellular signal-regulated kinase.

Conclusions.—Both HMGB1 and TLR4 protect against muscle necrosis after hindlimb ischemia. However, muscle regeneration does not appear to be tied to vascular density. HMGB1 likely activates angiogenic behavior in ECs in vitro, and this activation may be modulated by TLR4. The improvement in blood flow seen in mice with absent TLR4 and RAGE signaling may suggest anti-angiogenic roles for both receptors, or vasoconstriction induced by TLR4 and RAGE mediated inflammatory pathways.

▶ Peripheral artery disease causes significant functional disability and can result in limb loss within 6 months of diagnosis in 25% to 40% of patients who present with nonreconstructable disease. Some patients benefit from medical therapies that promote perfusion and muscle recovery. The growth of new vessels, by angiogenesis and arteriogenesis, is essential after ischemia; however, the signaling pathways involved are complex and not well characterized. Therefore, to identify potential therapeutic targets, it is important to characterize the signals that stimulate neovascularization and muscle regeneration to improve limb salvage rates. High-mobility group box-1 (HMGB1) is a ubiquitous nuclear protein that can be released by both necrotic and stressed cells in response to hypoxia and other insults and that signals through toll-like receptors (TLR) as well as the receptor for advanced glycation end-products (RAGE). This study evaluated the roles of HMGB1, TLR4, and RAGE in promoting neovascularization and muscle regeneration after limb ischemia using a murine hindlimb ischemia model. Their results demonstrate that TLR4 and HMGB1 appear to play a role in muscle protection and regeneration after muscle ischemia, and muscle regeneration is not dependent on angiogenesis. In addition, RAGE and TLR4 may mediate cutaneous vasoconstriction after injury, which may, in part, be a consequence of actions on endothelial and perivascular cells. The identification of the mechanisms involved in neovascularization and muscle regeneration is important in the management of peripheral artery disease, and given the high rate of limb loss, the potential of pharmacologic therapy using HMGB1/TLR4 as a target could be useful in the management of this disease process.

J. Cullen, PhD

Association between n-3 polyunsaturated fatty acid content of red blood cells and inflammatory biomarkers in patients with peripheral artery disease

Grenon SM, Conte MS, Nosova E, et al (Univ of California, San Francisco; et al)
J Vasc Surg 58:1283-1290, 2013

Objective.—The n-3 polyunsaturated fatty acids are dietary components derived from fish oil with beneficial cardiovascular effects that may relate in part to anti-inflammatory properties. Peripheral artery disease (PAD) is characterized by a marked proinflammatory state. We hypothesized that the n-3 polyunsaturated fatty acids content of red blood cells (omega-3 index) would be correlated with biomarkers of inflammation and vascular function in a PAD cohort.

Methods.—This was a cross-sectional study of subjects who presented to an outpatient vascular surgery clinic for evaluation of PAD. We used linear regression to evaluate the independent association between the omega-3 index, inflammatory biomarkers (C-reactive protein [CRP], intercellular adhesion molecule-1, interleukin-6, and tumor-necrosis-factor-α) and endothelial function (brachial artery flow mediated dilation).

Results.—64 subjects (61 claudicants and three with critical limb ischemia) were recruited for the study. The mean CRP level was 5.0 ± 5.0 mg/L, and the mean omega-3 index was 5.0% ± 1.8%. In an unadjusted model, the omega-3 index was negatively associated with CRP (38% increase in CRP for one standard deviation decrease in the omega-3 index; $P = .007$), which remained significant after adjustment for age, body mass index, smoking, ankle-brachial index, and high-density lipoprotein (33%; $P = .04$). There was also evidence for independent associations between the omega-3 index and IL-6 ($P = .001$). There were no significant associations between the omega-3 index and vascular function tests.

Conclusions.—In a cohort of patients with PAD, the omega-3 index was inversely associated with biomarkers of inflammation even after adjustment for covariates including the ankle-brachial index. Because patients with PAD have a high inflammatory burden, further studies should be conducted to determine if manipulation of omega-3 index via dietary changes or fish oil supplementation could improve inflammation and symptoms in these patients.

▶ Peripheral artery disease (PAD) affects approximately 20% of Americans aged 65 and older. Inflammation has been shown to play an important role in the initiation and progression of PAD, and increased circulating levels of proinflammatory makers, including C-reactive protein (CRP), have been demonstrated in patients with PAD. Indeed, inflammation has become a predictor of increased mortality in these patients. n-3 polyunsaturated fatty acids (PUFAs), which are found in fish oils, have been shown to decrease the production of inflammatory cytokines and adhesion molecules and can also improve endothelial function. The omega-3 index is a measure of the red blood cell (RBC) content of the 2 major long-chain n-3 PUFAs and is a valid marker of tissue n-3 PUFA content. In addition it is a strong reflection of dietary intake and an independent, graded risk factor for death from coronary artery disease (CAD). Proposed omega-3 index risk zones are high risk, $< 4\%$; intermediate risk, 4% to 8%; and low risk, $> 8\%$.

The present study examined the mean omega-3 index in a PAD cohort and correlated these values with biomarkers of inflammation and vascular function. The mean omega-3 index of the cohort of 64 subjects was 5.0% ± 1.8%, which actually places them at intermediate risk of death from CAD; however, one-third of the group's omega-3 indices fell in each of the 3 risk zones. Interestingly, the patients in the high-risk group were more likely to have been younger, have had history of smoking, and have a greater depression burden. There was also a significant inverse association between the omega-3 index and inflammation as measured with CRP and interleukin-6 which suggests that diet could play an important role in the inflammatory profile of patients with PAD based on their circulating proinflammatory biomarkers levels. These results are extremely interesting and, given that PAD affects such a large percentage of the population, the ability to manipulate the inflammatory pathways associated with it by simple dietary changes could be a favorable approach to the management of this disease.

J. Cullen, PhD

Cost analysis of endovenous catheter ablation versus surgical stripping for treatment of superficial venous insufficiency and varicose vein disease

Lin JC, Nerenz DR, Migliore P, et al (Henry Ford Hosp, Detroit, MI; Henry Ford Health System, Detroit, MI)

J Vasc Surg Venous Lymphat Disord 2:98-103, 2014

Background.—Due to its clinical efficacy and faster recovery, endovenous catheter ablation has become the treatment of choice over surgical intervention for patients with varicose veins secondary to saphenous vein reflux.

Methods.—A retrospective analysis of costs was performed on patients undergoing vein stripping, endovenous radiofrequency ablation (RFA), endovenous laser treatment (EVLT), and phlebectomy of varicosities at a community hospital and a tertiary care hospital in southeastern Michigan.

Results.—In 2010 to 2011, higher costs resulted in a net loss per case for vein stripping, RFA, and phlebectomy procedures performed in the operating room for the community hospital. In contrast, RFA, EVLT, and phlebectomy procedures performed in an office setting resulted in a net profit for the tertiary care institution.

Conclusions.—Treatment of saphenous vein reflux and varicose vein disease with vein stripping was associated with higher costs than RFA and EVLT. Endovenous RFA performed in the operating room is associated with net loss per case vs office-based interventions. At present, catheter-based interventions in an office setting can be considered the more cost-effective method for treating patients with superficial venous reflux and varicose veins (Tables 2 and 7).

▶ Endovenous ablative procedures for great saphenous vein insufficiency are a common practice. Although many endovenous procedures (endovenous laser ablation [EVLA], radiofrequency ablation [RFA], ultrasound-guided foam sclerotherapy [USGFS], mechanochemical ablation, and also ligation and stripping [HLS]) are performed in an office-based setting, the cost-effectiveness of such a procedure has not been appropriately tested. In this study, the authors sought to

TABLE 2.—Selected Treatment Strategies for Varicose Veins Evaluated in the Study

Strategy	CPT Code	Treatment Modality	Type of Hospital	Location	Type of Anesthesia
A	37722	HL&S of GSV	Tertiary	OR	General or regional
B	37722	HL&S of GSV	Community	OR	General or regional
C	36475	RFA	Tertiary	Office	Local
D	36475	RFA	Community	OR	General or IV sedation
E	36478	EVLT	Tertiary	Office	Local
F	37765	Phlebectomy	Tertiary	Office	Local
G	37765	Phlebectomy	Community	OR	General or regional

CPT, Current Procedural Terminology; *EVLT*, endovenous laser treatment; *GSV*, great saphenous vein; *HL&S*, high ligation and stripping; *IV*, intravenous; *OR*, operating room; *RFA*, radiofrequency ablation.

TABLE 7.—Comparison of Net Profit or Loss for Operating Room (OR)-Based Procedures vs Office-Based Procedures

	OR-Based Community Hospital			Office-Based Tertiary Hospital			
CPT Procedure	36475 RFA	37722 Stripping	37765 Phlebectomy	36475 RFA	36478 EVLT	37765 Phlebectomy	37766 Phlebectomy
2010 $	(1123)	(798)	(1370)	845	835	931	978
2011 $	(496)	(585)	(362)	1011	711	1217	2137

CPT, Current Procedural Terminology; *EVLT*, endovenous laser treatment; *RFA*, radiofrequency ablation.

determine from a retrospective analysis what is the cost-effectiveness of hospital-based versus office-based venous procedures for superficial venous disease. Importantly, cost-effectiveness is a critical outcome when comparing different modalities for treatment of varicose vein disease, especially in the current health care era of rising medical expenses. This is a retrospective analysis evaluating the costs of patients undergoing HLS, endovenous EVLA, and RFA between January 2010 and December 2011 at both tertiary and community-based hospitals and office-based versus hospital-based setting. The authors came up with 7 strategies, based on common procedural code terminology code, procedure type (HLS, EVLA, RFA, phlebectomy), hospital setting (community vs hospital), location of the procedure (operating room vs office), and anesthesia used (local vs general/regional; Table 2). Higher operating costs per case were consistently seen in vein stripping ($4280, $5626), RFA ($4884, $6267), and phlebectomy ($5458, $5910) performed in the operating room, compared with RFA ($1074, $1464), EVLT ($1534, $1402), and phlebectomy ($3217, $2463) performed in the office during the years 2010 and 2011, respectively. Higher operating costs resulted in net losses in procedures performed in the operating room at community hospitals, and in contrast, office-based procedures resulted in net positive profits for EVLA, RFA, and phlebectomy in both 2010 and 2011 (Table 7). This article is important for its careful cost analysis of common procedures performed for varicose veins and its demonstration that both RFA or EVLT performed under tumescent anesthesia in an office-based setting are more cost-effective and yield a higher net contribution margin for the institution. In addition, because of additional risks of general or regional anesthesia and the higher costs associated with the use of the operating room, operating room procedures for varicose veins cannot be justified in the current model of reimbursement. As the authors state, "In our current health care environment, physicians and hospital administrators should find ways to lower the costs of health care delivery without sacrificing patient care." How true and profound this statement is if we are to save our current health care system!

J. D. Raffetto, MD

Multicenter assessment of the repeatability and reproducibility of the revised Venous Clinical Severity Score (rVCSS)

Marston WA, Vasquez MA, Lurie F, et al (Univ of North Carolina, Chapel Hill; State Univ of New York at Buffalo; Jobst Vascular Inst, Toledo, OH; et al)

J Vasc Surg Venous Lymphat Disord 1:219-224, 2013

Background.—The Venous Clinical Severity Score (VCSS) was designed and validated as an objective measure of disease severity in patients with chronic venous disease (CVD). Recently, a revision of the VCSS (rVCSS) was performed to resolve ambiguity in the clinical descriptors and improve clarity and ease of use. This new revised VCSS requires validation to determine its repeatability and reproducibility in clinical evaluation of patients with varying levels of CVD.

Methods.—A prospective multicenter protocol was designed to enroll patients undergoing evaluation for CVD at venous practices with experience using the original VCSS. At the time of initial evaluation, two clinicians independently assessed both lower extremities to determine the rVCSS and the CEAP clinical score. Between 1 and 6 weeks, patients returned and received repeat assessment of the rVCSS by the same two clinicians independently. Patients were excluded if any venous intervention occurred between the two separate evaluation visits. Scores were compared to determine inter- and intra-observer variability overall and within each CEAP clinical class.

Results.—Seven centers enrolled a total of 136 limbs yielding 248 paired evaluations for interobserver variability and 258 paired evaluations for intraobserver variability. The mean interobserver rVCSS difference was 1.4 ± 1.7 and the mean intraobserver variability was 1.3 ± 1.6. Statistical assessment with weighted kappa yielded good repeatability ($\kappa = 0.68$; $P < .0001$) and good reproducibility ($\kappa = 0.72$; $P < .000001$) for the rVCSS. The rVCSS correlated well with the CEAP clinical class with significant differences between rVCSS in increasing classes. ($P < .0001$).

Conclusions.—In this multicenter evaluation, the rVCSS was demonstrated to be a reliable and reproducible instrument for documentation of the severity of symptoms in patients with lower extremity venous insufficiency.

▶ The Venous Clinical Severity Score (VCSS) is a useful and easy-to-use tool to assess the severity of disease and to determine how different therapies affect the VCSS. The Venous Severity Score (VSS) was developed to provide an objective measure of disease severity. It is an important tool for assessing longitudinal changes in chronic venous disease with treatment or when comparing different modalities of treatment. The VSS was designed to complement the CEAP classification by integrating elements from CEAP. Components of the VSS include the VCSS, which is the most widely used component, the Venous Segmental Disease Score (VSDS), and the Venous Disability Score (VDS). The original VCSS has been evaluated in clinical practice and validated as an important instrument with low variability for longitudinal research to assess outcomes after treatment.[1] In addition, it is an important instrument to use in daily practice, as was determined in a large series of patients undergoing endovenous radiofrequency ablation.[2] The VCSS is composed of 10 descriptors (pain, varicose veins, edema, pigmentation, inflammation, induration, number of ulcers, duration of ulcers, size of ulcers, compressive therapy) that escalate in severity with increased area of the limb involved and are graded 0 to 3 (absent, mild, moderate, severe). To provide clarification of the terms, less ambiguity, and better definition of the descriptors, a revised VCSS (rVCSS) was developed.[3] An important aspect of any instrument used in the assessment of disease severity and clinical outcomes is the validation of that instrument, so that the measured effects are specific to the disease being studied. In this article, the authors sought to validate the rVCSS, as was done for the original VCSS. The authors, from a multicenter study, found that the rVCSS was reliable and reproducible, had excellent interobserver variability (reproducibility) and intraobserver variability (repeatability), and correlated well with increasing clinical class in CEAP, indicating that patients with more advanced disease had higher VCSS scores, and hence increased severity of disease. The rVCSS has the 3 important and useful elements for clinical practice: 1) it is an objective measurement; 2) it includes all severities of chronic venous disease; and 3) it can be rapidly and efficiently performed by the clinician. Future studies should evaluate the responsiveness of the rVCSS, which would determine how well it is able to identify changes in a patient's clinical severity over time or after treatment.

J. D. Raffetto, MD

References

1. Meissner MH, Natiello C, Nicholls SC. Performance characteristics of the venous clinical severity score. *J Vasc Surg*. 2002;36:889-895.
2. Vasquez MA, Wang J, Mahathanaruk M, Buczkowski G, Sprehe E, Dosluoglu HH. The utility of the Venous Clinical Severity Score in 682 limbs treated by radiofrequency saphenous vein ablation. *J Vasc Surg*. 2007;45:1008-1014.
3. Vasquez MA, Rabe E, McLafferty RB, et al. American Venous Forum Ad Hoc Outcomes Working Group. Revision of the venous clinical severity score: venous outcomes consensus statement: special communication of the American Venous Forum Ad Hoc Outcomes Working Group. *J Vasc Surg*. 2010;52:1387-1396.

Compression Stockings after Endovenous Laser Ablation of the Great Saphenous Vein: A Prospective Randomized Controlled Trial

Bakker NA, Schieven LW, Bruins RMG, et al (Univ Med Ctr Groningen, The Netherlands; Scheper Hosp Emmen, The Netherlands)
Eur J Vasc Endovasc Surg 46:588-592, 2013

Objectives.—To determine if the duration of wearing compression stockings after endovenous laser ablation (EVLA) of the great saphenous vein (GSV) has influence on pain and quality of life.

Methods.—This was a prospective randomized controlled trial. Between December 2006 and February 2008, 109 consecutive patients with EVLA of the GSV were analyzed. Deep vein insufficiency, ulceration, more than one insufficient vein in one leg, and use of anticoagulants were exclusion criteria. Group A used compression stocking for 48 hours after therapy, group B for 7 days. Pain (visual analogue scale [VAS]) and quality of life (SF-36) were analyzed 48 hours, 1 week, and 6 weeks after therapy. Three months after treatment, duplex ultrasound imaging was performed to assess occlusion rates.

Results.—Both groups (group A, $n = 37$; group B, $n = 32$) where comparable at baseline. After 1 week, there was a significant difference in pain (VAS score 3.7 [±2.1] vs. 2.0 [±1.1], $p \leq .001$), and physical dysfunction (group A, 85.1 [±11.2] vs. group B, 95.7 [±10.1]; $p < .001$) as well as vitality (group A, 75 [±13.0] vs. group B, 83.7 [±13.4]; $p = .03$), all in favor of group B, which disappeared after 6 weeks. After 6 weeks, no significant differences in all endpoints were present. Duplex ultrasound imaging revealed complete GSV occlusion in all patients, while no cases of deep venous thrombosis had developed.

Conclusions.—Prescribing compression stockings for longer than 2 days after endovenous GSV ablation (without simultaneous phlebectomies) leads to reduced pain and improved physical function during the first week after treatment.

▶ Compression stockings are widely used in the treatment of chronic venous disorders. Their effectiveness has been shown in caring for patients with venous ulcers and to reduce ulcer recurrence. In addition, data on reducing the post-thrombotic syndrome appears to favor the use of compression versus no compression; however, the latter indication has recently been challenged in a randomized, controlled trial.[1] Nevertheless, even less is known about compression after endovenous procedures. It is common clinical practice for several compression modalities with different bandages followed by compression stockings to be applied after various types of endovenous ablative therapies. However, there are very little data to support a beneficial effect of compression for longer periods (beyond 48–72 hours after the procedure) in reducing pain and swelling. Although intuitive, it makes sense that longer duration of compression therapy after endovenous treatments of varicose veins would reduce symptoms related to the procedure itself, but needed are studies that show this with specified clinical endpoints. In this study, the authors evaluate 2 groups of patients undergoing endovenous laser ablation therapy for great saphenous vein insufficiency but without any concomitant ambulatory phlebectomies, or sclerotherapy. In group A, the patients wear compression stockings for 48 hours, whereas in group B, the patients wear compression stocking for 7 days. The compression applied was 35 mmHg, the entire lower extremity was treated (thigh high), and patients were instructed to wear them continually day and night until removal. The outcomes assessed are pain, physical dysfunction, and vitality. At the 1-week evaluation, patients wearing the compression for 1 week had improved physical function, vitality, and pain on the SF-36 and improved pain scores on visual analog scores. These differences were no longer apparent at 6-week follow-up. What is interesting in this study is that the dressing after the laser ablation was the full-length compression stocking and no other bandaging. It appears that in patients undergoing endovenous ablation of the great saphenous vein without any other concomitant procedures may benefit from compression stocking wear for an additional week after the surgery, with improved pain and physical function and vitality scores. It may be practical to adopt such a strategy, as many patients in the United States are advised to wear compression therapy before ablative procedures for varicose veins, hence, not adding much additional cost as long as they already have a full-length lower extremity compression garment.

J. D. Raffetto, MD

Reference

1. Kahn SR, Shapiro S, Wells PS, et al. Compression stockings to prevent post-thrombotic syndrome: a randomised placebo-controlled trial. *Lancet.* 2014;383: 880-888.

A plasma oxidative stress global index in early stages of chronic venous insufficiency

Condezo-Hoyos L, Rubio M, Arribas SM, et al (Universidad Autónoma de Madrid, Spain; Clínica Vascular Zurbano, Madrid, Spain)
J Vasc Surg 57:205-213, 2013

Background.—Chronic venous insufficiency (CVI) represents a social and health care problem because it affects working age populations, particularly in jobs requiring orthostasis, has no effective pharmacologic treatment, and requires surgery. Oxidative stress is present in varicose veins, but whether this is reflected in the plasma is controversial. We aimed to quantify plasma oxidative stress biomarkers in the early stages of CVI and calculate a global index of oxidative stress representative of the disease.

Methods.—Plasma was obtained from blood samples of nine patients with CEAP C_2 stage CVI and 10 healthy controls. Biomarkers related to antioxidant defense systems (total thiols, reduced glutathione, uric acid, total antioxidant capacity, catalase), oxidative damage (malondialdehyde-bound protein, protein carbonyls, advanced oxidation products, and 3-nitrotyrosine), and activity of enzymes producing key free radicals (xanthine oxidase and myeloperoxidase) were assessed.

Results.—Compared with the controls, CVI patients exhibited decreased catalase activity and thiol levels and increased malondialdehyde-bound protein and protein carbonyls. These parameters were used to calculate the global index of oxidative stress in CVI, which was significantly different between groups.

Conclusions.—It is possible to detect significant changes in plasma oxidative stress biomarkers in early stages of CVI and to calculate a global index representative of the oxidative status in an individual. This index, with the appropriate validation in a larger population, could be used for early detection or progression of CVI (Table).

▶ Chronic venous disease affects millions of individuals in Western and industrialized countries. Early disease, such as varicose veins, is a very common

TABLE.—Individual Standardized Parameters and the Indexes Calculated From Them in Patients With Chronic Venous Insufficiency and Controls

	Standardized variables				Index[a]		
Group	Log catalase activity	Protein carbonyls	Log protein-bound MDA	Total thiols	ANTIOX	OXY	OXyVen
Controls	−1.309	0.304	−1.444	−0.532			
(n = 10)	1.134	1.466	0.324	1.482			
	0.727	−0.238	1.561	−0.053			
	0.204	−1.023	−1.267	0.587			
	−1.890	−0.404	−0.206	1.838	0.000 (0.570)	0.000 (0.407)	0.000 (0.548)
	0.669	−0.149	−0.088	−0.028			
	−0.204	−1.919	−0.913	−0.998			
	0.785	1.023	0.619	−0.863			
	−0.669	0.857	1.208	−0.606			
	0.553	0.083	0.206	−0.828			
Patients	−2.123	4.319	2.386	−0.733			
(n = 9)	−2.673	4.175	2.033	−0.789			
	−1.250	2.173	1.090	−1.099			
	−2.007	8.268	−0.088	−1.420	−2.996[b] (0.841)	6.499[b] (0.203)	−9.495[b] (0.692)
	−1.832	5.281	1.326	−1.856			
	−1.948	4.728	1.620	−0.087			
	−2.763	8.732	1.915	−0.952			
	−1.716	3.091	2.799	−1.173			
	−1.658	2.848	1.797	−0.884			

ANTIOX, Antioxidant defense systems; *MDA*, malondialdehyde; *OXY*, protein oxidative damage; *OXyVen*, Oxidative Stress Global Index of chronic venous inssuficiency.
[a]Index values are expressed as mean (standard error of the mean).
[b]$P < .0001$ respect to controls.

disorder with unknown cause(s); however, genetic, physiologic, hemodynamic, and environmental factors all have a role. Currently, the mainstay of treatment for symptomatic varicose veins includes compression, pharmacologic venotonics, surgical, and endovenous therapies. Interestingly, not all patients who have varicose veins have symptoms referable to the disease, and an important aspect from both proper patient selection and cost effectiveness would be to identify patients with early venous disease who are at risk for progression. In this interesting study, the authors quantify plasma oxidative stress biomarkers that might already be changed in patients at early stages of chronic venous disease (clinical classification as CEAP C2, n = 9) compared with healthy controls (n = 10). Biomarkers that are studied are related to antioxidant defense systems (eg, thiols, reduced glutathione, catalase), and those involved with oxidative damage are related to proteins (eg, malondialdehyde [MDA]—bound protein, protein carbonyls) and activity of enzymes producing key reactive oxygen radicals (xanthine oxidase and myeloperoxidase). The elegance of this study is that the analysis of these oxidative stress markers is that they are easily measured with standard laboratory techniques; therefore, they are appealing in the clinical setting. The final product is a global index of oxidative stress related to early stages of chronic venous disease, called *OXyVen*, which is the mean difference of antioxidant defense systems (ANTIOX) and protein oxidative damage (OXY) (closer to 0 indicates balanced antioxidative/oxidative state, whereas the greater the deviation from control value the greater the global oxidative damage in the individual). The study determined that there was a decrease in plasma total thiols and catalase and increased damage to proteins by elevated levels of MDA and plasma carbonyls but no difference in enzyme related to production of reactive oxygen species in patients with varicose veins. There was a significant statistical difference in ANTIOX, OXY, and OXyVen between patients and control participants. The controls were balanced between oxidative and antioxidative processes (OXyVen = 0.00), while patients had significantly higher oxidative processes (OXyVen = −.49, Table). Several limitations of this study should be pointed out. The sample size for the patients with disease is only 9, and therefore further validation studies are required to show that increased oxidative index is indeed a characteristic of venous disease clinically. The disease patients have early venous disease, namely, varicose veins; therefore, generalizations that these findings apply to the spectrum of chronic venous disease cannot be made. As is well known, as the spectrum of chronic venous disease increases (skin changes and venous ulcers), the patients are also older. This is associated with other inflammatory conditions, including cardiovascular disease, tobacco use, and medication use. All of these factors may influence the oxidative stress of the individual, and therefore the utility of a OXyVen may be most applicable to early venous disease (as performed in this study), in which fewer metabolic stresses are present and decrease confounders, making the applicability of oxidative stress index appealing in guiding clinical severity of varicose veins, disease progression, and treatment.

J. D. Raffetto, MD

Postoperative pain and early quality of life after radiofrequency ablation and mechanochemical endovenous ablation of incompetent great saphenous veins

van Eekeren RRJP, Boersma D, Konijn V, et al (Rijnstate Hosp, Arnhem, The Netherlands; St Antonius Hosp, Nieuwegein, The Netherlands)

J Vasc Surg 57:445-450, 2013

Objective.—Thermal ablative techniques of varicose veins carry a risk of heat-related complications, including postoperative pain. Mechanochemical endovenous ablation (MOCA) might avoid these complications and reduce postoperative pain because of the absence of thermal energy. This study evaluated postoperative pain and quality of life after radiofrequency ablation (RFA) and MOCA for great saphenous vein (GSV) incompetence.

Methods.—Sixty-eight patients with unilateral GSV incompetence were treated with either RFA or MOCA in this prospective observational study. Patients monitored their pain for the first 14 postoperative days on a 100-mm visual analog scale (VAS). They also completed the general (RAND 36-Item Short-Form Health Survey) and disease-specific (Aberdeen Varicose Vein Questionnaire) quality of life questionnaires before and 6 weeks after treatment.

Results.—Patients treated with MOCA reported significantly less postoperative pain than patients treated with RFA during the first 14 days after treatment (4.8 ± 9.7 mm vs 18.6 ± 17.0 mm; $P < .001$) (mean VAS over 14 days). The lower postoperative pain score was associated with a significantly earlier return to normal activities (1.2 ± 1.8 vs 2.4 ± 2.8 days; $P = .02$) and work resumption (3.3 ± 4.7 vs 5.6 ± 5.8 days, respectively; $P = .02$). At 6 weeks, patients in both groups perceived an improved change in health status and an improved disease-specific quality of life.

Conclusions.—MOCA is associated with significantly less postoperative pain, faster recovery, and earlier work resumption compared with RFA in the treatment of GSV incompetence. MOCA and RFA are both related to a rapid improvement in quality of life (Fig 2).

▶ Endovenous therapies have become the mainstay of treatment for varicose veins and the refluxing great saphenous vein. The common treatment modalities to perform endovenous ablations involve laser, radiofrequency (RFA), and foam sclerotherapy. Laser and RFA utilize thermal energy to induce venous ablation, and both require tumescent anesthetic, whereas foam sclerotherapy does not. Although there are disadvantages with thermal ablation techniques (postoperative pain, superficial phlebitis, ecchymosis) and the use of tumescent anesthesia,

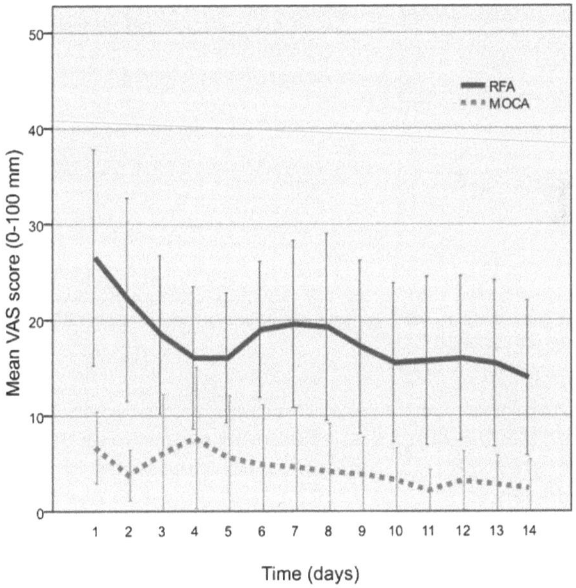

FIGURE 2.—Mean postoperative pain scores on a 0 to 100 mm visual analogue scale for 14 days after mechanochemical endovenous ablation (*MOCA*) and radiofrequency ablation (*RFA*). *CI*, Confidence interval; *VAS*, visual analog scale. (Reprinted from the Journal of Vascular Surgery. van Eekeren RRJP, Boersma D, Konijn V, et al. Postoperative pain and early quality of life after radiofrequency ablation and mechanochemical endovenous ablation of incompetent great saphenous veins. *J Vasc Surg*. 2013;57:445-450, Copyright 2013, with permission from the Society for Vascular Surgery.)

including pain and possible nerve paresthesias, the attractive aspect of foam is that it avoids these problems. However, foam sclerotherapy has increased failure rates of 16.3% of treated patients at 1-year follow-up vs 4% to 6% for laser and radiofrequency ablations, despite all modalities showing improved quality of life (QOL) at 1 year, but foam allows patients to return to normal activity sooner than laser ablation or surgical stripping.[1] Recently, mechanochemical ablation (MOCA), which combines endovenous mechanical damage of the venous intimal layer with the dispersion of a liquid sclerosant, has gained popularity in treating the incompetent great saphenous vein without the use of thermal energy or the need for tumescent anesthesia. MOCA appears attractive, but, as with any new treatment modality, randomized trials are critical to assess not only the efficacy but, more importantly, patient-perceived outcomes. In this study, the authors perform a prospective observational study to assess postoperative pain and quality of life in 68 patients treated with RFA or MOCA. At 6 weeks, the venous clinical severity score (VCSS) was decreased for both MOCA and RFA. Patients undergoing MOCA had significantly less pain at each day assessed and at 14 days postprocedure compared with RFA (Fig 2). In both groups treated with either MOCA or RFA, the QOL was significantly improved 6 weeks postprocedure, with no difference between MOCA and RFA. Patients undergoing MOCA had earlier return to normal activity and work than RFA-treated patients. Limitations of this study are the nonrandomized design, short duration, no ultrasound scan follow-up information, and small sample size, which the authors acknowledge as study limitations. For widespread acceptance of MOCA, randomized controlled studies will be required, with mid- and long-term follow-up evaluating technical efficacy, recurrent disease, venous clinical severity score, QOL measures, and cost effectiveness compared with other well-established treatment modalities.

J. D. Raffetto, MD

Reference

1. Rasmussen LH, Lawaetz M, Bjoern L, Vennits B, Blemings A, Eklof B. Randomized clinical trial comparing endovenous laser ablation, radiofrequency ablation, foam sclerotherapy and surgical stripping for great saphenous varicose veins. *Br J Surg*. 2011;98:1079-1087.

A randomized double-blind trial of upward progressive versus degressive compressive stockings in patients with moderate to severe chronic venous insufficiency

Couzan S, Leizorovicz A, Laporte S, et al (Clinique Mutualiste, Saint-Étienne, Lyon, France; Université de Lyon, France; Université Jean Monnet Saint-Étienne, France; et al)

J Vasc Surg 56:1344-1350, 2012

Background.—The present randomized double-blind multicenter study was designed to assess the efficacy of a progressive compressive stocking (new concept with maximal pressure at calf), compared to a degressive compressive stocking graded 30 mm Hg, evaluating the improvement of lower leg symptoms of chronic venous insufficiency (CVI) in ambulatory patients with moderate to severe chronic venous disease.

Methods.—Both gender outpatients presenting symptomatic moderate to severe CVI were eligible for a treatment by compressive stockings. Patients were randomly assigned to receive either degressive compressive stockings (30 mm Hg at ankle, 21 mm Hg at upper calf) or progressive compressive stockings (10 mm Hg at ankle, 23 mm Hg at upper calf). The primary outcome, evaluated after 3 months, was a composite success outcome, including improvement of pain or heavy legs without onset of either ulcer, deep or superficial vein thrombosis of the lower limbs, or pulmonary embolism. The ease of application of the compressive stockings reported by patients was one of secondary outcome.

Results.—Overall, 401 patients (199 in the progressive compressive stocking group and 202 in the degressive compressive stocking group) were randomized by 44 angiologists in France. Among them, 66% were classified in the C3 CEAP category. The rate of success was significantly higher in the progressive compressive stocking group compared to the degressive compressive stocking group (70.0% vs 59.6%; relative risk, 1.18; 95% confidence interval, 1.02-1.37; $P = .03$). This was mainly due to more frequent symptom improvement in the progressive compressive stocking group. The compressive stockings were considered easy to apply by 81.3% of patients in the progressive compressive stocking group vs 49.7% of patients in the degressive compressive stocking group ($P < .0001$). The rate of related serious adverse events was low and similar in both groups.

Conclusions.—This trial has demonstrated that progressive compressive stockings are more effective than usual degressive compressive stockings in the improvement of pain and lower leg symptoms in patients with CVI. Moreover, progressive compressive stockings were easier to apply, raising no safety concern at 3 months.

▶ Graded compression stockings have long been applied to patients with chronic venous disorders such as varicose veins, edema, and skin changes, including venous ulcers. Best medical evidence has clearly shown a benefit for patients with venous ulcers in healing and in decreasing the risk of recurrence of venous ulcers. There are many companies that manufacture and distribute compression hosiery for the treatment of chronic venous diseases, and the graduated compression is graded to have higher pressures at the foot and ankle and decreasing pressures in an ascending format at the midcalf and lowest pressure in the upper calf (degressive compression). A new concept has evolved with the development of progressive compressive stocking (with minimal pressure at the foot and ankle and maximal pressure at the calf). The progressive compression stockings used in this study had the pressure-graded sections of 10 mm Hg at the ankle and 23 mm Hg at the upper calf. Several reasons for developing and using progressive compression have been proposed. Progressive compression stockings are easier to apply because of less pressure around the foot and ankle; therefore, increased compliance should be observed. Additionally, the calf is the largest pump in the leg (the other 2 being the foot and ankle), making this the ideal section to have higher pressure and not less pressure. In this study, 401 patients with chronic venous disease (C2 to C5, 66% C3 disease) were randomly assigned to progressive compression stocking (10 mm Hg at the ankle and 23 mm Hg at the upper calf) or to a degressive compression stocking (30 mm Hg at the ankle and 21 mm Hg at the upper calf), and a composite outcome evaluated after 3 months of treatment (improvement of pain or heavy legs without onset of ulcer, deep or superficial vein thrombosis of the lower limb, or pulmonary embolism) was the primary endpoint. Secondary endpoints were ease of application and compliance. The results showed that at month 3, the rate of success was significantly higher in the progressive compressive stocking group (70.0%) than in the degressive compressive stocking (59.6%, risk-ratio = 1.18; 95% confidence interval [CI], 1.02–1.37; $P = .03$). This difference was mainly explained by a higher rate of symptom improvement in the progressive compressive stocking group and was significant in C3, C4, and C5. Interestingly, at 3 months the compliance was similar in both groups (72.2% progressive vs 71.1% in the degressive), but the reported ease to apply was greater for the progressive compression stocking group (86.2% vs 57.1%, $P < .0001$), despite that the compliance was the same. Several discussion points are worth mentioning. (1) It is unclear if all patients who were enrolled in the study had a duplex ultrasound scan evaluating the venous anatomy and valves/vein segments for reflux, how venous ultrasound studies were performed, or what parameters were set for superficial and deep vein reflux. This information is not provided. (2) Was the venous disease superficial, deep, perforator, or a combination, and what were the respective proportions in patients with progressive and regressive compression? (3) Were there any patients with combined venous and arterial disease? (4) What was the lowest allowable ABI to enroll patients in the study? (5) The follow-up of the study is short (6 months), and long-term evaluation will be necessary to determine equivalency or superiority. (6) Quality-of-life assessment with both general and disease-specific questionnaires was not assessed. (7) Both progressive and degressive compression stockings had around 20 mm Hg pressure at the calf, yet the results are better for progressive stockings for the primary endpoint in this study, despite no difference in compliance. (8) It is unclear what the physiologic effects are of having higher pressure at the ankle in regressive and lower pressure at the ankle in progressive stockings, when the calf pressure for each stocking is the same. (9) Patients with venous ulcers were not included in this study, and it is unclear if progressive compression has a clear benefit in this group, in which the current evidence-based data clearly have shown a benefit of graded compression. (10) What is the role of progressive compression stockings on deep vein thrombosis (DVT) prevention, DVT, and postthrombotic syndrome prevention? Before compression stocking manufacturers "reverse the mercury" in the gradation of pressure in the regions of compression of the leg, further data and studies with longer-term follow-up and patient-perceived validated quality-of-life questionnaires will be required before the current compression stocking will change.

J. D. Raffetto, MD

Great saphenous vein diameter does not correlate with worsening quality of life scores in patients with great saphenous vein incompetence

Gibson K, Meissner M, Wright D (Lake Washington Vascular Surgeons, Bellevue; Univ of Washington, Seattle; BTG PLLC, London, UK)

J Vasc Surg 56:1634-1641, 2012

Objective.—Previous studies have correlated increasing great saphenous vein (GSV) diameter with increasing CEAP clinical classification. Some insurance carriers are currently using specific GSV diameters to determine coverage for treatment of axial venous insufficiency. The aim of this study was to investigate the correlation of patient quality of life (QOL) measures with GSV diameters in varicose vein patients with GSV reflux.

Methods.—Data were collected from the records of 91 patients prospectively enrolled in two varicose vein trials. The patients had symptomatic varicose veins with saphenofemoral junction and proximal GSV reflux. Maximum GSV diameter was measured on duplex ultrasound imaging, with the patient standing, within 5 cm of the saphenofemoral junction. Chronic Venous Insufficiency Questionnaire 2 (CIVIQ-2; Servier, Neuilly-sur-Seine, France), Venous Insufficiency Epidemiological and Economic Study (VEINES) Symptom (Sym) and QOL assessments, and the Venous Clinical Severity Score (VCSS) assessment were completed before treatment of GSV insufficiency. Demographic information, patient weight, height, and body mass index were collected. Correlations between pairs of data were done using Pearson product-moment and Spearman correlation coefficients.

Results.—The 91 study patients (19 men, 72 women) were a mean age of 45 years (range, 18-65 years). The mean GSV diameter was 6.7 mm (range, 2.2-14.1 mm). The mean VCSS score was 7.8 (range, 3-12). There was a weak correlation between increasing GSV diameter and VCSS ($r = 0.23$; $P = .03$) and no correlation between GSV diameter and the CIVIQ-2 score ($r = 0.01$), VEINES-QOL ($r = -0.07$), and VEINES-Sym ($r = -0.1$).

Conclusions.—GSV diameter is a poor surrogate marker for assessing the effect of varicose veins on a patient's QOL; thus, using GSV diameter as a sole criterion for determining medical necessity for the treatment of GSV reflux is inappropriate. Further correlations between QOL measures and duplex-derived objective findings are warranted (Tables 3-5).

▶ Recently, insurance carriers have delineated the great saphenous vein diameter as a criterion for indication for ablation and remuneration. For example, United Healthcare requires that the diameters of the great saphenous vein (GSV) and the small saphenous vein (SSV) must each measure at least 5.5 mm to qualify for coverage. This indicates that GSV diameter is being used as a surrogate marker to indicate disease and to differentiate patients with medical necessity for vein treatment from those for whom the treatment is cosmetic. Intuition alone would dictate that setting a diameter size criterion on the refluxing GSV is a poor surrogate marker for patients' symptoms and quality of life (QOL) and that other factors (anatomic involvement of insufficient superficial, deep, and perforator veins;

TABLE 3.—Pearson Coefficient Correlations (*r* values) between Venous Clinical Severity Core (*VCSS*) and Quality of Life (*QOL*) Measures

Variable	VCSS	CIVIQ-2	VEINES-Sym	VEINES-QOL
VCSS	1	0.43	−0.37	−0.44
CIVIQ-2		1	−0.83	0.90
VEINES-Sym			1	0.96
VEINES-QOL				1

CIVIQ-2, Chronic Venous Insufficiency Questionnaire 2; *Sym*, symptoms; *VEINES*, Venous Insufficiency Epidemiological and Economic Study. $P < .01$ for all correlations.

TABLE 4.—Correlations (*r* values) between Great Saphenous Vein (*GSV*) Diameter and Reflux Time, and Assessments of Disease and Quality of Life

Assessment	GSV Diameter (n = 91)	Reflux Time (n = 82)
VCSS[a]	0.23[b]	−0.05
CIVIQ-2[c]	0.01	−0.01
VEINES-Sym[c]	−0.10	0.00
VEINES-QOL[c]	−0.07	−0.02

CIVIQ-2, Chronic Venous Insufficiency Questionnaire 2; *VCSS*, Venous Clinical Severity Score; *VEINES-Sym/QOL*, Venous Insufficiency Epidemiological and Economic Study-Symptoms/Quality of Life.
[a]Spearman correlation.
[b]$P = .02$, all other P values insignificant.
[c]Pearson correlation

TABLE 5.—Pearson Coefficient Correlations (*r* values) between Great Saphenous Vein (*GSV*) Diameter, Reflux Time, Patient Weight, Height, and Body Mass Index (*BMI*)

Variable	GSV Diameter (n = 91)	Reflux Time (n = 82)
Weight	0.26[a]	−0.04
Height	0.07	−0.19[b]
BMI	0.25[a]	−0.21[b]

[a]$P = .02$.
[b]$P < .10$.

above knee vs below knee venous insufficiency; calf muscle pump dysfunction) may be more relevant to the patients' symptoms and effect on quality of life. The primary objective of this study was to determine if the diameter of the GSV correlates with patient-derived rather than physician-derived measurements of disease severity. Secondary objectives included correlation of patient morphologic measurements (height, weight, and body mass index [BMI]) with Venous Clinical Severity Scores (VCSS) and QOL scores, and correlation of QOL scores with each other and with the physician-derived VCSS. In this study, the authors assessed retrospectively the data on 91 patients from 2 prospective trials. The study's main findings were the following. (1) A moderate, statistically significant correlation existed between the VCSS and the CIVIQ-2, VEINES-Sym, and

VEINES-QOL scores, but a strong correlation was present among the 3 QOL measures (Table 3). (2) There was a very weak correlation of GSV diameter and worsening VCSS (Table 4). (3) There was no correlation of the QOL scores and GSV diameter (Table 4). (4) There was no correlation of reflux time and VCSS or QOL measures (Table 4). (5). There was a statistically significant correlation between BMI and GSV diameter but no correlation of height and GSV diameter (Table 5). Further study with careful prospective design, appropriate and standardized methodology, specified outcome measures, balance of men and women, as well as the spectrum of chronic venous diseases (C2 to C6), balanced ethnic groups, and patient-derived QOL questionnaires is needed to determine the importance of refluxing great saphenous vein diameter and effect on global hemodynamics and the importance of clinical signs and symptoms.

J. D. Raffetto, MD

A multicenter randomized controlled trial evaluating balneotherapy in patients with advanced chronic venous insufficiency

Carpentier PH, Blaise S, Satger B, et al (Centre Hospitalier Universitaire, Grenoble, France; et al)

J Vasc Surg 59:447-454.e1, 2014

Background.—Apart from compression therapy, physical therapy has scarcely been evaluated in the treatment of chronic venous disorders (CVDs). Spa treatment is a popular way to administer physical therapy for CVDs in France, but its efficacy has not yet been assessed in a large trial. The objective was to assess the efficacy of spa therapy for patients with advanced CVD (CEAP clinical classes C4-C5).

Methods.—This was a single-blind (treatment concealed to the investigators) randomized, multicenter, controlled trial (French spa resorts). Inclusion criteria were primary or post-thrombotic CVD with skin changes but no active ulcer (C4a, C4b, or C5). The treated group had the usual 3-week spa treatment course soon after randomization; the control group had spa treatment after the 1-year comparison period. All patients continued their usual medical care including wearing compression stockings. Treatment consisted of four balneotherapy sessions per day for 6 days a week. Follow-up was performed at 6, 12 and 18 months by independent blinded investigators. The main outcome criterion was the incidence of leg ulcers at 12 months. Secondary criteria were a modified version of the Venous Clinical Severity Score, a visual analog scale for leg symptoms, and the Chronic Venous Insufficiency Questionnaire 2 and EuroQol 5D quality-of-life autoquestionnaires.

Results.—Four hundred twenty-five subjects were enrolled: 214 in the treatment group (Spa) and 211 in the control group (Ctr); they were similar at baseline regarding their demographic characteristics, the severity of the CVD, and the outcome variables. At 1 year, the incidence of leg ulcers was not statistically different (Spa: +9.3%; 95% confidence interval [CI], +5.6 - +14.3; Ctr: +6.1%; 95% CI, +3.2 - +10.4), whereas the Venous

Clinical Severity Score improved significantly in the treatment group (Spa: −1.2; 95% CI, −1.6 - −0.8; Ctr: −0.6; 95% CI, −1.0 - −0.2; $P = .04$). A significant difference favoring spa treatment was found regarding symptoms after 1 year (Spa: −0.03; 95% CI, −0.57 - +0.51; Ctr: +0.87; 95% CI, +0.46 - +1.26; $P = .009$). EuroQol 5D improved in the treatment group (Spa: +0.01; 95% CI, −0.02 - +0.04) while it worsened (Ctr: −0.07; 95% CI, −0.10 - −0.04) in the control group ($P < .001$). A similar pattern was found for the Chronic Venous Insufficiency Questionnaire 2 scale (Spa: −2.0; 95% CI, −4.4 - +0.4; Ctr: +2.4; 95% CI, +0.2 - +4.7; $P = .008$). The control patients showed similar improvements in clinical severity, symptoms, and quality of life after their own spa treatment (day 547).

Conclusions.—In this study, the incidence of leg ulcers was not reduced after a 3-week spa therapy course. Nevertheless, our study demonstrates that spa therapy provides a significant and substantial improvement in clinical status, symptoms, and quality of life of patients with advanced venous insufficiency for at least 1 year (Figs 3-5, Table 2).

▶ Compression therapy is a standard of care for chronic venous disease, especially for patients with ulcers and for the prevention of recurrent ulcers. Patients with advanced chronic venous disease are older and have increased complex patterns of venous insufficiency, and nearly always the superficial venous system is involved with incompetent valves. A variety of endovenous ablation therapies are available, including thermal (laser or radiofrequency); chemical, in the form of foam sclerosant; and mechanochemical ablation (the latter 2 do not require tumescent anesthetic).

When Conrad Jobst first discovered that the chronic venous disorder afflicting his lower extremities had significantly improved while in his pool with his

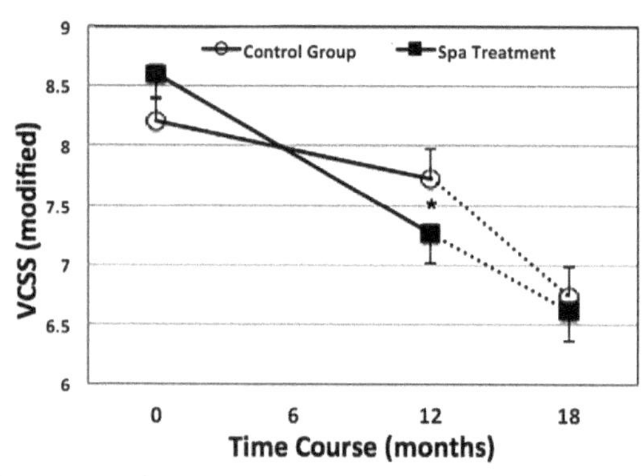

FIGURE 3.—Time course of variations in the Venous Clinical Severity Score (modified VCSS) (mean ± standard error of the mean) (*solid lines* = comparative period; *dotted lines* = follow-up) At *: $P < .05$ for the difference with M0. At the end of 1 year, the improvement in VCSS was significantly greater in treated patients than in controls. After 1 year, the control patients were given the spa treatment and their VCSS scores caught up with those of the other group. (Reprinted from Carpentier PH, Blaise S, Satger B, et al. A multicenter randomized controlled trial evaluating balneotherapy in patients with advanced chronic venous insufficiency. *J Vasc Surg*. 2014;59:447-454.e1, Copyright 2014, with permission from The Society for Vascular Surgery.)

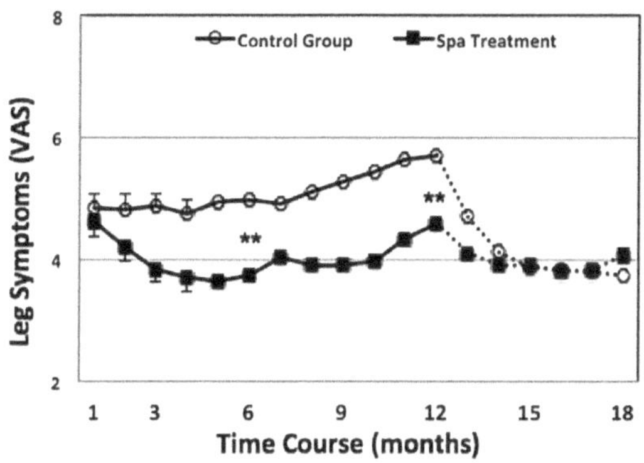

FIGURE 4.—Time course of variations in leg symptoms as assessed by monthly visual analog scale (*VAS*) (mean ± standard error of the mean) (*solid lines* = comparative period; *dotted lines* = follow-up). At **: $P < .01$ for the difference with M0. After spa therapy, the treated group soon experienced a reduction in leg symptoms, which reached a maximum at 4 to 6 months. The difference with the control group remained substantial and highly significant for the entire year. After month 12 and their own spa treatment, the control patients also showed a dramatic improvement in their symptoms. (Reprinted from Carpentier PH, Blaise S, Satger B, et al. A multicenter randomized controlled trial evaluating balneotherapy in patients with advanced chronic venous insufficiency. *J Vasc Surg*. 2014;59:447-454.e1, Copyright 2014, with permission from The Society for Vascular Surgery.)

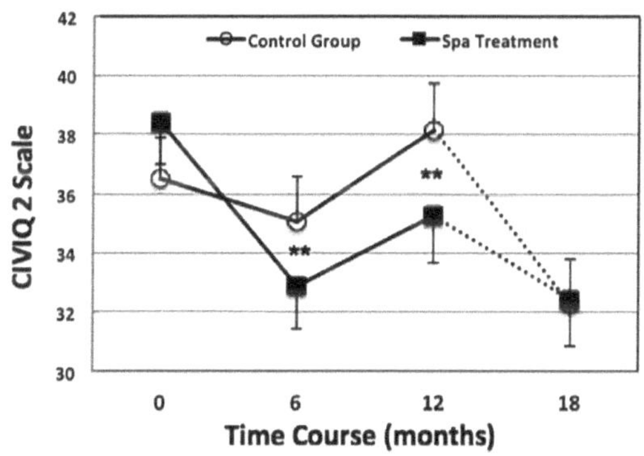

FIGURE 5.—Time course of variations in the venous-related quality-of-life scale Chronic Venous Insufficiency Questionnaire 2 [*CIVIQ2*] (mean ± standard error of the mean). Higher scores are related to larger changes in quality of life (*solid lines* = comparative period; *dotted lines* = follow-up). At **: $P < .01$ for the difference with M0. In spite of seasonal variations (the spa treatment is performed mostly during summer months), the treated group showed a substantial and significant improvement vs the control group, with the difference remaining significant at month 12. Again, after the control patients were given spa treatment, their CIVIQ2 scale reached the same level as the other group. (Reprinted from Carpentier PH, Blaise S, Satger B, et al. A multicenter randomized controlled trial evaluating balneotherapy in patients with advanced chronic venous insufficiency. *J Vasc Surg*. 2014;59:447-454.e1, Copyright 2014, with permission from The Society for Vascular Surgery.)

limb submerged, he determined that pressure was important in reducing symptoms. He rationalized that the pressure exerted by the water at different depths created a gradient that exerted external pressure on his legs. This was the beginning of the development of compression stockings.

TABLE 2.—Incidence of Leg Ulcers at 1 Year in Both Groups, and in the C4 and C5 Subgroups

Incidence of Leg Ulcers at 1 Year	Controls, No. (%) [95% CI]	Spa Treatment, No. (%) [95% CI]	*P*
Total population	(n = 197)	(n = 193)	.231
Ulcers	12 (6.1) [3.2-10.4]	18 (9.3) [5.6-14.3]	
C4 subgroup	(n = 120)	(n = 115)	1.0
Ulcers	3 (2.5) [0.5-7.1]	3 (2.6) [0.5-7.4]	
C5 subgroup	(n = 77)	(n = 78)	.194
Ulcers	9 (11.7) [5.5-21.0]	15 (19.2) [11.2-29.7]	

CI, Confidence interval.

In various areas of France, spa therapy is a common modality for treating the symptoms of chronic venous disease. However, the actual effects of spa therapy are poorly defined. In this randomized trial of 425 patients with chronic venous disease (C4ab and C5), subjects were randomized to two groups: the treatment group, which received 3 weeks of spa therapy and, the control group, which did not receive spa therapy. (After 12 months, the control group also received balneotherapy to decrease the dropout rate.) Balneotherapy consisted of an intense and sophisticated 15-minute walking session in a specially designed pool with tracks in semideep (80 cm), cool (28°C) water; training of muscle pump function under water compression; a 20-minute whirlpool bath session with automatic air and water massage cycles aimed at relaxation and mobilization of the superficial skin volume flow; and a 10-minute bath session with customized underwater strong massaging jets, intended to mobilize and soften the sclerotic subcutaneous tissues. In addition, it included a 10-minute massage session of legs and ankles by a registered physiotherapist under a light spray shower (also intended to soften the sclerotic subcutaneous tissues) or a 15-minute joint mobilization session in a deep (50 cm), warm (34°C) pool under the supervision of a physiotherapist for the improvement of ankle, knee, and hip mobility for better ambulation and muscle-pump function. Therapy comprised 4 balneotherapy sessions per day, 6 days a week, for a total of 3 weeks. All patients wore compression stockings. To remain enrolled in the study, study and control patients could not receive any endovenous or surgical treatment for their venous insufficiency.

The primary end point was development of venous leg ulcer at 12 months; secondary outcomes included the Venous Clinical Severity Score, a visual analog scale for leg symptoms, as well as the Chronic Venous Insufficiency Questionnaire 2 and the EuroQol-5D quality-of-life questionnaires. The hypothesis was that there would be a reduction of venous ulcers at 1 year with balneotherapy.

The main findings were that there was no statistical difference in the primary end point (Table 2), but the balneotherapy group had significantly improved in all 3 aspects of the secondary end points (Figs 3-5). Importantly, when the control patients also received their therapy after 12 months, they had the same benefits in secondary outcomes. Some unanswered question are the following: (1) Would increasing the length of time of balneotherapy reduce venous ulcer rates? (2) What are the hemodynamic benefits of balneotherapy?

(3) Do the venous filling index, residual volume fraction, and ejection fraction improve? (4) Should this form of therapy be offered to patients with primary and/or secondary disease, and who benefits most? (5) What is the cost-effective analysis of such a therapy?

I must admit that it would be very nice to be able to enjoy a pool and spa resort in the beautiful country of France, especially given that balneotherapy is partly reimbursed by the French National Health insurance system!

J. D. Raffetto, MD

16 Technical Notes

Transealing: A Novel and Simple Technique for Embolization of Type 2 Endoleaks Through Direct Sac Access From the Distal Stent-Graft Landing Zone

Coppi G, Saitta G, Coppi G, et al (Baggiovara – Univ of Modena and Reggio Emilia, Italy)

Eur J Vasc Endovasc Surg 47:394-401, 2014

Objective.—Type 2 endoleak (T2EL) is the Achilles' heel of endovascular abdominal aortic aneurysm repair. Experience with transealing, an alternative technique for the treatment of T2ELs, is described.

Methods.—The outcome of a group of patients treated with transealing has been reviewed. Femoral access was obtained with a 9-Fr sheath. A super-stiff guide wire and a stiff hydrophilic wire were placed inside the stent-graft and a Piton GC catheter inserted. The stiff hydrophilic wire was retrieved to allow the catheter to regain its curvature and the catheter tip was placed against the iliac wall, at the edge of the stent-graft. The hydrophilic wire was then forced between the stent-graft and arterial wall into the sac. A 5/6-Fr introducer was inserted inside the sac and angiography was performed to evaluate the leak. Coils, cyanoacrylate, or fibrin glue were deployed. After removal of the catheters, the iliac limb was ballooned.

Results.—Seventeen patients were treated between February 2009 and April 2013. It was possible to access the aneurysm in 16/17 attempts. One patient treated with acrylic glue suffered from colon ischemia. One intraoperative secondary type 1b endoleak was treated with an iliac extension. Mean follow-up was 21.5 months. Three months of follow-up were completed in 14 patients with a 53% freedom from endoleak rate. At 1 year, the rate was 45%. During the study period, there was one surgical conversion, one aneurysm growth, and one re-embolization procedure. The remaining leaks remained stable.

Conclusions.—This study shows that transealing is feasible and represents a valid alternative in selected patients. The advantages of this technique are mainly its low invasiveness, reduced costs, and ease of use (Figs 1 and 3).

▶ This is a nice little technique article describing a method for the treatment of type 2 endoleaks after endovascular aneurysm repair (EVAR). I have actually used this technique in the past but never reported on it, and there are some important technical aspects described in this article.

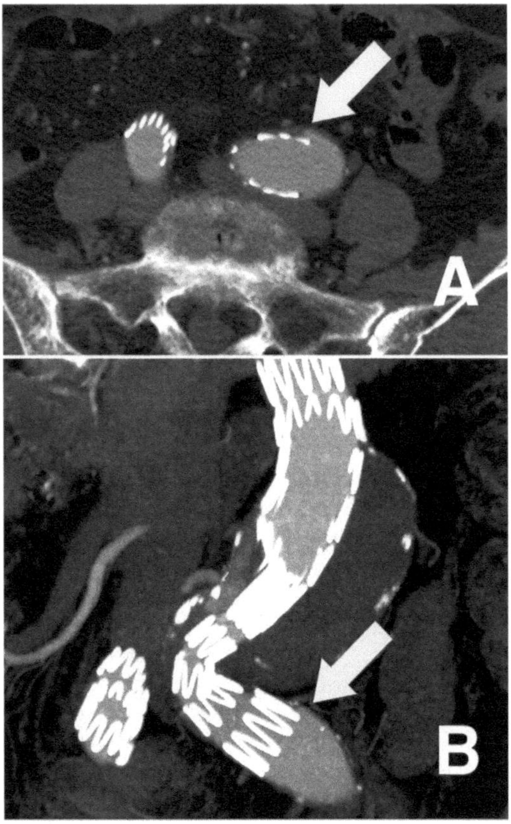

FIGURE 1.—(A) Pre-operative computed tomography angiography showing the presence of a minor gap between the distal edge of the left iliac limb and the arterial wall (arrow). (B) The remaining limb shows good apposition to the artery wall, without type 1b endoleak. Note. *Type 2 endoleak with feeding lumbar arteries. (Reprinted from Coppi G, Saitta G, Coppi G, et al. Transealing: a novel and simple technique for embolization of type 2 endoleaks through direct sac access from the distal stent-graft landing zone. *Eur J Vasc Endovasc Surg*. 2014;47:394-401, Copyright 2014, with permission from European Society for Vascular Surgery.)

Type 2 endoleaks are fairly benign with approximately 70% to 90% resolving within a year of the EVAR procedure. Described herein is a method of getting outside the stent graft, along one of the limbs identified ahead of time. The access site (right or left) was chosen if a minor gap between the common iliac artery and the stent graft could be detected on computed tomographic angiography (Fig 1). If no gap was detected, the side with the shortest iliac limb was used.

Once inside the endoleak, blood is aspirated from the sheath to verify successful entrance into the leak. If there is no backflow, a multipurpose catheter is used to reach the nidus. Saccography is then performed to identify the endoleak.

Important technical considerations are that the authors abandoned cyanoacrylate because of complications and used a technique of fibrin sealant injection

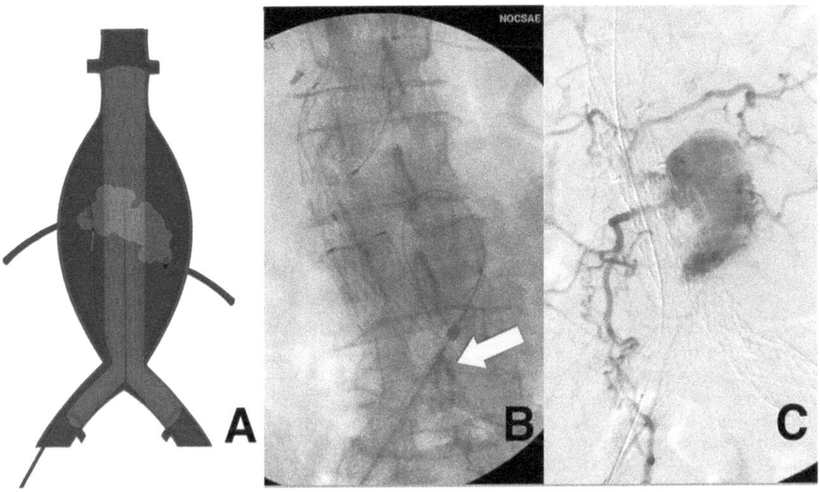

FIGURE 3.—(A) Schematic depiction of the position of the introducer sheath between the stent-graft and aortic wall, inside the aneurysm sac. (B) Fluoroscopic image showing the sheath (yellow arrow) inside the sac. (C) Saccography showing the leak nidus with two feeding vessels (lumbar arteries). For interpretation of the references to color in this figure legend, the reader is referred to web version of this article. (Reprinted from Coppi G, Saitta G, Coppi G, et al. Transealing: a novel and simple technique for embolization of type 2 endoleaks through direct sac access from the distal stent-graft landing zone. *Eur J Vasc Endovasc Surg*. 2014;47:394-401, Copyright 2014, with permission from European Society for Vascular Surgery.)

by placing a 4F catheter through the sheath and injecting thrombin and fibrinogen through both the sheath and catheter separately to avoid mixing in the sheath and sheath occlusion (Fig 3).

B. W. Starnes, MD

Direct sonographic-guided superior gluteal artery access for treatment of a previously treated expanding internal iliac artery aneurysm

Herskowitz MM, Walsh J, Jacobs DT (State Univ of New York Downstate Hosp, Brooklyn)

J Vasc Surg 59:235-237, 2014

Isolated internal iliac artery aneurysms are relatively uncommon compared with all aortoiliac aneurysms. Transcatheter treatment with coil embolization is an attractive noninvasive alternative to surgical resection. However, if the aneurysm is insufficiently treated with only proximal coil embolization without concurrent embolization of distal runoff vessels, there is a risk of aneurysm expansion from retrograde collateral flow. We present a case of previously treated internal iliac aneurysm that underwent late rapid expansion. Due to occlusion of the internal iliac artery, direct sonographic-guided puncture of the superior gluteal artery was

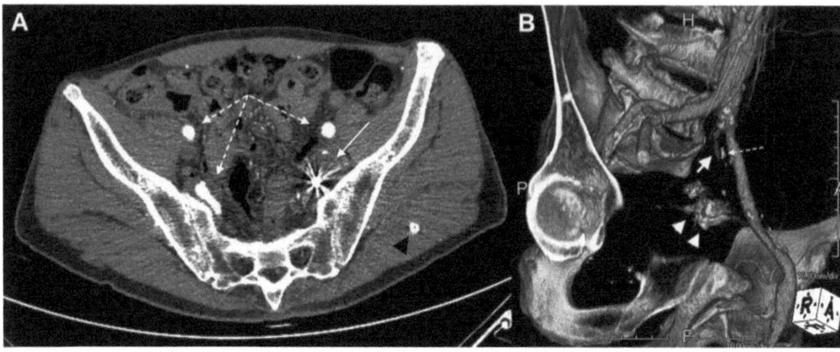

FIGURE 3.—A, Axial image from pelvic computed tomography (CT) angiogram several months after embolization demonstrates thrombosed, partially calcified left internal iliac artery aneurysm (*white arrow*). There is significant beam hardening artifact due to the presence of numerous metallic coils within the aneurysm sac. The left and right external iliac and right internal iliac arteries are normally opacified (*dashed arrows*). Also seen is a coil within the left gluteus maximus, near the superior gluteal artery access point (*black arrowhead*). B, Three-dimensional reconstruction of pelvic CT angiogram (*oblique view*) demonstrates residual stump of the left internal iliac artery (*arrow*), coil from the first embolization procedure (*dashed arrow*), and coil nest and thrombosed aneurysm (*arrowheads*). (Reprinted from Herskowitz MM, Walsh J, Jacobs DT. Direct sonographic-guided superior gluteal artery access for treatment of a previously treated expanding internal iliac artery aneurysm. *J Vasc Surg*. 2014;59:235-237, Copyright 2014, with permission from The Society for Vascular Surgery.)

made in order to access the aneurysm. We believe this is the first reported case of such treatment (Fig 3).

▶ Technical advances have made transcatheter embolization an attractive alternative to open surgery. Appropriate treatment via embolization involves both proximal and distal coil embolization, including all runoff branches. The description provided in this case report, along with review of 3 existing case reports, presents us with an elegant technique for retrograde embolization of type 2 endoleaks arising from internal iliac arteries after endovascular aneurysm repair. The technical description in this case report is excellent.

In the prone position, a point is marked fluoroscopically just lateral to the superior aspect of the left sciatic foramen, at the expected location of the superior gluteal artery. The artery is located sonographically, verified with color Doppler mode by the presence of pulsatile flow and punctured with a Neff 21-gauge by 15-cm micropuncture needle (Cook, Inc, Bloomington, IN). A wire is advanced and the needle replaced with a 5Fr angiographic sheath. After the embolization procedure, an additional 8-mm coil is placed at the gluteal artery entry point by the sheath (Fig 3).

This may serve as a nice technique to gain access to the internal iliac artery after "the door has been closed," so to speak, from standard approaches.

B. W. Starnes, MD

Static contrast technique for creating transpedal arterial access in patients with tibioperoneal occlusions

Chang JC-H, Lin L-S, Chiu C-H (Buddhist Dalin Tzu Chi General Hosp, Chiayi County, Taiwan)

J Vasc Surg 58:1120-1122, 2013

Transpedal arterial access is a useful but challenging technique for patients with tibioperoneal occlusions. It is associated with a long learning curve, requires the administration of a large amount of contrast media, and exposes patients and interventionists to additional radiation. Here we present a new technique by which it is easier and faster to create a transpedal arterial access (Figs 1 and 2).

▶ Transpedal access is a technique that can salvage technical success when antegrade lesion crossing fails during attempted endovascular treatment. This case report describes a technical description of an alternative to ultrasound-guided access, which (as the authors point out) can be challenging because of the lack of depth and small diameter of the dorsalis pedis artery. Inflation of a long balloon in the distal superficial femoral artery using this technique permits ongoing visualization during fluoroscopy-guided access without the need for repeated contrast injections (Figs 1 and 2); a potential disadvantage of this technique versus ultrasound-guided access is that it wastes a long balloon in

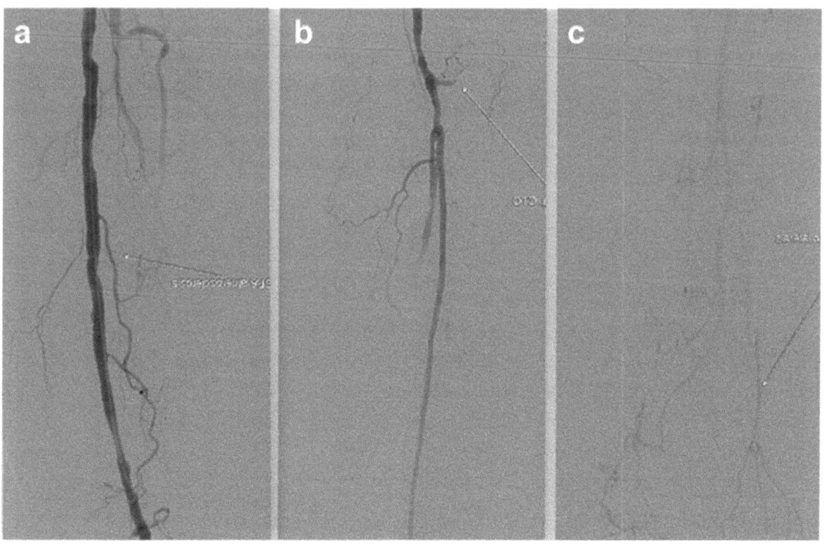

FIGURE 1.—Baseline angiography of the left lower leg showed superficial femoral artery (SFA) atherosclerosis without significant stenosis (a), chronic total occlusion (CTO) of the anterior and posterior tibial arteries (b), and the dorsalis pedis (*arrow*) reconstituted by collaterals (c). (Reprinted from Chang JC-H, Lin L-S, Chiu C-H. Static contrast technique for creating transpedal arterial access in patients with tibioperoneal occlusions. *J Vasc Surg*. 2013;58:1120-1122, Copyright 2013, with permission The Society for Vascular Surgery.)

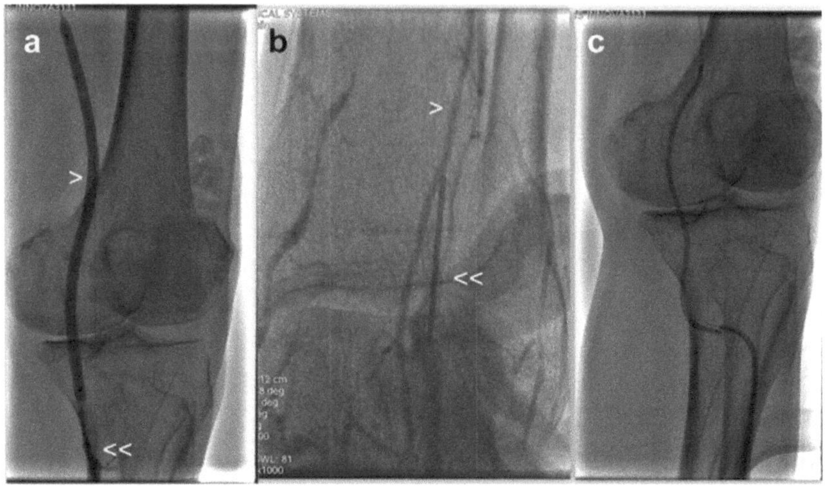

FIGURE 2.—A 5- × 150-mm balloon (Rival; Bard, Murray Hill, NJ) was inflated to 8 atm to occlude the distal superficial femoral artery (SFA) and popliteal artery (**a**, *arrow*), and 10 mL diluted iohexol contrast media was injected via a balloon catheter (**a**, *double arrow*). The contrast media was static in the pedal arteries, and the dorsalis pedis was punctured (**b**, *arrow*) with a 20-gage, 4-cm needle (**b**, *double arrow*) according to real-time roadmapping. After a subintimal approach to the anterior tibial artery, a double-balloon technique with two 2.5- × 120-mm balloons (Ampherion; Medtronic-Invatec, Roncadelle, Italy) was used, and the anterior tibial artery (**c**) was successfully revascularized. (Reprinted from Chang JC-H, Lin L-S, Chiu C-H. Static contrast technique for creating transpedal arterial access in patients with tibioperoneal occlusions. *J Vasc Surg*. 2013;58:1120-1122, Copyright 2013, with permission The Society for Vascular Surgery.)

the setting of technical failure (with associated increases in cost). Although the authors have used this technique in a small cohort of patients, no comparisons with ultrasound-guided access are provided (among which technical success, time to establish access, and fluoroscopy time would be of greatest interest). A no-contrast technique to fluoroscopy-guided access is another alternative in patients with pedal artery calcification (which is highly prevalent among individuals with occlusive tibial disease).

M. Corriere, MD, MS

Clinical and Economic Evaluation of Ambulatory Endovascular Treatment of Peripheral Arterial Occlusive Lesions

Albert B, Davaine J-M, Chaillet M-P, et al (CHU Nantes, France)
Ann Vasc Surg 28:137-143, 2014

Background.—Ambulatory management of patients is an alternative to conventional hospitalization. In this study we evaluate the results of a prospective cohort study of patients receiving ambulatory endovascular treatment for peripheral arterial lesions.

Methods.—From June 2008 to October 2010, ambulatory management was proposed for endovascular treatment of peripheral arterial lesions. An arterial closure device (Angio-Seal®; St. Jude Medical) was used. For ambulatory treatment, patients were prohibited from driving a vehicle at discharge, had to be accompanied the first night after the procedure, had to live <1 hour from a medical facility, had to be reachable by telephone the day after the intervention, and had to remain hospitalized in the event of a complication. The principal criterion was morbimortality at 1 month. Secondary criteria were clinical improvement, patency, complications related to the arterial closure, and costs evaluation at 1 month.

Results.—Forty-five patients were included and 50 ambulatory procedures were carried out. The patients presented with claudication (92%) or a critical ischemia (8%) of the lower extremities. All procedures were carried out by femoral puncture (retrograde in 94% and anterograde in 6% of the cases). The patients presented with iliac (68%) and femoropopliteal (64%) lesions. Lesions included stenoses (70%), thromboses (16%), and intrastent restenoses (14%). The rate of failure of ambulatory hospitalization was 16% ($n = 8$) without a serious undesirable event: 2 patients were hospitalized after a surgical conversion for iliac rupture and disinsertion of stent; 3 patients developed a hematoma during the intervention at the point of puncture; and in 3 cases the system of percutaneous closure failed. The mean duration of hospitalization was 1.36 ± 1.33 days. At 1 month, clinical improvement was observed in 97.5% of cases, with a primary patency of 100%. No perioperative rehospitalization or puncture site complications were observed. Ambulatory management made it possible to save 42 days of hospitalization, with associated costs of 10,971€, compared with conventional hospitalization. The additional costs related to use of the Angio-Seal amounted to 7427€.

Conclusion.—Ambulatory endovascular treatment of patients presenting with peripheral arterial lesions is reliable and effective and may contribute to savings in healthcare spending.

▶ This prospective study with the use of a closure device after endovascular procedures shows the feasibility of same-day discharge in select patients. Obviously, careful patient selection is essential. The authors list sensible but restrictive criteria that their patients had to meet before they allowed same-day discharge. All of the patients who failed same-day discharge were identified before discharge. During the study period, however, only 10% of the patients who underwent an endovascular procedure were included in the analysis, and the mean age of the patients included was only 60.4 years. The degree of selection bias this suggests points to the need for a well-designed prospective and randomized study of this practice. If one considers that many patients are discharged after a diagnostic endovascular procedure in which similar sizes sheaths are used, the key question is whether it is safe to discharge a patient after arterial puncture and a loading dose of Plavix. As economic pressure increases to reduce the need for hospitalizations, a better answer to this questions would be helpful.

P. White, MD, FACS

17 Miscellaneous

Cannabis-Associated Arterial Disease

Desbois AC, Cacoub P (AP HP Goupe hospitalier Pitié-Salpêtrière, Paris, France)

Ann Vasc Surg 27:996-1005, 2013

Background.—The aim of this study was to describe the different arterial complications reported in cannabis smokers.

Methods.—This study was a literature review.

Results.—Cannabis use was found to be associated with stroke, myocardial infarction, and lower limb arteritis. Arterial disease involved especially young men. There was a very strong temporal link between arterial complications and cannabis use for stroke and myocardial infarction episodes. Patient outcome was closely correlated with cannabis withdrawal and relapses associated with cannabis rechallenge. Cannabis use was associated with particular characteristics of arterial disease. The increased risk of myocardial infarction onset occurred within 1 hour of smoking marijuana compared with periods of non-use. Strokes occurred mainly in the posterior cerebral circulation. Compared with cohorts of thromboangiitis obliterans patients, those with cannabis-associated limb arteritis were younger, more often male, and had more frequent unilateral involvement of the lower limbs at clinical presentation.

Conclusion.—Cannabis use is associated with arterial disease such as stroke, myocardial infarction, and limbs arteritis. It appears essential to investigate cannabis use in young patients presenting with such arterial manifestations, as outcome is closely correlated with cannabis withdrawal.

▶ With the recent legalization of recreational marijuana use in some states, this timely article looks at cannabis-associated arterial disease. The authors performed a review of the literature via a PubMed search and identified 3 potential arterial manifestations of cannabis use with specific clinical manifestations. First, they report an increased incidence of myocardial infarction within 1 hour of cannabis use. Second, this review reports that strokes associated with cannabis use typically involve the posterior circulations. Finally, they report that arteritis associated with cannabis use differs from thromboangiitis obliterans in that unilateral involvement is more common, and patients are younger and more commonly male. The authors suggest that in patients with these clinical presentations, cannabis use should be investigated. It is yet to be determined what impact the legalization of marijuana will have on the overall prevalence of its use, but studies regarding the medical implications of cannabis use may now be easier to conduct.

B. Peterson, MD

Delayed presentations of popliteal artery entrapment syndrome in a middle-aged military population

Radowsky J, Patel B, Fox CJ (Walter Reed Natl Military Med Ctr, Bethesda, MD)

Ann Vasc Surg 27:1184.e1-1184.e6, 2013

Popliteal artery entrapment syndrome (PAES) is a rare but significant cause of disability usually diagnosed in young, healthy adults. Advancements in diagnostic imaging modalities have prompted a current report of our recent experience with PAES in a middle-aged military population at the Walter Reed National Military Medical Center. The addition of computed tomographic angiography (CTA) and magnetic resonance angiography (MRA) permit accurate and facile diagnosis of this complex syndrome.

▶ Popliteal entrapment syndrome (PAES) is a serious condition compromising lower extremity perfusion, yet it can be very difficult to diagnose. This report analyzes the presentation and diagnosis of popliteal entrapment in a military population, which represents the young patient population often afflicted with this problem. These authors present the clinical scenarios, diagnostic course, and clinical interventions in 5 classic patients experiencing disabling claudication. Although all 4 patients had similar symptoms of claudication, one of the patient's exercise treadmill test result did not show a reduction in ankle brachial index. Because of a high index of suspicion, computed tomographic angiography (CTA) and magnetic resonance angiography (MRA) were performed and both results were consistent with type 1 PAES. This patient was treated with arterial reconstruction. Another patient's diagnosis was delayed because of the assumption that the pain was neurogenic. The presence of a moderately diminished ankle–brachial index (ABI) was seen at rest, which did decrease with exercise. A CTA found short-segment occlusion of the popliteal artery, which was treated with an interposition graft. Another patient with exercised-induced claudication and decreased ABI with exercise had a completely normal MRA. A CTA performed with provocative maneuvers did show a mildly deviated popliteal artery. Because of the equivocal noninvasive imaging studies, a digital angiogram was performed with provocative maneuvers, which showed complete occlusion of the artery. At exploration, the patient was found to have a fibromuscular band along the popliteal artery. This band was excised without resection of the artery or interposition graft. This resulted in complete alleviation of symptoms and normalization of the exercise treadmill test. The take-home message of this report is that a multimodal approach needs to be utilized in diagnosing popliteal entrapment—no single test is totally reliable to include or exclude the diagnosis.

M. T. Watkins, MD

Comparison of open and endovascular treatment of acute mesenteric ischemia

Beaulieu RJ, Arnaoutakis KD, Abularrage CJ, et al (Johns Hopkins Med Inst, Baltimore, MD; Johns Hopkins Hosp, Baltimore, MD)

J Vasc Surg 59:159-164, 2014

Introduction.—Acute mesenteric ischemia (AMI) is a commonly fatal result of inadequate bowel perfusion that requires immediate evaluation by both vascular and general surgeons. Treatment often involves vascular repair as well as bowel resection and the possible need for parenteral nutrition. Little data exist regarding the rates of bowel resection following endovascular vs open repair of AMI.

Methods.—Using the National Inpatient Sample database, admissions from 2005 through 2009 were identified according to International Classification of Diseases, Ninth Revision codes correlating to both AMI (557.0) and subsequent vascular intervention (39.26, 38.16, 38.06, 39.9, 99.10). Patients with a diagnosis of AMI but no intervention or nonemergent admission status were excluded. Patient level data regarding age, gender, and comorbidities were also examined. Outcome measures included mortality, length of stay, the need for bowel resection (45.6, 45.71-9, 45.8), or infusion of total parenteral nutrition (TPN; 99.10) during the same hospitalization. Statistical analysis was conducted by χ^2 tests and Wilcoxon rank-sum comparisons.

Results.—Of 23,744 patients presenting with AMI, 4665 underwent interventional treatment from 2005 through 2009. Of these patients, 57.1% were female, and the mean age was 70.5 years. A total of 679 patients underwent vascular intervention; 514 (75.7%) underwent open surgery and 165 (24.3%) underwent endovascular treatment overall during the study period. The proportion of patients undergoing endovascular repair increased from 11.9% of patients in 2005 to 30.0% in 2009. Severity of comorbidities, as measured by the Charlson index, did not differ significantly between the treatment groups. Mortality was significantly more commonly associated with open revascularization compared with endovascular intervention (39.3% vs 24.9%; $P = .01$). Length of stay was also significantly longer in the patient group undergoing open revascularization (12.9 vs 17.1 days; $P = .006$). During the study time period, 14.4% of patients undergoing endovascular procedures required bowel resection compared with 33.4% for open revascularization ($P < .001$). Endovascular repair was also less commonly associated with requirement for TPN support (13.7% vs 24.4%; $P = .025$).

Conclusions.—Endovascular intervention for AMI had increased significantly in the modern era. Among AMI patients undergoing revascularization, endovascular treatment was associated with decreased mortality and shorter length of stay. Furthermore, endovascular intervention was associated with lower rates of bowel resection and need for TPN. Further research is warranted to determine if increased use of endovascular repair could improve overall and gastrointestinal outcomes among patients requiring vascular repair for AMI.

▶ This review of data from the National Inpatient Sample (NIS) on endovascular versus open therapy for acute mesenteric ischemia (AMI) indicates how much more we still have to improve in the treatment of AMI but also the promise of endovascular therapy in treating this disease. Of nearly 24 000 admissions for AMI in the NIS, not even 5000 received surgical or interventional therapy. As the authors point out, a query to the NIS for only 1 *International Classification of Diseases, Ninth Revision,* code probably greatly over estimates the true incidence of a disease, but the disparity between admissions for AMI and definitive therapy for AMI is concerning. Also troubling was the nearly 2-day delay between admission and surgery in both the open and endovascular groups. As the authors point out multiple times, reducing the time from onset of symptoms to surgical therapy reduces the morbidity and mortality associated with AMI. Endovascular therapy outperformed open surgery with regard to length of stay, mortality, need for bowel resection, and need for total parenteral nutrition. This is most likely because of the increased severity of the disease in those patients treated with open surgery as evidenced by increased rates of lactic acidosis and acute respiratory distress syndrome. Perhaps the greatest advantage of endovascular therapy is that the consequences of an endovascular procedure in the case of a false-positive diagnosis are relatively minor. By advertising the benefits of endovascular therapy and its less invasive nature, vascular surgeons may be able to shorten the critical time from disease onset to definitive therapy.

P. White, MD, FACS

The risk of carotid artery stenting compared with carotid endarterectomy is greatest in patients treated within 7 days of symptoms

Rantner B, for the Carotid Stenting Trialists' Collaboration (Innsbruck Med Univ, Austria; et al)

J Vasc Surg 57:619-626.e2, 2013

Objective.—Among patients with symptomatic carotid artery stenosis, carotid artery stenting (CAS) is associated with a higher risk of periprocedural stroke or death than carotid endarterectomy (CEA). Uncertainty remains whether the balance of risk changes with time since the most recent ischemic event.

Methods.—We investigated the association of time between the qualifying ischemic event and treatment (0–7 days, 8–14 days, and >14 days) with the risk of stroke or death within 30 days after CAS or CEA in a pooled analysis of data from individual patients randomized in the Endarterectomy vs Angioplasty in Patients with Symptomatic Severe Carotid Stenosis (EVA-3S) trial, the Stent-Protected Angioplasty versus Carotid Endarterectomy (SPACE) trial, and the International Carotid Stenting

Study (ICSS). Data were analyzed with a fixed-effect binomial regression model adjusted for source trial.

Results.—Information on time of qualifying event was available for 2839 patients. In the first 30 days after intervention, any stroke or death occurred significantly more often in the CAS group (110/1434 [7.7%]) compared with the CEA group (54/1405 [3.8%]; crude risk ratio, 2.0; 95% confidence interval, 1.5-2.7). Patients undergoing CEA within the first 7 days of the qualifying event had the lowest periprocedural stroke or death rate (3/106 [2.8%]). Patients treated with CAS in the same period had a 9.4% risk of periprocedural stroke or death (13/138; risk ratio CAS vs CEA: 3.4; 95% confidence interval, 1.01-11.8; adjusted for age, sex, and type of qualifying event). Patients treated between 8 and 14 days showed a periprocedural stroke or death rate of 3.4% (7/208) and 8.1% (19/234), respectively, for CEA and CAS. The latest treatment group had 4% complications in the CEA group (44/1091) and 7.3% in the CAS group (78/1062).

Conclusions.—The increase in risk of CAS compared with CEA appears to be greatest in patients treated within 7 days of symptoms. Early surgery might remain most effective in stroke prevention in patients with symptomatic carotid artery stenosis.

▶ One of the major changes in carotid artery revascularization, specifically carotid endarterectomy (CEA), is the shortening of the interval between symptoms and surgery. Traditional practice was to wait about 6 weeks after an ischemic event. Now that time has been shortened to 7 to 14 days because of a decline in intervention benefit with an accompanying increase in the likelihood of a recurrent ischemic event. The crux of this study was to determine whether this timing can be extrapolated to carotid artery stenting. The current data on carotid artery stenting (CAS) points to an increased risk of periprocedural stroke and death compared with CEA. This study looked at the first 30 days after CAS and different time points: less than 7 days, 8 to 14 days, and greater than 14 days after the initial ischemic event. The data used were pooled from several of the recent CAS vs CEA trials. Clearly demonstrated in this analysis was that the risk of CAS is increased within 7 days of the neurologic symptom onset compared with CEA, thus, leading the authors to conclude that CEA should remain the first choice in the early days and thereafter. Surgery had better results at each treatment interval. The outcomes were poorest in CAS patients within 7 days of the ischemic event. Despite all of the trials comparing CAS and CEA and determining CAS as a "reasonable alternative," more data are being published showing the superiority of CEA.

R. L. Bush, MD, JD, MPH

Vascular surgery, self-awareness, and the University of South Carolina School of Medicine Greenville

Taylor SM (Greenville Hosp System, SC)

J Vasc Surg 58:1106-1114, 2013

Background.—If more surgeons were available for leadership and engaged in those pursuits, better solutions might arise and physicians would have less reason to feel under-represented in important decision-making events. Surgeons tend to be intelligent, disciplined, and able to lead teams to achieve complex objectives, but few make lasting contributions in areas beyond surgery. The traits that make surgeons successful surgical leaders should be adapted to help them lead successfully in other situations.

Surgical Personality Traits.—Evidence supports the existence of a surgical personality. Surgeons tend to be extroverted, open-minded, and conscientious. They hold in low regard those who avoid harm and reward dependence. Surgeons tend to be assertive, welcome conflict, and embrace being in control, usually to avoid feeling vulnerable. Surgeons—whether men or women—like being the captain of their ship.

Emotional Intelligence and Leadership.—Personality is largely set by adulthood, but leaders can nurture emotional intelligence through conscious leadership tasks. This promotes authentic communication, which is essential for high-performing teams. Among the personality styles that exist are low-functioning, medium-functioning, and high-functioning types. The surgeon's desire to be the one in charge can manifest in various ways depending on his or her level of emotional maturity. The personality traits identified in surgeons are equally found among prison inmates. The difference is the degree of emotional maturity, which can be trained in the right or wrong direction.

The central element in effective leadership is self-awareness. People tend to experience the world in one of four ways. The most common way is in a victim mentality, or "to me." The activities of the world are viewed as happening to these individuals. These persons tend to lack self-awareness and blame others for their feelings and actions. A second way of experiencing the world is using a "by me" mentality. In this insight, people have a strong sense of self-awareness and take healthy responsibility for what they contribute to situations. They understand that the source of their feelings is found in themselves, not others. These individuals are challenged to reveal rather than conceal themselves, to be present rather than always right, to participate and not just control, to be curious rather than defensive, and to be appreciative rather than feel entitled. With further evolution, people can experience the world in a "through me" mindset that requires intense awareness and total surrender. They accept that something is trying to emerge through them and can surrender so it can happen.

The personality styles can be expressed in low, medium, or high functioning ways. Low performing personalities are stuck in "to me" approaches, but medium and high performing personality styles can experience the

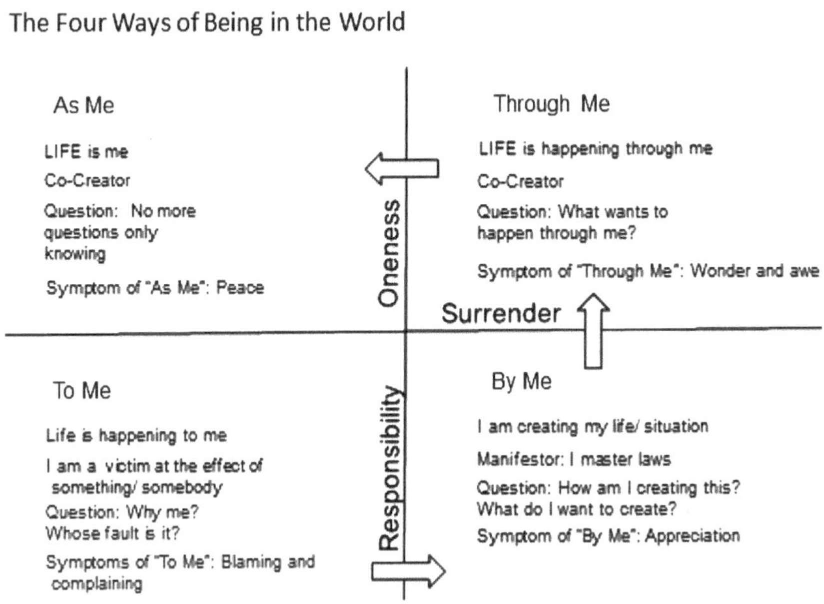

FIGURE 3.—The four ways people experience the world according to our Corporate Teacher. (Reprinted from Taylor SM, Vascular surgery, self-awareness, and the University of South Carolina School of Medicine Greenville. *J Vasc Surg*. 2013;58:1106-1114, Copyright 2013, with permission from The Society for Vascular Surgery.)

world in "by me" or even "through me" approaches. The key element to achieve evolution of personality style is self-awareness, which is seeking to understand how we show up in a situation to outside observers.

Conclusions.—To be successful leaders outside of the operating room, surgeons must understand more about why they are the way they are. They also need to be willing to step outside of their comfort zone and become more self-aware (Fig 3).

▶ I thoroughly encourage every surgeon reading this edition of YEAR BOOK OF VASCULAR SURGERY to read this excellent Southern Association of Vascular Surgery Presidential Address by Spence Taylor, MD. Dr Taylor delves into the surgical personality and how it relates to leadership or the lack thereof . . .

"The surgical personality, he explained, can be found with equal prevalence in the operating room as it can in the federal prison system." Perhaps the most enlightening piece of this address was the "Four Ways of Being in the World" (Fig 3) and how we, as leaders in our field, need to lead by moving away from the "To Me" mentality, to the "As Me" mentality.

This is an interesting read for anyone interested in modern medical education and the Herculean effort necessary to start a program like that of the University of South Carolina School of Medicine, Greenville. It stands as the only medical school in existence founded as a consequence of the actions of 4 southern vascular surgeons—Edward Floyd, MD; Jerry Youkey, MD; Spence Taylor, MD; and Richard Dean, MD.

B. W. Starnes, MD

Feasibility and safety of endovascular treatment for chronic cerebrospinal venous insufficiency in patients with multiple sclerosis

Lupattelli T, Bellagamba G, Righi E, et al (Istituto Clinico Cardiologico (ICC) Gruppo Villa Maria (GVM) Sanità, Rome, Italy; Salus Hosp GVM Sanità, Reggio Emilia, Italy; et al)

J Vasc Surg 58:1609-1618, 2013

Objective.—Chronic cerebrospinal venous insufficiency (CCSVI) is a recently discovered syndrome mainly due to stenoses of internal jugular (IJV) and/or azygos (AZ) veins. The present study retrospectively evaluates the feasibility and safety of endovascular treatment for CCSVI in a cohort of patients with multiple sclerosis (MS).

Methods.—From September 2010 to October 2012, 1202 consecutive patients were admitted to undergo phlebograpy ± endovascular treatment for CCSVI. All the patients had previously been found positive at color Doppler sonography (CDS) for at least two Zamboni criteria for CCSVI and had a neurologist-confirmed diagnosis of MS. Only symptomatic MS were considered for treatment. Percutaneous transluminal angioplasty was carried out as an outpatient procedure at two different institutes. Primary procedures, regarded as the first balloon angioplasty ever performed for CCSVI, and secondary (reintervention) procedures, regarded as interventions performed after venous disease recurrence, were carried out in 86.5% (1037 of 1199) and 13.5% (162 of 1199) of patients, respectively. Procedural success and complications within 30 days were recorded.

Results.—Phlebography followed by endovascular recanalization was carried out in 1999 patients consisting of 1219 interventions. Balloon angioplasty alone was performed in 1205 out of 1219 (98.9%) procedures, whereas additional stent placement was required in the remaining 14 procedures (1.1%) following unsuccessful attempts at AZ dilatation. No stents were ever implanted in the IJV. The feasibility rate was as high as 99.2% (1209 interventions). Major complications included one (0.1%) AZ rupture occurring during balloon dilatation and requiring blood transfusion, one (0.1%) severe bleeding in the groin requiring open surgery, two (0.2%) surgical openings of the common femoral vein to remove balloon fragments, and three (0.2%) left IJV thromboses. The overall major and minor complication rates at 30 days were 0.6% and 2.5%, respectively.

Conclusions.—Endovascular treatment for CCSVI appears feasible and safe. However, a proper learning curve can dramatically lower the rate of adverse events. In our experience, the vast majority of complications occurred in the first 400 cases performed.

▶ The focus of this large retrospective experience with endovascular treatment for patients with chronic cerebrospinal venous insufficiency (CCSVI) was on technical success, intraprocedural complications, and short-term risks, and, in this regard, it is no surprise that feasibility and safety were supported with a low rate of adverse events. However, this study was not designed to evaluate outcomes of angioplasty in patients with CCSVI from the perspective of improvement of symptoms of multiple sclerosis and, therefore, adds nothing to the controversial evidence to support that endovascular treatment should be a treatment consideration. Yes, the procedure can be done safely with a proper learning curve in experienced hands, but whether it is the correct therapy has yet to be definitively proven. Until comparative evidence from a properly conducted prospective, randomized trial is performed, any assumed connection between multiple sclerosis and CCSVI or endovascular treatment and clinical outcomes needs to be tempered.

M. A. Passman, MD

A nationwide survey of vascular surgery trainees reveals trends in operative experience, confidence, and attitudes about simulation

Duran C, Bismuth J, Mitchell E (The Methodist Hosp, Houston, TX; Oregon Health and Sciences Univ, Portland)

J Vasc Surg 58:524-528, 2013

Objective.—There is mounting evidence supporting the benefit of surgical skills training in a simulated environment. However, the use of simulation in vascular surgery has been limited, and its value has been poorly understood. Access to simulation is presumed to be a major barrier to its widespread implementation. While a great deal of discussion is taking place at the national level, input from current trainees has not been obtained.

Methods.—The Association of Program Directors in Vascular Surgery Committee on Education and Simulation sent a survey to all vascular surgical trainees assessing access to vascular simulation, the perceived value of simulation, and expectations for the future. Data were analyzed for junior (postgraduate year $\leq$4; n = 73) and senior (postgraduate year $\geq$5; n = 110) level and program type (traditional = 5 + 2/4 + 2; integrated = 0 + 5).

Results.—A total of 183 of 326 (56%) trainees completed the survey, 72 (0-5), 5 (4+2), 111 (5+2), respectively. Of the respondents, 86% believe there is educational value in simulation. Cadaver dissections, followed by peripheral endovascular simulators and endovascular aortic aneurysm repair simulators, were ranked the most valuable tools by seniors, while anastomotic models are valued most by juniors, followed by cadavers and endosimulators. Fifty-six percent of programs currently offer simulation training, most commonly in the form of peripheral endovascular simulators (70%), anastomotic models (58%), or endovascular aortic aneurysm repair simulation (53%). Senior residents are more likely than juniors to have attended outside simulation courses (37% vs 19%). Overall, 57% of trainees expect that technical skills assessment will be incorporated into the certification process, and 52% endorse skills assessment for certification.

Conclusions.—Trainees report limited operative experience and confidence, and confidence levels are improved for a number of index procedures among those trainees with access to simulation. Trainees endorse the use of simulation to augment their surgical training, and a significant proportion of them already have access to it. These data support a perceived need and utility for implementation of a standardized simulation curriculum in vascular surgical training.

▶ This survey of residents conducted by the Association of Program Directors in Vascular Surgery appraised trainee confidence as affected by operative experience and the use of simulation in training. The authors point to 4 of the many factors that have affected significant change on surgical training over the past decades: (1) the 80-hour workweek, (2) shorter training pathways (0 + 5 integrated residencies), (3) decreased resident autonomy caused by greater public scrutiny and an increasing emphasis on patient safety, and (4) increases in outpatient endovascular procedures. Each of these changes has led to a decrease in the operative experience (especially in open surgeries) of trainees. Simulation may be one of the solutions to this problem. Gauging trainees' current attitudes toward and experience with simulation is clearly a first step in assessing the value of simulation, and this article does an excellent job of providing an initial look at these perceptions of simulation. It was encouraging that trainees have the common sense and good judgment to value those simulation modalities that best address their individual needs. Junior residents prefer simulators that help them achieve basic technical skills, and senior residents favor more complex models that incorporate many different and higher-order skills.

As surgical training adapts to the changes mentioned and faces new challenges, novel approaches to training must be found. There is no substitute for operative experience, but, perhaps, simulation, surgical videos and other methods can enhance the value of each operative experience for residents. As a resident, I found that I was much better prepared for and learned more from each surgery if I had the opportunity to view a detailed video of a given operation before performing it in the operating room. Maximizing the educational value of limited operative experience is a necessity as the opportunities for that experience shrink.

P. White, MD, FACS

A randomized comparison of a 3-week and 6-week vascular surgery simulation course on junior surgical residents' performance of an end-to-side anastomosis

Robinson WP III, Schanzer A, Cutler BS, et al (Univ of Massachusetts Med School, Worcester)

J Vasc Surg 56:1771-1781, 2012

Objective.—We assessed the effect of an open vascular simulation course on the surgical skill of junior surgical residents in performing a vascular end-to-side anastomosis and determined the course length required for effectiveness. We hypothesized that a 6-week course would significantly increase the surgical skill of junior residents in performing an end-to-side anastomosis, while a 3-week course would not.

Methods.—We randomized 37 junior residents (postgraduate year 1 to 3) to a course consisting of three (short course, n = 18) or six (long course, n = 19) consecutive weekly 1-hour teaching sessions. Content focused on instrument recognition and performance of an end-to-side vascular anastomosis using a simulation model. A standardized 50-point vascular skills assessment (SVSA) measured knowledge and technical proficiency. Senior residents (postgraduate year 4 to 5) were tested at baseline. Junior residents were tested at baseline and at 1 and 16 weeks after course completion, and their scores were compared with baseline and senior resident scores. Residents and faculty completed a standardized anonymous evaluation of the course.

Results.—Baseline scores between short-course and long-course participants were not different. At baseline, junior residents had significantly lower SVSA scores than senior residents (36 ± 7 vs 41.4 ± 2.5; $P = .002$). One week after course completion, SVSA scores for short-course (43.5 ± 2.9 vs 34.2 ± 7.5; $P = .008$) and long-course (43.9 ± 5.6 vs 38.3 ± 5.9; $P = .006$) participants were significantly improved from baseline. SVSA scores decreased slightly at 16 weeks but remained above baseline in short-course (39 ± 6.2 vs 34.2 ± 7.5; $P = .03$) and long-course (40 ± 4.5 vs 38.3 ± 5.9; $P = .08$) participants. Long vs short course length did not affect improvement in SVSA scores at 1 or 16 weeks. In short-course and long-course participants, SVSA scores at 1 and 16 weeks were not significantly different from senior resident scores. Course ratings were high, and 95% of residents indicated the course "made them a better surgeon." Residents and faculty felt the educational benefit of the course merited the investment of resources.

Conclusions.—An open vascular simulation course consisting of three weekly 1-hour sessions increased the surgical skill of junior residents in performing a vascular end-to-side anastomosis to that of senior residents on a standardized assessment. A 6-week course provided no additional benefit. This study supports the use of an open vascular simulation course to teach vascular surgical skills to junior residents. A course consisting of three 1-hour sessions is an effective and efficient component of a simulation program for junior surgical residents in a busy surgical center.

▶ Graduate medical training has undergone dramatic changes in the past decade, and training for vascular surgery in particular has changed. The 80-hour workweek, the endovascular revolution, 0 to 5 vascular surgery residencies, increasing oversight, increasing societal emphasis on patient safety, and a decreasing acceptance of trainee independence all propose new challenges to the specialty of vascular surgery. Simulation in surgical training is becoming a necessity to meet some of these challenges. It offers an approach to overcome decreasing case numbers and enables trainees to demonstrate some degree of proficiency before they are performing procedures on human patients. Additionally, simulation offers program directors and attendings the opportunity to assess trainees with objective, quantifiable metrics. As the Accreditation Council for Graduate Medical Education moves forward with milestones and the next accreditation system, I expect that these quantifiable metrics will need to be recorded and tracked with increasing frequency.

This article describes a simple, straightforward simulation program and elucidates several key facts about simulation. First, simple technical tasks can be mastered with as few as 3- or 4-hour-long sessions. Second, gains in technical proficiency degrade with time, and, therefore, recurrent training for reinforcement is necessary. As the authors acknowledge, simulation will require the investment of time and effort by training programs. Nevertheless, simulation will become an integral part of surgical training. General surgery already strongly emphasizes laparoscopic surgery simulation in its training programs. Vascular surgery must quickly follow suit and develop useful, straightforward, and realistic simulation programs.

P. White, MD, FACS

A Single-institution Experience: The Integrated Vascular Surgery Residency's Effect on Fellowship and General Surgery Resident Case Volume and Diversity

Carroll MI, Downes K, Miladinovic B, et al (Univ of South Florida, Tampa, FL)
Ann Vasc Surg 28:253-259, 2014

Background.—To determine whether the formation of an integrated vascular surgery residency (0 + 5) has negatively impacted the case volume and diversity of the vascular surgery fellows (5 + 2) and chief general surgeons at the same institution.

Methods.—Operative data from the vascular integrated (0 + 5), independent (5 + 2), and general surgery residencies at a single institution were retrospectively reviewed and analyzed to determine vascular surgery case volumes from 2006–2012. National operative data (Residency Review Committee) were used for comparison of diversity and volume. Standard statistical methods were applied.

Results.—During this period, the 5 + 2 fellows at our institution performed on average 741 (range, 554–1002) primary cases and 1091 (range, 844–1479) combined primary and secondary cases for the 2-year fellowship. Our integrated residency began in July 2007. Our fellows' primary case volumes remained relatively stable between 2006 and 2011, with a 4% increase in the number of cases, although their total (primary and secondary) case volumes fell 15%; by comparison, the equivalent national 50th percentile rates rose 16% during this time frame. Our institution's general surgery residents performed an average of 116 (range, 56–221) vascular cases individually during their 5-year residency from 2005–2011. From 2006–2011, the total case volume fell only 5%, while the national 50th percentile rate fell 24%. Across all years, however, resident and fellow volumes both continue to be above Accreditation Council for Graduate Medical Education minimum requirements, and the major vascular case volume at our institution in all groups studied remained statistically greater than or equal to the national 50th percentile of cases. Our first integrated resident to graduate finished in June 2012 with 931 total vascular cases and 249 general surgery cases for a total operative experience of 1180 cases during the 5-year residency. Finally, after an 8-year period (2003–2010) in which none of our general surgery residents pursued vascular training, 1 resident in each of the 2011, 2012, and 2013 graduating years has now done so.

Conclusions.—At our institution, the introduction of a 0 + 5 vascular residency has correlated with a modest drop (15%) in overall case volume for the 5 + 2 fellows, but the number of primary cases have actually increased slightly and they continue to meet or exceed Accreditation Council for Graduate Medical Education requirements and national 50th percentile rates. General surgery residents' vascular volumes, by contrast, have remained stable, and interest in vascular surgery by residents has increased. Our integrated vascular residents are projected to exceed the fellows' 50th percentile case volume and diversity targets during their residency experience (Figs 1 and 2).

▶ This article presents an analysis of the operative experience of vascular surgery trainees at an academic medical center as an integrated 0 + 5 vascular residency was added to an institution with an existing 5 + 2 vascular surgery fellowship and an existing general surgery residency. The authors claim that little effect was noted over the study period, but I do not believe they fully elucidate the apparent stability in case numbers. First, the institution is clearly a high-volume center and may have had the cases needed to support the new 0 + 5 residency already. Smaller volume centers might experience much greater disruption in trainee case volume. Second, as the authors admit and as Figs 1 and 2 show, the graphs of case volume for 5 + 2 fellows show a clear inflection point around the time that the 0 + 5 residents reach the postgraduate year-3 and could be expected to compete for senior-level cases. It would be helpful to extend the collection of data to earlier and later time periods. (The fellowship did transition from a 1-year to a 2-year fellowship just before the study period, but cases per

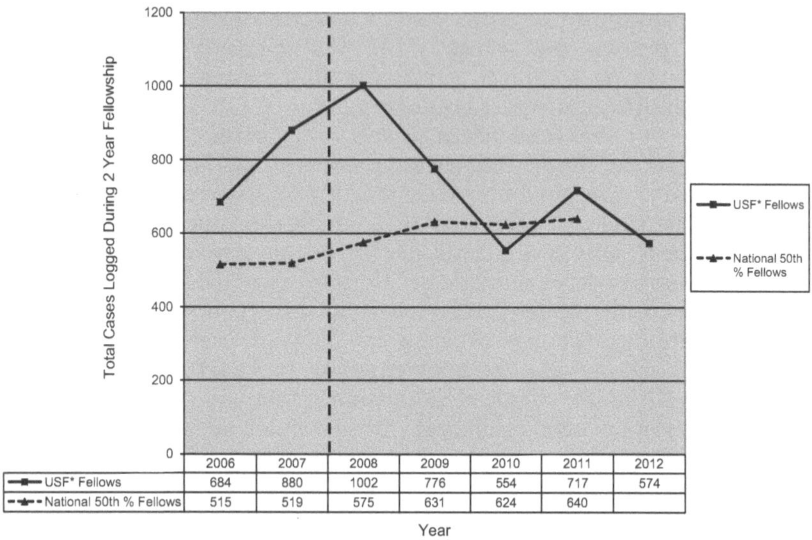

	2006	2007	2008	2009	2010	2011	2012
USF* Fellows	684	880	1002	776	554	717	574
National 50th % Fellows	515	519	575	631	624	640	

FIGURE 1.—Total primary cases performed by vascular fellows per graduating year with comparison of University of South Florida (USF; $N = 1$ per year) and Resident Review Committee published data on the national 50th percentile of vascular fellows. The inaugural year of integrated vascular residency is indicated by the vertical *dashed line*. (Reprinted from Carroll MI, Downes K, Miladinovic B, et al. A single-institution experience: the integrated vascular surgery residency's effect on fellowship and general surgery resident case volume and diversity. *Ann Vasc Surg*. 2014;28:253-259, Copyright 2014, with permission from Annals of Vascular Surgery, Inc.)

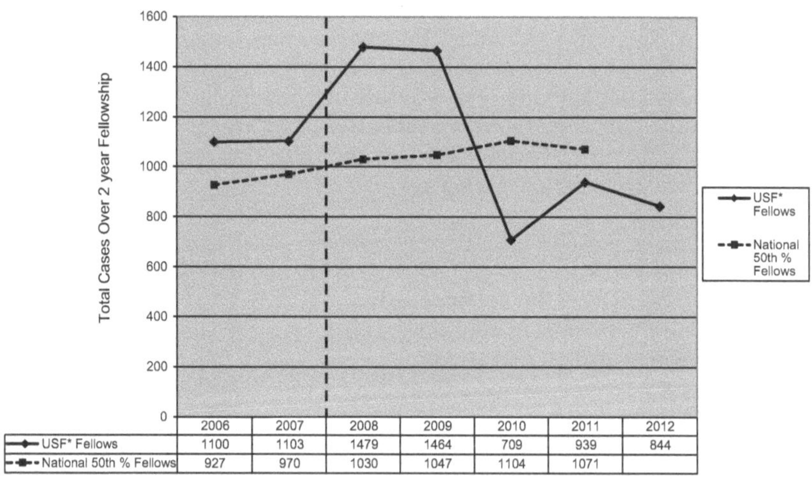

	2006	2007	2008	2009	2010	2011	2012
USF* Fellows	1100	1103	1479	1464	709	939	844
National 50th % Fellows	927	970	1030	1047	1104	1071	

FIGURE 2.—Total combined primary and secondary cases performed by vascular fellows per graduating year with comparison of University of South Florida (USF; $N = 1$ per year) and Resident Review Committee published data on the national 50th percentile of vascular fellows. The inaugural year of integrated vascular residency is indicated by the vertical *dashed line*. (Reprinted from Carroll MI, Downes K, Miladinovic B, et al. A single-institution experience: the integrated vascular surgery residency's effect on fellowship and general surgery resident case volume and diversity. *Ann Vasc Surg*. 2014;28:253-259, Copyright 2014, with permission from Annals of Vascular Surgery, Inc.)

year might be a useful substitute for total cases.) Third, as the authors also admit, the Accreditation Council for Graduate Medical Education has begun to allow for partial coding of cases; that is, the junior resident is given credit as primary resident surgeon for a femoral artery exposure, whereas a fellow is given credit for an endovascular aneurysm repair for the same operation (previously, only 1 trainee could claim credit). This clearly would inflate case numbers.

Perhaps the most disturbing aspect of this article is that overall vascular case numbers for 5 + 2 fellows are nearly identical to vascular case numbers for 0 + 5 residents. (Very similar numbers were presented at the 2014 Meeting of the Association of Program Directors in Vascular Surgery.) In other words, fellows in 2 years obtain the same operative experience as residents in 5 years, and fellows have the added experience and maturity gained over a 5-year general surgery residency with 3 to 4 times the number of general surgery cases as 0 + 5 vascular surgery residents. I worry that the 0 + 5 pathway is producing less experienced surgeons.

Admittedly, as laparoscopic and endovascular techniques continue to advance, general surgery and vascular surgery will drift farther apart as specialties. A dedicated vascular surgery residency may reduce the amount of unnecessary training to produce a competent, safe vascular surgeon, but much of the experience needed to be a safe vascular surgery is, to paraphrase one of my partners, "knowing how to operate." This experience can only be gained by hours in the operating room and in the hospital. Hours it appears our 0 + 5 trainees might not be getting. Moreover, as the authors point out in the first paragraph of the body of the article, reducing the length of training was the chief reason the 0 + 5 residencies were initiated. The 7- to 9-year period traditionally required to train a vascular surgeon was viewed as an obstacle to recruiting the "best" medical students. That old paradigm of training being not conducive to "quality of life" was perceived as repellant to the younger generation of medical school graduates. I think we must continue to look closely at operative experience in all the vascular surgery training pathways, and we must be prepared to make significant changes if needed.

P. White, MD, FACS

Article Index

Chapter 1: Basic Considerations

Chapter 2: Epidemiology

Chapter 3: Vascular Laboratory and Imaging

Chapter 4: Perioperative Considerations

Chapter 5: Grafts and Graft Complications

Chapter 6: Aortic Aneurysm

Chapter 7: Abdominal Aortic Endografting

Chapter 8: Thoracic Aorta

Chapter 9: Aortoiliac Disease and Leg Ischemia

Chapter 10: Upper Extremity Ischemia/Dialysis Access

Chapter 11: Carotid and Cerebrovascular Disease

Chapter 12: Carotid and Endovascular Disease

Chapter 13: Vascular Trauma

Chapter 14: Venous Thrombosis and Pulmonary Embolism

Chapter 15: Chronic Venous and Lymphatic Disease

Chapter 16: Technical Notes

Chapter 17: Miscellaneous

Author Index

G

H

I

J

K

L

M

N

O

P

Q

R

S

T

U

V

W

X

Y

Z

FSC
www.fsc.org
MIX
Papier | Fördert
gute Waldnutzung
FSC® C083411

Kolibri 360 GmbH
Ferdinand-Jühlke-Straße 7
99095 Erfurt, Deutschland
produktsicherheit@kolibri360.de